GUT-BRAIN SECRETS

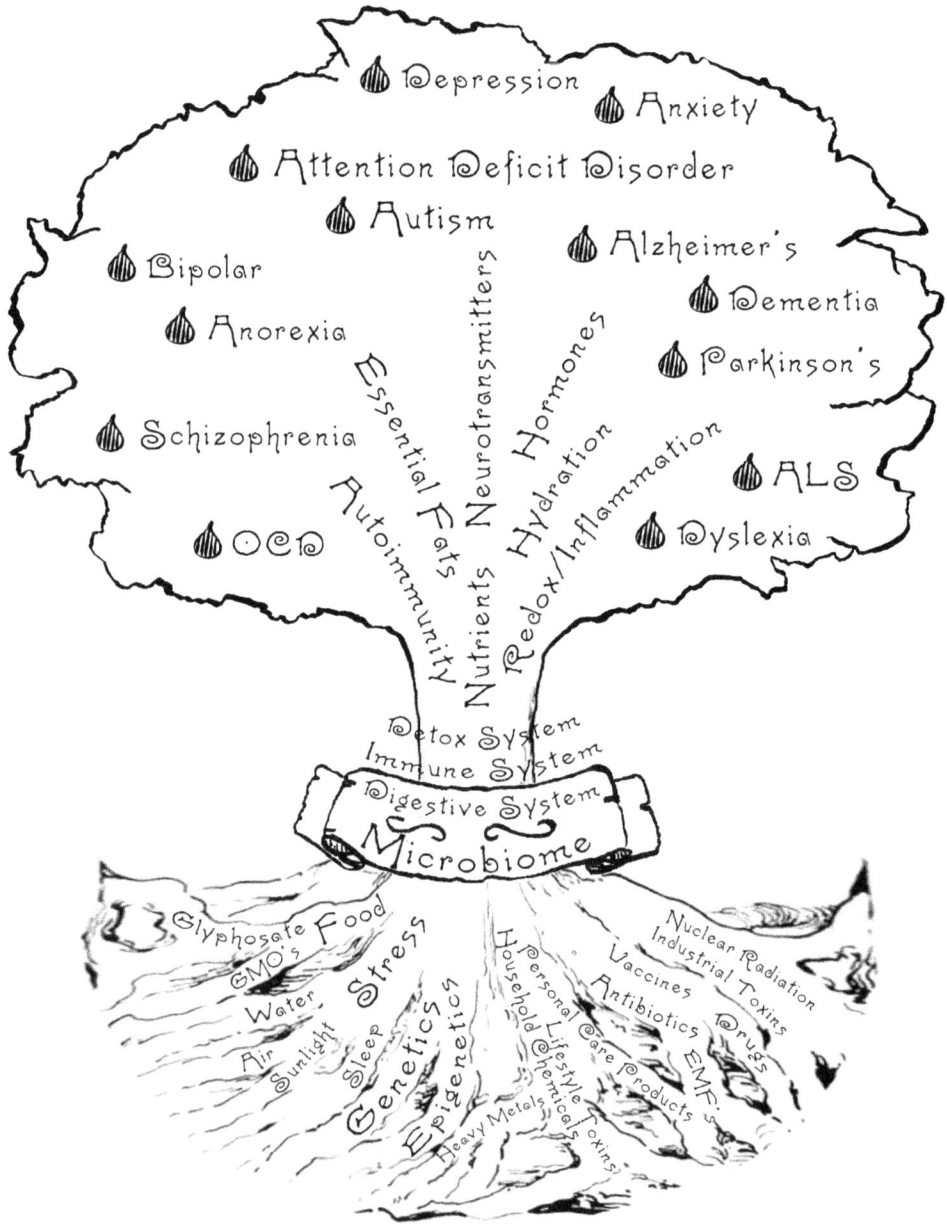

GUT-BRAIN SECRETS
R. D. Lee

DISCLAIMER

IF YOU'RE NEW TO THIS SORT OF INFORMATION, IT MAY SERIOUSLY SHAKE UP YOUR WORLDVIEW. IF YOU HAVE THE SLIGHTEST BIT OF HUMANITY, SENSIBILITY, AND URGE FOR SELF-PRESERVATION, THIS INFORMATION WILL MAKE YOU UNCOMFORTABLE AND PROBABLY UPSET. IT MAY EVEN CAUSE YOU TO RETHINK EVERYTHING YOU THOUGHT YOU KNEW ABOUT THE NATURE OF YOUR REALITY AND EVERYTHING IN IT.
…FAIR WARNING.

IT IS NOT INTENDED TO BE USED AS A SUBSTITUTE FOR PROFESSIONAL MEDICAL ADVICE, DIAGNOSIS OR TREATMENT. THE AUTHOR(S) MAKE NO REPRESENTATIONS, AND ASSUME NO RESPONSIBILITY, CONCERNING THE ACCURACY, SAFETY, EFFICACY, OR APPROPRIATENESS OF THE PRODUCTS, PROCEDURES, TESTS, TREATMENTS, SERVICES, OPINIONS, OR OTHER INFORMATION CONTAINED HEREIN.

CONSULT YOUR HEALTH PROFESSIONAL BEFORE UNDERTAKING A NEW DIET, TREATMENT, OR LIFESTYLE CHANGE. IF YOU SUFFER A LIFE-THREATENING EMERGENCY WHILE YOU'RE READING THIS BOOK, RESIST THE URGE TO CONTINUE READING. PUT THE BOOK DOWN IMMEDIATELY AND DIAL 911.

Contents

Part 4: Solutions to Gut-Brain Problems

Additional Material

ACKNOWLEDGEMENTS

Gut-Brain Secrets is based on the work of the following educators, followed by my description of their field of expertise.

1. **Dr. Natasha Campbell-McBride** connection between a corrupted gut microbiome and disturbed psychology. How good food nourishes and protects the brain and body, and bad food does the opposite.
2. **Dr. Zach Bush** redox molecules, oxidation and reduction.
3. **Dr. Elaine Ingham** soil food web and natural farming practices.
4. **Dr. Don Huber** glyphosate, plant pathology/physiology.
5. **Gary Samuelson, PhD** redox molecules, oxidation and reduction.
6. **Dr. Christopher Shade** therapeutic detoxification.
7. **Kerri Rivera** parasites and autism.
8. **Barbara O'Neill, ND** traditional healing techniques.
9. **Dr. Russell Blaylock** vaccines.
10. **Dr. Fereydoon Batmanghelidj** water's role in health or sickness.

The teachings of these subject matter experts also contributed to the creation of this work: Ken Rohla, Jeffrey Smith, Sally Fallon Morell, Dr. Daniel Amen, Donna Gates, Weston A. Price, DDS, Ryan Dougherty, Dr. Derrick MacFabe, Dr. Garry Gordon, Gary Null, Dr. David Getoff, Brittany Auerbach, Dr. Michael Antoniou, Hippocrates, Steven Druker, Dr. Thierry Vrain, Stephanie Seneff, PhD, Sofia Smallstorm, Bruce Lipton, Vaughn Lawrence, Winston Kao, Dr. Eric Berg, Berny Dohrmann, Izabella Wentz, PharmD, Dr. John Bergman, Dr. Gary Kaplan, Dr. Alessio Fasano, Dr. Joseph Mercola, Dr. Hal Huggins, David Hudson, Jim Humble, Dr. Andreas Kalcker, Dolores Cannon, Paul Chek and David Wilcock.

FOREWORD
by Stephanie Seneff, PhD

If you've been paying attention to nutritional advice coming from mainstream media and medicine, you're probably utterly confused by what's true and what's not at this point. You may have been tricked into believing that saturated fat and cholesterol should be avoided at all cost, and that vegan, casein-free and gluten-free diets are the healthiest way to support your heart, nutritional needs, immunity and longevity. You may be caught on the slippery slope of eliminating more and more foods from your diet to the point that you hardly have anything left to eat.

Contributing to the confusion, mainstream media seldom talks about the toxic contaminants in our food, or the depletion of micronutrients and biologically active molecules from real food to make the "factory foods" on our store shelves today. These toxic, chemical-laden pseudo-foods are, in my opinion, the main reason most of the Western world is suffering crippling rates of mental health problems, degenerative diseases, and autoimmune conditions.

If you want to know how to take control of your health through what you eat or don't eat, you need to read this book

Based on my thousands of hours of research, the understandings and assessments Mr. Lee presents in *Gut-Brain Secrets* are, unfortunately, all-to-accurate. Even more revealing, he's not afraid to talk out about the small group of people operating behind the scenes who are manipulating our food and medical systems for their own benefit, at the expense of us all.

At the heart of the matter – despite the fact that medical schools devote precious little time to nutrition – food is undoubtedly the most important factor in our health. Yet, the food widely available in America today is not only depleted of nutrients, it's also unacceptably toxic from all the chemicals recklessly sprayed on the plants that go into making that food.

For these reasons, eating a 100% certified organic diet has become far more conducive to producing good health than eliminating certain foods from a person's diet. And, contrary to what you may have heard, dietary cholesterol is not bad for you. Rather, it's essential.

Randy tells it like it is: "At its deepest level, the real source of our health and environmental problems is the agenda, profits and control of a small group of people at the top." This is so true! A great deal of their profit comes not only from the cheap foods made with these chemical-filled and genetically-modified agriculture, but also from treating all the diseases and dysfunctions that develop from eating these unnatural foods. As a result, the United States spends the least of any First World country on food, and by far the most on health care per capita.

This thought-provoking exposé gives you a thorough understanding of the gut-brain connection

It links attention deficit disorder, and other neurological conditions, to gut dysbiosis brought about by toxic foods. It starts the discussion by showing how the killing of soil bacteria by agricultural chemicals leads to disruption of plants' ability to absorb nutrients. It describes how nutrients power the body's biochemistry, its defenses, and genetic expression.

The scope broadens to show how agro-chemicals wipe out microorganisms in the atmosphere, leading to alterations in the electromagnetic/light frequencies hitting the earth, and in climate change that could soon make our planet uninhabitable. Presciently, he writes: "Glyphosate and the heavy metal/chemical cocktails they're aggressively spraying in stratospheric aerosol injections have killed off beneficial microbes in the atmosphere that used to filter the sun's light, making it perfectly attuned to the needs of life on earth."

The most destructive, yet sneaky, chemical in the whole mess is glyphosate, the active ingredient in the weed killer Roundup. Glyphosate is by far the most widely-used herbicide in the world. And the US uses far more than any other country. Fundamental to all life, the sequestration of carbon, nitrogen and sulfur into organic matter is a wondrous process that forms the basis of all life on earth. But, to our detriment, toxic chemicals are disrupting this process and wreaking havoc on biological systems, from the smallest and simplest bacteria to the most advanced and complex, such as humans.

That's why the US spends more on health care than any other country

I'm thrilled to see considerable attention paid to glyphosate. Mr. Lee has clearly articulated how glyphosate harms life at every scale. Glyphosate creates microbial imbalances in the gut of all higher life forms, chelates minerals, and interferes with detoxification in the liver. Indeed, the scientific evidence is clear: Microbes in the gut, soil, and atmosphere are all adversely affected by glyphosate, with devastating consequences.

However, I would like to add one crucial concept about glyphosate toxicity not covered in the book and not yet widely known: **Glyphosate,**

My update 2022: Dr. Seneff's contention from ~2017 appears to be correct. The glyphosate molecule looks similar to glycine (a major building block of collagen). So the body wrongly inserts glyphosate into tendons and cartilage, thereby reducing their terminal elasticity/ breaking strength. Mitochondriacs believe this is partly responsible for the striking rise in sports injuries lately.

acting as an analogue to the amino acid glycine, may get inserted in place of glycine in the construction of proteins. This disrupts a plethora of biochemical processes that I feel will ultimately prove to be the defining mechanism by which glyphosate does most of its damage in the body.

While not proven definitely yet, I believe the evidence is overwhelming. Together with colleagues, I have published several papers explaining how this effect alone can account for the strong correlations we are seeing between glyphosate usage on core crops and the alarming rise in a long list of debilitating diseases, including autism, AD(H)D, dementia, diabetes, obesity, inflammatory bowel disease, pancreatic cancer, thyroid cancer, bladder cancer, liver disease, kidney failure, sleep disorder, and many others.

The ideas and solutions in *Gut-Brain Secrets* will help you improve your health for a lifetime

It provides a wealth of information on what's wrong with our food supply, many ways you can choose your lifestyle influences more wisely, and the path forward to a new era in which humans become wise stewards of the planet we live on as guests – for instance, renewing the nutritional value of soil through sustainable biodynamic agriculture, and reversing the damage done by climate change.

The foods produced from this newly-enriched soil will be far healthier in terms of micronutrients, and free of toxic chemicals. Ultimately, these sustainable growing practices will not only bring humanity to a new plane of sustained well-being, but also renew the vitality of planet earth itself. If you care about your health, your longevity and the ecology, you simply must read *Gut-Brain Secrets*.

———————— ❧ ————————

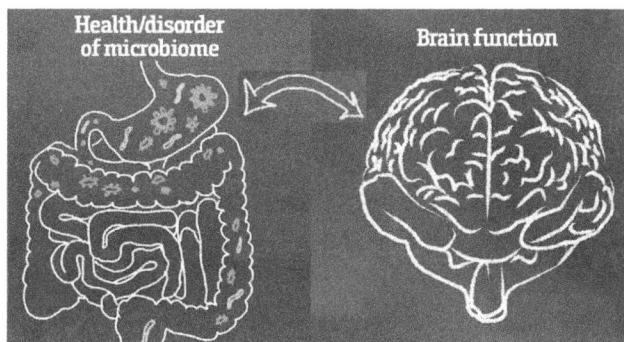

Health/disorder of microbiome   Brain function

PREFACE
What Gut-Brain
Secrets *is all About*

This material focuses on the physical origins of attention deficit disorder, rather than behavioral, social or developmental causes

This book's main purpose is to explain how a disordered gut leads to a dysfunctional brain. It examines the many factors that go into the inception and perpetuation of ADD, as well as the many ways in which the root cause of ADD – a corrupted gut – affects the individual biochemically, physically and immunologically.

A corrupted gut is my umbrella term to describe unhealthful, imbalanced conditions in the gut. In medical terms, this "gut dysbiosis" is one or more of the following conditions: (1) too many pathogenic microorganisms in the gut; (2) too few good, probiotic bacteria (they're opposite sides of the same coin); (3) broken tight junctions causing leaky gut and leaky membranes; (4) improper digestion and mal-absorption; and (5) usually immune system problems.

When your gut's a mess, that's a corrupted gut. And when your gut falls into dis-ease, that opens the door for psychological disturbances to occur. In other words, disordered thinking and problematic behavior are *physical* in nature first, *psychological* in origin second or third. Many patients and practitioners all over the world now refer to these gut-brain conditions as "Gut and Psychology Syndrome" conditions (GAPS for short), based on Dr. Natasha Campbell-McBride's book and diet protocol by the same name.

Tight junctions: Filaments between cells of the gut lining that open and close on-demand to let food particles and immune cells through. When these break, undigested food particles enter the bloodstream and cause food sensitivities, autoimmunity, and toxicity issues.

Our once sturdy and supportive guts are now hurting us as much as they're helping

Around 2010–2015, I feel we passed the tipping point where the average person could ignore this material and have some hope of living their lives without experiencing substantial ill effects. Unfortunately, none of us have that choice anymore. The sources and severity of damage are expanding too rapidly to expect, or even hope, to be one of the lucky few to escape side effects for long.

You simply must understand how gut health works, or fails to work, along with its downstream effects, if you're to get healthy and stay healthy into the future. It's no longer an option because the damage is already upon us. We've just failed to recognize the ways that our corrupted guts are draining the health right out of us and activating states of disease.

Anyone who's up to speed on toxicity, the microbiome, and mental health can now say with 99% certainty you are currently being affected by a corrupted gut. You just don't know which symptoms that you have are being caused by environmental factors that people have blamed on scapegoats such as genes and bad luck.

We also explore how the mind itself works

We'll uncover many mysteries behind the non-physical aspects of the mind as we explore how thoughts, consciousness and compulsions are formed, as well as how the brain is connected to spirit. In dissecting and examining the causes of ADD, I hope to give you and your medical providers insight into why ADD individuals think and act in ways that society views as anti-social, counter-productive, or just plain odd.

Demystified within: The sources and inner workings of: (1) gut dysbiosis, (2) neurological disorders, (3) mysteries of the mind, (3) immune system dysfunction, as well as (4) chronic, degenerative physical diseases. By bringing specificity and connections to the ADD enigma, you and your providers can unravel the mystery that ADD is. Over time, we can reverse the explosive rise in ADD and GAPS, and reduce the damage they do everywhere.

This information is collected straight from the cutting edge

According to mainstream medicine and nutritional science, this material is speculative and unproven. As far as holistic healing is concerned, it is simply ancient wisdom being rediscovered and explained scientifically. Big Food and Big Pharma oppose this information because it explains how their products harm people and planet, while exposing their reckless disregard for humanity in their ways of doing business. It reveals their ugly intentions. This book shows you many of the lies and deception that plague our print and airwaves. And it gives you big heaping doses of reality.

As of 2018, only the most blatantly obvious concepts have become common knowledge, such as the microbiome's role in health or sickness. Most of the views are still not widely accepted or practiced yet. Most still believe this information to be quackery.

Real world experience *vs.* the scientific method

Although scientific studies and publishing are core components of the scientific method, intelligent people know "the science" is only as valid and trustworthy as the morality of the people paying the researchers. There's good material you can rely on or, just as frequently, there's dishonest literature meant to deceive and confuse.

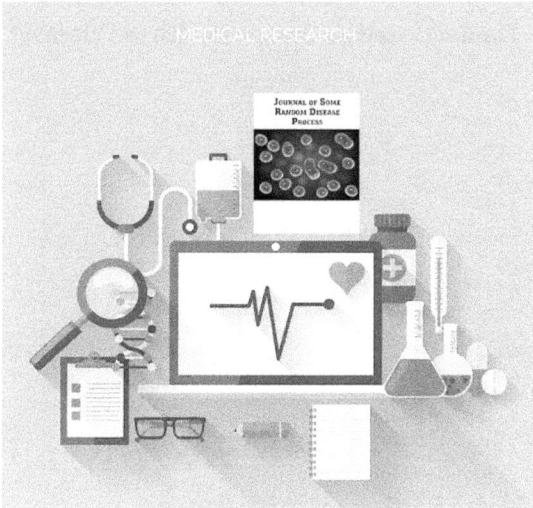

Just because a paper is coming from a reputable source doesn't mean a thing. I repeat, "science" is only as honest and reliable as the intention of the parties funding the research. That means most formal research is biased from conception all the way to dogma, in order to support some group's predetermined conclusions. Whatever you want your research to show, if your wallet and will are large enough, there are many ways to make research appear to support your preplanned outcome. You can setup studies, and perpetuate ideas, that prove almost anything that you want, because it's a simple, straight-forward process to manipulate study criteria, experiments, and conclusions that make it seem like the data supports any preconceived conclusion, no matter how far from the truth they may be. Deceit and trickery in science is easy when you know how to do it and you've got deep pockets.

Dr. Natasha Campbell-McBride: Pioneer in connecting gut health with brain function – particularly autism, attention deficit, and what she calls "GAPS" conditions (short for Gut and Psychology Syndrome).

Dr. Natasha Campbell-McBride:

"I diagnose by a clinical picture. I believe in clinical experience and clinical picture, much more than I believe in science. Our science has lost its way. More than 90% of scientific studies are commercially funded. They are deceptive. And the majority of us have no tools, and no training, to really decipher whether the study was designed properly, conducted properly, and then analyzed properly. It's very difficult.

So there's a huge amount of information that leads you away from the truth. So I work with real people on a daily basis. I see what works and what doesn't work in real life. And if I need some scientific backing for any of those truths that I've discovered, I will find it. And, usually, those scientific studies are kosher… are correct. I believe in Mother Nature. I believe in real life, and real people."

Gut-Brain Secrets is not some miracle cure or fad diet. It is the very foundations of human health, as seen through the gut and brain

I don't believe there is a one-size-fits-all diet, drug, or treatment protocol to reversing gut-brain problems. As the wellness community is becoming more keenly aware every day, people's outcomes with any particular wellness effort is now as varied as their biochemistry, environmental exposures, and lifestyle choices. **If you want to get healthy and stay healthy for good, you have to at least "suffice" in these basic areas of biology:**

- support the barriers of the body
- increase hydration in cells
- evict toxins from their hiding places

Fundamentals of Human Health (or Disease)

- minimize new toxin exposure
- enhance nutrient levels
- expand your energy supply
- restore communication networks of the body (e.g., neurotransmitters, redox signaling and hormones)
- bring the microbiome into balance.

Lifestyle
Sleep, Rest, Stress, Exercise, Body weight

Microbiome
Diversity of species, Pro-life balance

Nutrition
Minerals, Vitamins, Essential Fats, Fiber, Antioxidants, Moisture, Digestive Enzymes, Phytonutrients

Toxins
Get toxins out, Cut toxin intake

Mindset
Thought patterns, Beliefs, Expectations, Permission

Communication Networks of the Body

Community Connection

Energy
Mitochondria quantity + production

Redox Signaling Neurotransmitters Hormones

Protection & Repair
Tight junctions, Gut lining, Immune system

Hydration
Phase angle, T.E.E.R., Water intake, Electrolytes

Genetic expression
Epigenetics, MicroRNA, Genetics

When you get a handle on these fundamentals of human health, disease is simply not needed or welcome in the body. Dysfunction is just totally out-of-place in a body that's well-supported, clean, and in a great state of tune. In other words, fix the real source of your problems, and the symptoms that bother you cease to exist… instead of chasing symptom after symptom with "band-aids" and short-term solutions.

Gut-Brain Secrets is your travel guide to learning the fundamentals of admirable gut-brain health. It's your roadmap to help you get to wellville and stay there. Strive not for perfection, though. Few will make it. A more sensible approach is simply to be better informed, and act more purposefully, than the day before. *Gut-Brain Secrets* will get you started in the right direction. We're going to cover a lot of ground because the health hazards we encounter daily demand it. You have to be prepared to fight for your own health because the deck is becoming ever-more stacked against the health of us all. Just ask any long-time practitioner. They'll say the symptoms and diseases they're treating on a daily basis are vastly more complex and stubborn than they were just a few decades ago.

Fortunately, there are plenty of juicy secrets to tell, straight from the cutting edge, about why the body needs nourishment, how it adapts to problems, and what you can do to recover from diseases generally thought to be incurable. Knowledge and solutions are growing as fast as the threats are. However, truth travels slowly when it prevents money from landing in Big Pharma pockets. So don't expect to get the truth, the whole truth, and nothing but the truth from mainstream sources. For them, getting you hooked on medical care is a higher priority than any of your concerns.

The real source of our health and environmental problems is a small group of people at the top

As you dig in, you may ask why so much ink is devoted to the politics, corruption, control, and reckless profiteering of puppet-masters operating behind the scenes. Can't we just focus on nutrition, biology and psychology, and forget the unpleasant things that seem to be outside our control?

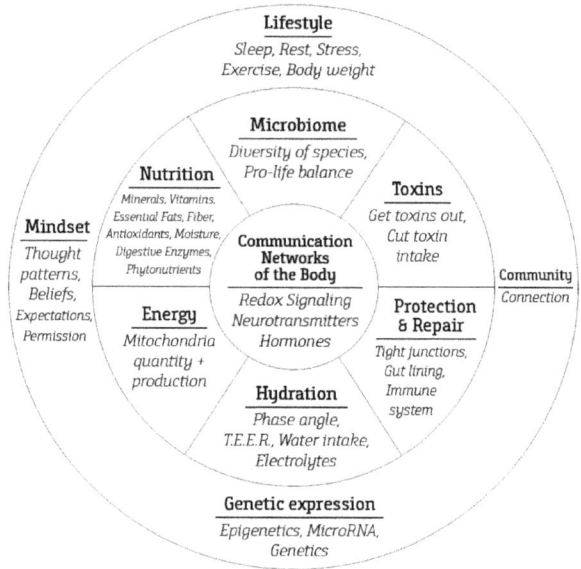

The reason is simple: This book is about the underlying causes of gut-brain problems. And you can't fully comprehend the true source of your problems, and what might be required to fix them, unless/until you understand who created them, and why they designed your problems the way that they did. That's where most efforts fall short in our manufactured reality. Until you understand: (1) who is behind the system, (2) how they create dysfunction, disease and destruction, and (3) why they do what they do, you're basically trying to solve symptom after symptom, while the root cause remains.

No matter how effective your nutritional and lifestyle changes are in reversing your GAPS condition, if you don't fix the real problem, you'll be spinning your wheels a little to a lot. You'll be putting out fire after fire in every aspect of your life, while the arsonist remains at-large, wreaking havoc wherever he sees opportunity to exert more control over your health, life and pocketbook.

Along the way, new, more menacing hazards and "solutions" will continue popping up and expanding as long as the real source is allowed to persist – as we're seeing today. As plainly as I can put this, globalists and their plans are the real source of our health and environmental problems. Until you understand that, and we all put a stop to it, our problems will not only continue, they'll grow and multiply.

2022 update

For the Third Edition of *Gut-Brain Secrets,* I reformatted the layout and heavily polished the content. However, I kept the gist of what was written from 2014–2018 largely unchanged, only cleaning up obvious errors. In other words, it's 2016 material, in today's words, if that makes sense.

For example, genetic modification has advanced a great deal since then, but I did not update the essence of the content to reflect the current state of the art in 2022. My knowledge base, and that of the wellness community, has also grown considerably in the areas of biophysics (including light, water and magnetism), mitochondria, and seasonal cycles of the body, giving us the second half of the composition.

Actually, I'm surprised how well the material has held up. It's even more timely and desperately needed than it was five years ago. With *Gut-Brain Secrets* and *The Mitochondriac Manifesto* cluing us into what's happening in our minds, bodies and surroundings, we now have a more complete story of biology to arm our efforts going forward. Fitting together somewhat by accident, they form Part I and Part II of a virtual user guide/repair manual for the human body.

PART I

———— ⚬ ————

How Nature Nurtures and
Man Manipulates

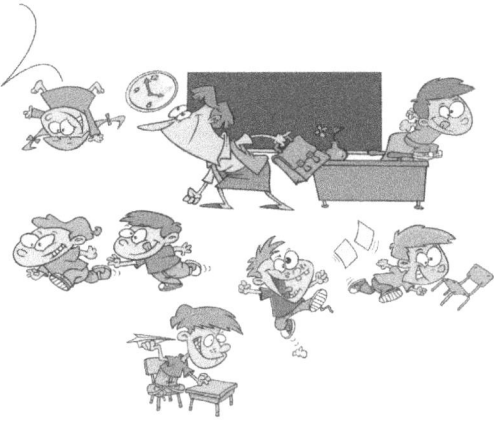

I

ADD NOW TOUCHES EVERYONE
(Whether you know it or not)

Attention deficit disorder (ADD) has become so common, people now think it's normal

If you have ADD, others in your family probably do too. Odds are, your coolest friends have it. Almost all the celebrities you follow have it. And, unless you work in a mundane industry, the marketers, creatives, owners and salesmen around you have ADD as well. In fact, you're surrounded by people who have attention deficit. Yet many don't know it because ADD has become so common, society thinks it's normal.

Many of those affected don't know it because very few people know what it's like to have ADD <u>and</u> to not have ADD. Only a miniscule portion of the population knows from personal experience what it's like to have their brain working at 100% *vs.* what it's like to live with altered brain function. Both groups – affected *vs.* unaffected – go through life getting only occasional glimpses into the other's daily norm.

Meaning, most individuals either know what it's like to be able to put their attention wherever they want, for as long as they want. *Or else* they constantly go from one extreme to the other: bored and discontent to fixated and pacified for the moment. Few have seen the world through both lenses, and thus a great deal of confusion and controversy ensues.

Outside observers can't easily tell who's affected by ADD, and who isn't, until you analyze the individual's thought patterns and behaviors. The symptoms are just too subjective and varied in milder cases, unless you know exactly what to look for. Affected individuals often appear perfectly functional and unimpaired one moment – which they indeed may be – then a slave to their impulses the next. So unless you're aware of the symptoms and observant, it's hard to recognize the signs through casual interaction.

Which leads affected individuals to say things like the following:

- I think I might have ADD.
- I was tested for ADD as a child.
- I didn't even know I was fidgeting.
- I just can't concentrate unless I have a coffee or Red Bull.
- Oh, that's normal; everyone does it.

A lot of people say their attention span isn't always the greatest. But they can't say for sure whether they have ADD or not because their basis for comparison is limited. They haven't been diagnosed by a medical professional. And they've never done a brain scan to prove it to themselves and others. So only severe cases of hyperactivity or misbehavior lead untrained observers to suspect some form of ADD may be involved.

Short of that, mildly anti-social behavior appears for all the world to be lack of discipline, defective personality, bad parenting, or innate character flaws – not a clinical disorder stemming from compromised gut health. In fact, prior to the groundbreaking work of Dr. Natasha Campbell-McBride, Donna Gates, Dr. Daniel Amen, and others in the mental health field, almost everyone thought ADD was purely psychological in origin, not physical in nature. Now we know better.

Before the gut-brain connection was made, people thought bad behavior and poor brain function were products of the mind, not the body

This book explains how these common misconceptions have persisted for so long. We're going to talk about how the present state of our food supply, societal constructs, and system of sick care have contributed to the health challenges threatening us all today. This is groundwork to understand the ADD enigma and other GAPS conditions.

Specifically, I show you why a shocking percentage of modern humans have disturbed brain function, nutrient deficiencies, chronic, degenerative diseases and autoimmune conditions. We examine the exact mechanisms of action by which environmental exposures turn into biochemical imbalances impacting learning, behavior and social interaction, as well as which influences deplete the body's defenses, enabling attention deficit disorder to occur.

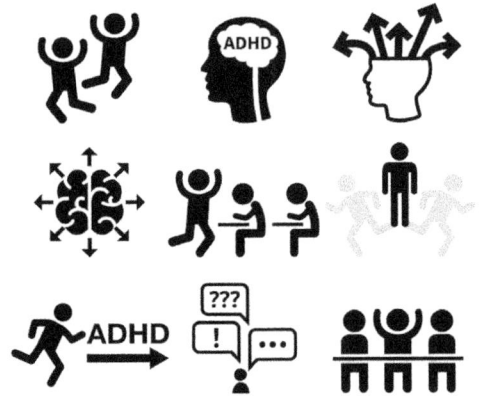

I say, a much higher percentage of the general population has attention deficit than the 5% of school children diagnosed as "hyperactive." So the questions we need to ask ourselves are: 'Have we learned enough about the causes and solutions of ADD and GAPS to turn it around? Can we change how we grow our food, how we support our mental and physical health, and how we live our lives in time to stop the alarming trends in disease, dysfunction and infertility? Can we be saved?'

Frankly, it's debatable. For now, we'll have to settle for changing one life and family at a time, while we expand our results and reach. In our time together, we'll systematically unpack the ADD puzzle to under-stand what might be required to fix, manage, and even prevent it.

Disease rates are out of control

And we're not talking just a few diseases, places or population groups, but in every single disease we know by name, everywhere. Present day numbers are alarming enough. But when you examine their growth curves – that's what's really scary – because skyrocketing disease is caused by a net loss in our rate of recovery. That is, we're adding to our "health bank accounts" slower than ever before, while our environments deplete us increasingly faster with each new generation of technology.

Clearly, human health is no longer sustainable. But, to date, the explanations we're given for these problems are just as inadequate as the solutions offered. So who can blame those living in a state of denial or learned helplessness? I have to admit, in some respects, you're better off not knowing the truth when you can't do anything about it. No knowledge + no power to change = no responsibility.

COSTS OF SICKCARE

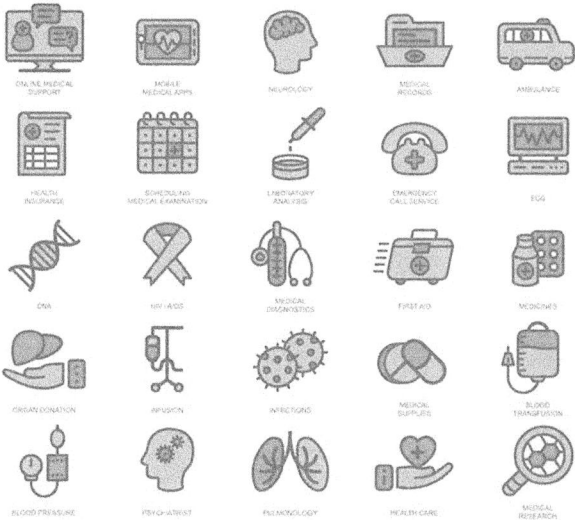

Well, what a coincidence. That's exactly what the system is designed to do: keep the public ignorant and disempowered, often in fear, yet always believing that you're receiving the best health care in the world. Treat people like mushrooms and you get obedient consumers that believe anything you tell them. Oh, the masses will complain from time to time. But most people end up doing very little to help themselves until their situation gets desperate and the body runs out of resources to heal itself. Here are the real-world results:

In the Western world

- **Diabetes.** Diabetes is absolutely out of control. Nearly 10% of the US population has it. Fifteen years from now, one-third to one-half of certain population groups are predicted to be affected. As a real-life cautionary tale, India already has 72 million diabetics in 2019, and is projected to top 200 million by 2050.
- **Autism.** In 1990, 1 in 10,000 was affected. **In 2021, it's 1 in 27 boys, and rising fast.** By 2025, Dr. Stephanie Seneff (senior research scientist at MIT) projects 25% of all children born in the US will eventually be diagnosed on the autism spectrum… 50% of all children by 2032.

- **Heart disease.** Before 1920, heart disease was very rare. Now it's competing with cancer as our leading killer.
- **Cancer.** Recent stats say about half the male population born today will get cancer in their lifetime. If that stat doesn't jar your senses, I don't know what will.
- **Alzheimer's.** Alzheimer's is now believed by many to have overtaken both cancer and heart disease as America's #1 killer. However, you won't see its full statistical effect until after 2030.
- **Allergies.** About 33% of people have allergies, 50% of school children.
- **Infertility.** Fertility of men in America has dropped by more than 50% in the last 10–15 years.
- **Autoimmunity.** Some 95% of teenage girls show clinical markers of autoimmunity to their own thyroid. Most don't know it.

ADD

Public health experts estimate ADD affects 1 in 20 school-age children. But, although kids may grow out of hyperactivity, the root causes of ADD seldom go away on their own. So, my guess is, ADD affects closer to 20–40% of the population to the point of true gut and brain disorder, with an additional 20–40% shortening their attention spans through environmental exposures such as blue light and social conditioning.

nnEMF: Non-native electromagnetic frequencies (i.e., man-made electromagnetic frequencies).

ADD is far more common than estimated or diagnosed because mental health professionals still look mostly for observable symptoms such as hyperactivity when diagnosing AD(H)D, instead of altered brain function. Incredibly significant in the way we perceive affected individuals, **every disease on the list has visible effects** (with the possible exception of depression). Some are even quantifiable with testing. But not ADD.

Because its effects can vary moment to moment, ADD is not obvious to observers, short of a SPECT brain scan. That's one reason ADD is severely underdiagnosed, indeed denied, by many as being made up by marketers and bad parents in order to try and get away with something.

Dozens of environmental threats become mental health problems

Science and medicine have failed to adequately explain that dozens of environmental threats we encounter every day damage the body in serious, yet invisible ways – particularly the health of our gut bacteria. This damage to the microbiome causes subtle, sometimes unnoticeable, brain dysfunction. And that brain dysfunction is the root cause of inability to think and behave "normally."

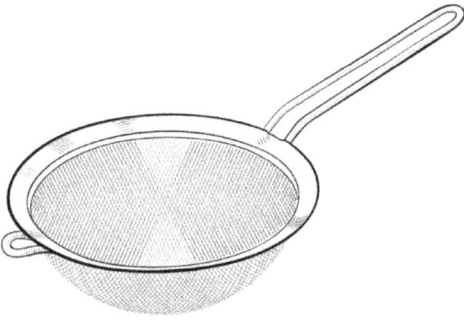

An unhealthy digestive tract is a foundational disturbance of disease in general

A primary way by which a corrupted gut causes mental and physical disorders is that the "glue" holding cells of the gut wall together gets dissolved by certain chemicals and foods, causing leaky membranes which would otherwise block these exposures from entering the bloodstream and contaminating brain and organ function. This "leakiness" can manifest itself in wide variety of ways throughout a person's lifetime, depending on toxin exposures, diet, genes, detox capacity, and general state of health. For example:

- From the age of 4–6 weeks, leaky gut and leaky membranes can cause discomfort around the digestive tract and inconsolable crying in babies called **colic.**
- After that, sensory processing deficits can occur that we categorized as **autism spectrum disorders,** from about 18–24 months onward.
- Shortly thereafter, if the individual's vulnerabilities, constitution and exposures are tipped a little more in their favor, they might instead develop **attention deficit disorder.**
- By ten years to the early teens, we start to see **anxiety disorders.**
- Into their teens, many people develop **irritable bowel syndrome or headaches.**
- Starting in the late teens, **depression, suicidal or homicidal behavior** is becoming disturbingly common.
- Starting in the early 20s, we see skyrocketing **infertility.**
- By the late 20s to early 30s, we're seeing increased **metabolic syndrome** and **type 2 diabetes.**
- By the 40s and 50s, shocking percentages of the population have **cardiovascular disease** and **kidney failure.**
- If you survive that, by your 40s, 50s and 60s, about half the population will be diagnosed with some form of **cancer.**
- And, if you're lucky enough to make it unscathed past your 60s, we're statistically likely to suffer **Alzheimer's, dementia or neurological degeneration** to one degree or another.

Which is all to say that leaky gut is far more than just gluten and casein intolerance, celiac disease, Crohn's disease, or irritable bowel syndrome. It's a much broader story of injury to the protective membranes of the body initiating a cascade of health-robbing effects throughout the body at different stages of life. It's a big deal that mainstream medicine is just now beginning to acknowledge and treat.

Sound far-fetched that so many diseases could come from a single source? It does until you learn all the amazing things that our good gut microbes do to nourish the body, protect us from harm, and regulate the brain. It all makes perfect sense when you know how food gets converted into brain function, well-being and longevity.

Join us on a journey to uncover how a corrupted gut causes attention deficit disorder and other GAPS conditions, as well as contribute to almost every chronic disease known to man. It's one of the biggest stories affecting our individual lives today, our healthcare systems, and the world in which we live. As Hippocrates, the father of modern medicine, said two thousand years ago, "All disease begins in the gut." Now you're going to learn the how and the why, so you can do something about it. Welcome to *Gut-Brain Secrets*.

Update 2022: Homosexuality and gender dysphoria originate from baby's brain being subjected to altered hormone levels in the womb

Since ~2000, there appears to be a sharp rise in the percentage of people who do not think and feel the same as their biological sex. Gender disharmony is causing millions of Gen Zs and millennials to go through life deeply conflicted/confused about their sexuality. It causes immense pain and suffering as the individual tries to cope as best they can with life-long compromises and can't-win scenarios. The phenomenon is truly an elephant in the room that the mental health field refuses to talk about.

Brain development basics: Fetal brain development is an extremely rapid and delicate process, with neural pathways being formed in mere weeks. A specific hormonal balance needs to be present in utero for a baby's brain to develop normal male or female characteristics. Whereas slight variations can incorporate flaws into the brain's operating system that cannot be revised once they're established. Anomalies are baked in permanently.

This cognitive/emotional priming process is designed to run on infinitesimally small hormonal parameters. Unfortunately, mothers and babies today are acutely and chronically overexposed to estrogen mimics from soy in foods, bisphenol-A and phthalates leeching from plastics, birth control pill residue in our water, artificial hormone replacements, and the herbicide atrazine. Environmental contaminants such as these wire the brain in a way that does not match a person's chromosomal blueprint – resulting in feminized male brains and masculinized female brains.

These people then experience lifelong gender dysphoria or sexual preference incongruities which are virtually impossible to resolve or even understand. Many or most become tortured souls. NWO puppet masters then harness the rampant depression and discontent for their own political gain. And that's how society devolves into the state that it's currently in.

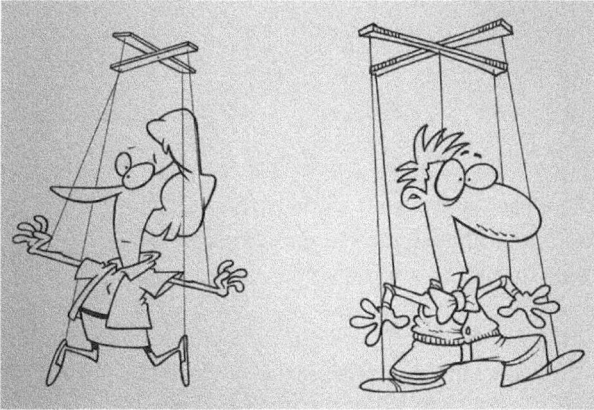

2

WE'RE IN A MATRIX OF A MESS

Productive action starts with accurate thinking

When skillful manipulators want to control your actions, habits and outcomes, they start at the source and influence your thoughts, beliefs, values and behaviors. First, they condition you to think in binary terms of *on or off, good or bad*, so they can divide and conquer. Then, they feed you half-truths so you think you know what's what, while important distinctions – the stuff that really matters – slips right by you. That's how propaganda works.

To illustrate what a profound difference that root mentality makes in a person's perspective, let's examine cultural biases. Westerners have been trained to think that the world is black or white, right or wrong, good or bad. It's been ingrained into us by all facets of society since the moment we were born. For example, an answer to a math problem is either right or it's wrong. Vegetables are good for you, and smoking is bad. A foreign country is good, or it's evil. But, you may be surprised to learn, much of the rest of the world does not think the way that Westerners do. The majority of the world's population, particularly in Asian countries, doesn't think in terms of either one *or* the other. Instead, they think in terms of black-*and*-white, good-*and*-bad, yin-*and*-yang.

Their way of thinking accepts the notion that "heads" and "tails" are two sides of the same coin, co-existing simultaneously. This side-by-side co-existence is the one of the foundational concepts of Asian culture. It's how they view the world, and the things in it. And they're better off in many respects for having this perspective… some others, not so much. This is an important concept to embed in your consciousness because it lays the foundation for accurate thinking and intelligent action when present. Or, it plants seeds for flawed thinking, indecision, apathy, and subjugation when absent. A confused mind has a hard time making decisions and taking action.

Real-life example of propaganda in action: Health educators tell you that calcium is good for you. They say you need calcium to keep your bones and teeth strong, so you should increase your dietary intake, and/or supplement with it. But do they tell you that you need potassium to balance out that calcium (they go together)? Do they tell you most calcium supplements are made from calcium carbonate, which does you very little good because the body can only convert a small percentage of it into usable form?

Do they tell you that you need vitamin K$_2$ to direct calcium into bones and teeth where it needs to go, instead of into soft tissues such as the blood vessels, where it calcifies and causes problems? Do they tell you most Westerners get plenty of calcium in their diet and don't need to supplement? Nope, nope, and nope.

One-dimensional thinking such as "calcium is good for you" gives you tunnel vision. Like going through life with blinders on, it makes you think what "they" want you to think, do as they desire, and buy what they want to sell you – including products, ideas and agendas. In this case, the dairy industry is the force operating behind the scenes to make us believe half-truths about calcium. Now, to be clear, the concept of "calcium is good for you" is not incorrect. It's just incomplete and borderline deceptive.

Unfortunately for us, half-truths like this can hurt you more than complete falsehoods, because you think you know how the world works when, in fact, you're living your life corrupted by false premises and assumptions. That's what happens when your foundational beliefs are built upon misdirection. As you're beginning to see, partial truths are one of the Establishment's favorite ways to control what you think and do. And until you wake up, you'll be living a life based on lies.

Social engineering

We've been trained to believe that the people in power have all the answers – while religion, arts, feelings, family ties, and personal experience are somehow less legitimate. Unfortunately, we the people automatically and unconsciously accept that context as our personal reality. And we do it without question because our hive minds want to think of ourselves as being good citizens in polite society.

Our social firmware wants so desperately to fit in with the program, that we'll believe anything we're told, so long as it comes from an authority figure and is repeated frequently. But it's just a construct. And it's not the only way you can organize your thoughts. It's just one way that you can, if you choose, think about a subject. You can alter the lens through which you see a subject, and that mode of thinking can completely change your perspective about it.

Unfortunately, most people never realize when they're being psychologically manipulated, because Edward Bernays' methods of propaganda are built on human nature and unspoken social rules. Remember, we may be human, but we're still part animal. You may think you're in control of your own thoughts and decisions but, the reality is, salesmen and politicians have been actively molding human behavior quite successfully for more than a century now. Special interest groups have got their indoctrination and gaslighting techniques dialed in to such a degree that they now tell truths or monumental lies with equal fluidity.

Edward Bernays: The father of public relations (PR), originator of propaganda and author of book by the same name (Propaganda, 1928).

Conclusion: If an evil-doer has got a huge budget, and lots of time to indoctrinate, he can make people believe anything he wants them to believe. Don't fall for it. The mediums of indoctrination evolve over time – including the Internet, social media, and traditional channels such as publishing and education. But the techniques invented by Edward Bernays in the 1920s and '30s to create authority and craft public opinion change very little. The process of getting groups to think in a certain way is very expensive and time consuming. But brainwashing is a well-defined, straightforward process to implement that's being used with shocking success by the elite and their foot soldiers today.

Groups are led by emotion

Groups are controlled by a reactionary, pack-like, mentality – rather than individual thought and rational choice. That's why it takes monumental effort, organization and, usually, money to get a group to accomplish something constructive. It's like herding cats. Yet people can be coaxed into supporting the most heinous acts of indecency by triggering their emotions. Spin doctors and PR people know this. Hitler and Goebbels knew it.

Joseph Goebbels: Reich Minister of Propaganda for the Nazi party.

These are the personality types that have (rightly) proclaimed: 'The bigger the lie, the easier it is fool people into believing it.' Why is this? Because individuals have some ability to think for themselves. Whereas groups have none. Groups are led by "groupthink." Therefore, most big ideas and achievements – both good or bad – are conceived, paid for, and propagated to promote some organization's agenda.

On the other hand, individuals that enjoy serving others seldom have the strategy, organization, money and, most important, the will to build consensus and effect large-scale change. The people that truly support freedom and humanity rarely have the resources and technique to fight The Powers That Be. Their good nature prevents them from even believing that globalists would hurt people in pursuit of their goals. The result: do-gooders usually get slaughtered taking on the Establishment. This is why most people believe, in error, that 'if a remedy were good, I would have heard about it already.' Normies underestimate the amount of coordination it takes for a big idea to succeed, as well as the lengths to which the Establishment will go to defend their positions of power.

Conclusion: We know healthcare is a business – a business masquerading as science and a profession. Indeed, healthcare is the biggest industry in the world. Likewise, food is a business. Big Food controls most of the nutrition education we receive today. We also know that globalists are motivated by profit and control. Nothing inherently wrong with profit or control; it's the methods and moral compass of the rule-makers that do the damage.

The problem is, we so badly want to believe that the world is a fair place, and that our leaders care about us, we'll gladly think what they want us to think, and do what they want us to do, despite all evidence that we are nothing more than livestock to most of them. Knowing that, it's up to you to seek the knowledge, and raise your responsibility, to the point that you can take care of yourself, because no one cares more about your health and well-being than you do. Through this process of self-enlightenment, we'll take you off the path that leads to disease and chronic dysfunction, and put you back in alignment with the life-giving forces of Nature.

The elite don't want you knowing the truth because it robs them of power

The drug companies, and those they influence, don't like it when people know the real reason that disease happens. They hate it when people learn the root causes of chronic disease, find ways to treat it, and tell others about it. They hate people knowing the truth, because it takes power away from them and gives it to you. This does more than just threaten their income; it robs them of control.

The ugly truth is, the drug companies don't want you dead, and they don't want you completely well either. Both are bad for business. Instead, they want to put you and keep you in a state of partial health – somewhere in between full health and death. So they do everything in their power to ignore, deny, distract, obstruct, ridicule, regulate, legislate, suppress, buy-out, bury, or otherwise defeat treatments that *they* can't monetize. They love partial solutions that keep you chronically ill and dependent on them.

So, most important to recognize, drugs don't cure. **They just change the expression of imbalance and disease in the body to another form, a different place, or a later time.** In doing so, mainstream medicine partially solves some of your problems (or tries to convince you that they did), and gives you a new set of problems in their place.

Mainstream medicine and agricultural science leads us astray

With several decades of "science" influencing our food, medicine, schools and media, we should have seen rates of ADD and autism decline, or at least stay the same. But the exact opposite has occurred: they've skyrocketed. Why is this? Hint: It's not a more sedentary lifestyle, bad parenting, or a lack of willpower. Our physiology is still the same as it's always been. Genetics are the same. Human nature is the same.

The problems we're experiencing have more to do with the information we're fed, lifestyle choices we make, foods we eat, toxins we ingest, and medical treatments we receive. Whether through omission or commission, coercion or subversion, we have been misguided. We've been led astray by the very organizations we've entrusted to run many aspects of our life.

But that is what it is. "They've" done what they've done. And they're going to continue doing what they're doing until they're forced to stop. Try as they may to convince us that they're on our side when it comes to supporting our health and finances, **they are not**. Their motivations are aligned with ours only to the extent that it affects their image and profits. The health and happiness of their customers may indeed be one of their considerations. It's just lower down their list of priorities than most of us would care to admit.

But now it's up to *us* to take our power back. We must realize there are reasons that mental health disorders like ADD, autism, anxiety, depression and dementia are occurring at records rates. It's no accident that physical diseases such as heart disease, diabetes, cancer and autoimmunity are accelerating in the population. It's not bad luck in the genetic lottery. And it's not unknown. When you take responsibility for your own beliefs and outcomes, you will find answers and solutions to diseases of modern man.

As the one person who is most interested in your success, you must fight for your right to make your own choices. Don't give away your power to choose to anyone. It's your right – should you choose to exercise it – to live your life in the best health possible. With new insights into biochemistry and biophysics pouring into the public consciousness over the last two decades, health or sickness is rapidly becoming a choice we all have to make – either proactively or unintentionally.

Ken Rohla on how "the system" is rigged against us

"The medical system is really good at dealing with acute injury, but they're horrible at dealing with degenerative injury because their industry has been manipulated by the drug industry, the medical technology industry, and others. So I saw all these very well-intentioned people who were completely ignorant of natural methods of healing – nutrition and things like that. It was by design. For example, nutrition is kept out of medical doctors' training. Herbology and natural methods have historically been kept out of the medical system since its founding because those methods are viewed as not as profitable as conventional medical techniques using drugs and surgery.

So there's this lack of awareness among well-meaning people who are perpetuating a system that's not sustainable and doesn't work well for degenerative illness. And yet they all believe that they're doing good for the population because of their programming and their beliefs… and so that's kind of a metaphor for what's going on on this planet.

You've got people at the upper echelons of power throughout history who have a better understanding of the nature of our reality… of matter, energy, science and physics. They've intentionally kept the masses misdirected through systems they've put in place, that have evolved over time, and become more sophisticated, to keep people's awareness limited in a paradigm that benefits them, they can profit off of, that they can feed off of, and that they can control."

Comparing two paths to wellness: Man's Way *vs.* Nature's Way

Examining two different approaches to nutrition and disease, side-by-side, can revolutionize your understanding of human health. One approach is based on top-down principles supporting the profit and politics of big business. This way – Man's Way – is all about centralized control. The other approach is one in which man cooperates with the extremely sophisticated, but subtle, finesse of Nature. This way – Nature's Way – is unimaginably intelligent and experienced.

Most important to this discussion, the first paradigm has been deliberately crafted to create disease and manage it. It's all about "what's in it" for people at the top and those that "play ball" with them. Conversely, the second paradigm focuses on respecting the body's healing ability, removing unfriendly influences, and increasing the resources with which the body can restore balance.

Approach #1: Man's Way

First, let's invent a fictional world where people in power like to control and manipulate the masses for fun and profit. In this fantasy land, anything goes so long as the people don't know what makes them sick or well, don't take responsibility, and trust those in power because they wear nice suits and look good on TV. Here, you can get away with anything so long as the people can't tell when they're being tricked, and evildoers aren't held accountable. In this paradigm where elected and appointed officials know what's best for We The People, multi-national corporations engage in malfeasance that normies automatically label as conspiracy theory, without actually looking at the facts.

Hypothetically, how would these power- and profit-hungry parties go about convincing the public that their offering is safe and effective – even when it's not, while at the same time maligning things that *are* good for you? For example, let's say an entity such as agriculture company wanted to convince consumers that a crop amendment such as glyphosate, a food additive, or a genetically modified organism is safe. Or let's say they wanted to show that a food or nutritional component that comes from Nature, and that man has eaten for thousands of years, all of a sudden is bad for you (e.g., saturated animal fat).

Puppet masters might use "scientific research," publishing, higher education, PR, news media, grants, status, and official accolades to create a perception of reality. What they could do is find research scientists who have impressive-sounding credentials, and/or who are associated with

Normies: Unawakened member of the general public who believes official narratives because they trust authority figures more than themselves.

well-respected institutions, and ask them if they want to accept 2, 10 or 50 million dollars to go study their X, Y or Z hypothesis.

The money will pay for laboratory expenses, support staff, publishing PR and, most important, income of the researchers. Remember, scientists have families to feed, just like everybody else. And, let's not forget, the reputation and career path of research scientists is measured by the papers they publish and the studies they participate in. Their worth and legacy is closely tied to the recognition they get, and the projects they're associated with.

So, the special-interest party finds their people and offer them big bucks to design, conduct, analyze and, hopefully, publish the study. All the while, the scientists – presumably interested in their own survival – understand implicitly or explicitly which results benefit the special-interest party that gave them the money, and which ones do not.

How to brainwash the masses, Step 1: These hand-picked scientists are "flexible" enough to: (1) devise study criteria, (2) conduct studies, (3) analyze data, and (4) summarize conclusions in a way that favors the predetermined outcomes of their "sugar daddies." Generally speaking, if you make your living off of grant money, you know you might have bend over backwards to protect the interests of your benefactors, or else your career might be over sooner, rather than later. So, with money to drive the project forward, the study proceeds.

Next, what might happen in this imaginary world is that follow-up studies, articles, press releases, marketing messages, and academic curriculums (e.g., books teaching the researchers of tomorrow) could all reference the first study's results, and confirm its findings. Whereas the studies that failed to support the initial study's findings could be re-written, redone, spun, buried in obscure publications, or simply never published.

Through repetition over time, special-interest groups like these could build what appeared to be a consensus of opinion throughout the industry on the subject. With lots of money and power at stake, as well as abundant means and opportunity to influence the prevailing paradigm, they could all chip in to drown out the voices of skeptics. They could silence dissenters through tried-and-true methods such as these.

Examples of myths built on lies:
- Disease is genetic. Food quality is irrelevant. The USDA Food Pyramid.
- Cholesterol and saturated (animal) fats cause heart disease and stroke.
- Fluoride is good for your teeth.
- UV light causes cancer.
- "Everything in moderation." The idea sounds reasonable, but inaccurate thinking leads you into viewpoints with which you're easy to fool. Mercury, aluminum and glyphosate are perfect examples. No amount of them is safe.

How to build apparent consensus for ideas – whether valid or not.
For even greater impact, influential entities such as health agencies, prominent universities, and health associations may amp-up the fear and anxiety
by repeatedly warning consumers of dire consequences should they fail to
heed the entities' recommendations. Their giant commercial and PR
engines could traumatize the psyche of the people by broadcasting messages
of impending doom should people not reduce their "X," or do more "Y."

Our educational system could be deployed to indoctrinate leaders from
many fields into that way of thinking. They would repeat the message as
gospel in textbooks, government guidelines, news outlets, speaking engage-
ments, books and lifestyle magazines. Unwitting participants, out to make
a buck, would undoubtedly get swept up in the hype and design programs
that avoid the dreaded "X" or give you more of the miracle supplement "Y."

Regulatory agencies, medical boards, and private foundations could
regulate, investigate, smear, and load up competing ideas with expenses
and regulations to drive them out of business. Meanwhile, special-interest
groups could heighten the perceived credibility of their own
spokespeople by fast tracking them into prominent positions,
commendations, collaborations, and lots of airtime.

You think this could actually happen? You really think people could
be so uncaring as to lead humanity astray like that? And what would this
imaginary world be like to live in? What would happen if situations like
this were allowed to operate more or less unhindered?

A: We'd be brainwashed into believing that, out of the goodness of
their hearts, our institutions were looking out for the interests of "the
people," and not the puppet masters paying the bills of those in the
system. We would find ourselves in a complex web of influence and
control that spends 99% of its research and marketing budget on a
paradigm of disease and dysfunction, instead of teaching people how the
body supports itself with food and lifestyle choices.

We would have a population so backwards in its thinking, so perverse
in its lifestyle choices, that it actually thought Nature is stupid, fragile, and
does not know what it's doing. We would have the most educated
people on earth believing Nature made a bunch of mistakes in its billions
of years of experience, and that man's science and industry can beat
Nature at its own game.

Back to reality. When you examine the level of intelligence inherent in
human biology – its sophistication, adaptability, and abuse tolerance – you
realize that we as a society are getting *more things wrong* with our agriculture
and food supply, healthcare, commerce, and societal ways *than we're getting
right*. Virtually every aspect of the way we live now depletes us of health
– yet life, currently under attack from all angles, is still in the fight. Remove
harmful exposures, provide good resources, and life usually prevails.

But we're not examining mass mind-control techniques and identifying problems just to vilify any particular group. It's to show you how, given the opportunity, certain people and groups might use their positions of power for their own benefit. "They" might not place your health and happiness at the top of their priority list. They might tend to spend more time worrying about their own interests, than you and I, once they've gotten drunk off of the power, privilege and control that comes from running other people's lives. I'm just saying, it might be a temptation.

But, believe it or not, the long list of catastrophes we're now facing – they're all related to a corrupted gut in some way. Interestingly consistent with what we just talked about, gut dysbiosis causes man to act out more of his animal instincts by suppressing higher brain functions that would normally control his base impulses. Corruption of the gut is increasing the very conditions in the brain, and in our actions, that are problematic for individuals, groups, and the entire planet. It's the perfect storm of man's lust for power and control, meeting man's primitive urges coming from the hind (reptilian) brain.

Approach #2: Nature's Way

A perfect example of how working with Nature, rather the against it, can help mankind (re)discover practical knowledge we can use: Weston A. Price, DDS was a dentist and prominent health researcher who travelled the world in the 1920s and '30s, studying the relationship between nutrition, dental health, and physical health in indigenous peoples 'before' and 'after' they were introduced to a Western diet.

Among the fascinating discoveries he cataloged in his travels, native Eskimos told Dr. Price that their sled dogs could not work all day long when they fed them plain, fresh fish. On the other hand, their dogs happily pulled hard all day long when the fish was fermented first.

The Eskimos concluded that if fermenting increases a dog's stamina, then it must be enhancing the nutritional value of food, which benefitted a dog's physiology in some way. They didn't know how or why fermenting worked, but it did. They also didn't notice any side effects. It never failed to work. It seemed to be in alignment with Nature. So they stuck with it. This is the miracle of Nature in action – a way of thinking that corporate interests have been trying to discredit for decades.

The Eskimos didn't need to pay someone to study the science behind their observations. They didn't need to know the mechanisms of action in the body. They didn't look to a government agency to certify the process safe and grant its approval. They just made the assumption that 'if it's good for our dogs' it must be good for us too. They trusted that this was no accident; Nature knew what it was doing. So they went with it.

Likewise, seeing what works and what doesn't in the real world is a more direct route for the holistic community to take when they haven't got millions or billions to back their ideas, like Big Food and Big Pharma do. Much of the material that follows gives you example after example of Man's Way getting it dead wrong over the past century, and Nature having the truth, and the way, all along.

Our saving grace: For every problem, there is a solution

The good news is, you don't have to live in a state of fear, hopelessness, or dependency when you learn about the challenges we face in our modern world. The way the universe works, each disease or problem must have an equal and opposite force counterbalancing it. It's a foundational rule of Nature that our universe is built upon, which is closely related to polarity. For the negative to exist, there must be positive. There is both light and dark. There's hot and cold. Highs can't exist without lows. For every yin, there is a yang.

So, the moment a problem comes into existence, the universe simultaneously creates a solution to that problem. Whether that deals with health, society, personal or business, a problem cannot exist without a way to solve it. Of course, problems are usually planned, executed and promoted better than solutions because most problems are (intentionally) concocted by The Powers That Be to serve their master plans. But, as bad as a situation appears to be, you can be sure there is a solution for every problem, for those who seek it. That means you don't have to accept someone else's plan for the way your health is, or will be. You don't have live in someone else's reality. You can create your own outcomes, starting with the decision to be your own health boss.

You will need knowledge and a few new tricks

Solving chronic health challenges will take some discovery, trials and tribulation on your part. But take comfort in the understanding that the universe never makes you experience any more than you can handle. So when you're ready for answers, and seek them out, the right information will find you. It's long been said that, 'When the student is ready, the teacher will appear.' You can do your part to bring that into being by acting in agreement with it. What's more, the universe is not bound to the same time restrictions that we humans are. The universe can (re)arrange events that we perceive to be in our past, or future, so that we find our present to be different than what we expected.

Staying in the right frame of mind is crucial to keep us from obsessing over problems and accidentally attracting more of them into your life.

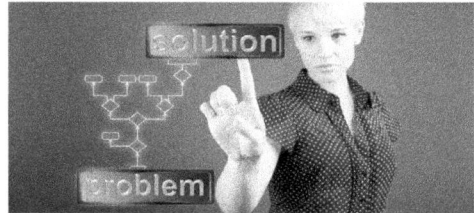

Instead, learn everything that you can about the problem and solution in as detached a manner as possible. Don't dwell on the negativity of the situation. Instead, work the problem and then release any anxiety you have of its emotional charge. Let go of any fear you have, and it loses its power over you. Then, redirect your attention and positive energy toward finding a solution. That draws health and prosperity into your life, like a magnet.

Now, I should note, I'm not a big fan of keeping a positive attitude just for its own sake (i.e., without doing the homework and being ready spiritually to receive the lessons). Gratitude is great, but I'd start with focusing your attention and energy on finding answers and solutions to your own problems. You need to help you. Don't rely on positivity alone to heal you. With new understandings of biochemistry and biophysics coming into practical use, I can tell you: it is now possible.

Ken Rohla on the importance of mindset

"Great masters throughout time have taught this concept of being unattached. And the reason is, when you create your reality, yes, you're responsible for everything in it. And you can take that to a great degree with things like ho'oponopono, which is a Hawaiian kahuna concept of taking responsibility for everything in your life that you encounter, and asking forgiveness for it. When you do that, everything around you changes with great effect.

On the flip side of the coin, you've got this New Age concept of everything's just love, light and angels. And, of course, the Law of Attraction says you should focus only on what you want to attract. Therefore, you shouldn't look at the dark side. The problem with that is, you don't want to be dwelling on the dark side of things. But you need to be aware of it, so you can navigate through this reality. And if you truly 'get' at a deep, emotional level that you create your reality, and that you're empowered, and that you're living consciously, then the dark side can't affect you.

You will always have a counter to whatever things the dark side is coming up with. And so it's very important to face your dark side, or whatever these negative things are in your reality, and to understand them. And, through understanding them, then you can do what you need to do to counteract any possible effects they may have on you, while not dwelling on them. You can be aware of them. You can understand the nature of them. And then you can focus on the positive. Focus on what you want to create, and you'll attract that. But **living in denial of the dark side is every bit as disempowering as just focusing on the positive.** You've got to be aware of it, but not focus on it.

When you create your reality, and you have the power, then these negative things don't have power over you. For example, someone asked me on an interview yesterday: 'Don't all these negative things in the world make you depressed?' Absolutely not, because I know the solutions are out there. I've seen them. I've witnessed them. So I'm not depressed at all. I think, in the end, we're going to pull everything out just fine. I'm out there in the world sharing with people these solutions, so that we can all change it."

Knowing what causes health or disease is rapidly becoming the most valuable knowledge a person can have

It's one of the greatest assets in life – especially for ADDers. The truth about what causes mental dysfunction can change your life, because without physical health AND a well-functioning brain, you're going to get a fraction of what you can out of life. Without a brain that works right, your life is one big compromise.

One of the goals I had in creating this book is to give you a brand-new perspective about how the body works, so you can reverse your psychological and physical health challenges, and build better health for yourself and those around you. Knowing what enhances brain function, and what impairs it, starts right now.

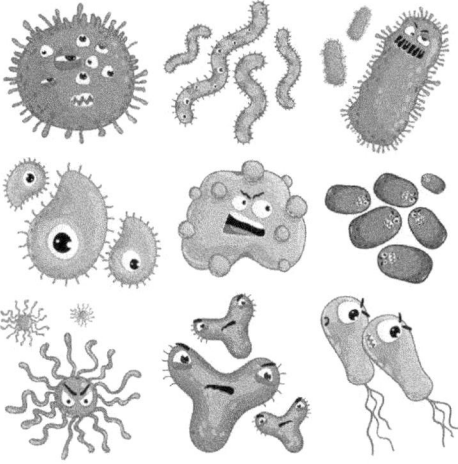

3

THE WISDOM OF NATURE *VS.* THE FALLIBILITY OF MAN

"Illnesses do not come upon us out of the blue. They are developed from small daily sins against Nature. When enough sins have accumulated, illnesses will suddenly appear." —Hippocrates

Every type of microorganism on this planet is here for a reason

They each have an important role to play in keeping the earth's ecosystem balanced and prosperous. That includes microorganisms we traditionally think of as disease-causing, such as molds, fungi, yeasts, viruses and bacteria. Bacteria, in particular, play far more pro-life roles in the food chain than we've traditionally given them credit for. Bacteria regulate the health of the entire food chain from start to finish.

- **Nutrient cycling in soil.** The growth and sustenance of naturally-grown plants are run by bacteria.
- **Short chain fatty acid production in pasture-grazing animals (e.g., cows).** Bacteria convert fibrous plant material into fat in the stomachs of pasture animals.
- **The digestion of carnivores that eat the herbivores.** Bacteria control the digestion of most creatures on earth.
- **The health of apex consumers.** Bacteria are essential to nutrient production and absorption, immune system modulation, and the gene expression of omnivores atop the food chain.

Beneficial bacteria play many roles in nourishing the food chain

Not so many know that so-called "disease-causing" pathogens have their own roles to play too. Their purpose in life is to decompose plants and animals after they die. Pathogens are the garbage collectors and recyclers of the planet. They return the nutrients of dead plants, animals, and toxic materials back to the earth so they can be used again in the next cycle.

This second half of the food cycle – the recovery phase – is not-so obvious, because it's not celebrated in the way that nutrients make their way *up* the food chain. Death and decay are not sexy topics for marketing departments or media to spotlight. Nor are they as profitable for science to study. Death isn't pretty, and decay doesn't sell. So neither receive the attention that happier topics do. However, death and decay do create raw material for the next cycle, so it's crucial to understand why pathogens exist in the first place. This is a very important point:

Pathogens are called to duty when disease conditions are present

Degenerative conditions, such as an acidic environment, invite pathogens out to play. It's an ancient understanding that modern humans must relearn. But, hiding within that concept, is the fact that pathogenic organisms are always present in small numbers on every scoop of soil, piece of fruit, and surface of biology. All animals host pathogens all over their insides and outsides. They're in the rivers and seas. They're in the air. They're everywhere. In a healthful environment, pro-life organisms predominate. And while pathogens are always present, they keep such a low profile that you might never know they're there.

However, there are two situations where pathogens make their presence known: When disease-promoting conditions tell the microbes that it's time to recycle dead plant and animal matter. And when the probiotic flora that keep pathogens in check are suppressed. They usually go hand-in-hand, because when an animal dies, its probiotic populations shrink and pathogens swell. When pathogens increase, you become nutrient deficient, and the environment shifts to suit pathogen populations. This is the present state of most Americans. To our microscopic housekeepers, our internal environment increasingly looks like it's dying and in need of decomposition.

Disease conditions that trigger pathogen overgrowth
- Poor oxygenation/high CO_2 of blood and tissues.
- Acidic conditions. The first two usually go together.
- Buildup of positive charge and chronic inflammation. (i.e., too much oxidation, not enough antioxidant activity).
- Slow removal of toxic metabolic waste products.
- Environmental toxin exposure, such as heavy metals, industrial chemicals, crop amendments, hormone mimics and pollution.
- Lack of diversity in the microbiome.
- Nutrient deficiencies.

In general, degenerative conditions fall into the following categories: (1) digestion or metabolism, (2) detoxification, or (3) gut dysbiosis. They are the blueprint by which disease materializes. Conversely, when you get the nutrients you need, eliminate waste properly, and are biochemically balanced, you're naturally free of disease. For example, cancer can't survive in the presence of plenty of oxygen, good nutrition, a clean environment, and cells that are repairing and replacing themselves.

To sum up, pathogens can only take over your inner terrain when they are invited to do so. This occurs when your life force is low and conditions indicate that it's time to decay the organism back to the earth. Pathogens then go to work decomposing matter back to its original form.

Pathogens proliferate when friendly flora isn't there to protect you
For example, after a round of antibiotics, major illness, or bad infection like cholera. The reason being, probiotic life is inherently superior to pathogens. Probiotics are a higher life form because the universe favors life. In living systems, probiotic organisms evolved as the stronger life form. They can out-compete pathogens with more powerful antimicrobial substances. Seems obvious when you think about it: for decomposers to exist, you first must have builders.

Unfortunately, man's interventions have upset this delicate balance of Nature ever since Big Business hijacked our food and medicine. That's why you usually don't see pathogens take over a space as a result of a so-called "infection." Instead, they proliferate because your good bacteria are weak, pH is off, immune system is dysregulated, or you're malnourished.

So, you see, pathogens are not the bad guy. Even though we think of them as disease-causing, they don't exist to do us harm. They're simply the back side of the cycle of life that we don't like to think about, talk about, or research. Disease-causing microorganisms are Nature's way of culling weak and infirm cells and organisms, and removing them from the food chain, so their resources can be put back into the ecosystem.

But, just as valuable, most pathogens do some good things in the body. They have special skills that only they can do, such as synthesizing certain vitamins; producing antibiotic substance to suppress more harmful pathogens; or detoxing heavy metals, chemicals, and even radioactive substances. Which all goes to show: Nature knew what it was doing when it designed probiotics, pathogens, and a delicate balance between the two. So when pathogens show up in your life prematurely, consider it a wakeup call to change your diet and exposures, to put the good guys back in charge.

Microbes transform themselves according to their environment
Royal Rife and others have shown that microbes can transform themselves from bacteria to fungi to virus, and back again, in response to their environment – called "pleomorphism." That is, when an organism is healthy, its microbes will take one form. And when the organism dies and is in decay, the microbes' role will change from a supporter of life into a microscopic housekeeper/recycler. Microorganisms sense their surroundings and change to a structural form that's needed in their environment. This is how Nature promotes the circle of life and death.

However, this metamorphosis does not happen instantly. And it's not discernable to the casual observer, thus medical science has nothing to say about pleomorphism. As a concept, the whole idea of pleomorphism conflicts with their agendas – particularly their model of infection and contagion – so anything they know about the subject is kept quiet.

More and more hospitals are feeling the pain of opposing Nature, as they become breeding grounds for drug-resistant germs

We now live in a germaphobic culture (no thanks to those pushing hand gel, antibiotics and sanitizing practices). No one is more infatuated by this idea than hospitals. They obsessively, compulsively try to sterilize every touched surface with chemical disinfectants. But the problem is, pathogens are the first to grow back after each cleaning. Without good guys there to protect surfaces against pathogens, all they succeed in doing is creating unguarded territory for nasty pathogens to breed as best they can in the relatively infertile grounds of furniture, fixtures, office equipment, and workers' clothing.

The medical system seems slow to realize that killing everything, over and over again, carries substantial risks. They think more frequent use of hand sanitizer, and more thorough sterilization of surfaces, will eradicate drug-resistant organisms from their facilities. But that approach may not solve rising MRSA rates, because the paradigm competes with Nature by trying to smother life. As a result, some hospital systems have even been forced to shut down, demolish, and rebuild facilities because all attempts to exterminate multiple-drug-resistant pathogens have failed. Efforts to reduce infection rates among patients were unsuccessful, so they basically had to hit the reset button and start over from scratch.

Infectious diseases of old, and modern-day syndromes, may have a common cause

Many diseases feared in past centuries were caused by an overgrowth of infectious microorganisms. Plagues and such were caused by microbes that thrive(d) in unsanitary conditions, along with poor nutrition. On the other hand, most modern diseases are a collection of symptoms we put into a diagnostic box and call "disease." Not knowing their origins, more and more diseases are becoming a bunch of observations such as hyperactivity, or effects such as poor circulation – some of which are associated with microbial overgrowth, but most are not.

Point being, something upstream from diseases, both old and new, is causing illness to occur. Often, the root cause is not a pathogen alone. Instead, it's unhealthful conditions that allow(ed) the disease to take place. Cancer and heart disease are two examples of multi-factor imbalances leading to breakdown of the body's compensation mechanisms. Therefore, pathogen overgrowth and observable symptom clusters, are not driving forces that create disease. They are consequences of an imbalanced internal environment, and exhaustion of protective (rebalancing) mechanisms. For this reason, a diagnosis these days tells you little to nothing about the source and solution to each situation, at least from a mainstream doctor's perspective.

Update 2022: My new way of describing how microbes cause infections
It will revolutionize your understanding of infections and pandemics. For context, *the germ theory* contends that when microbes outside of your body get inside, they multiply and cause an infectious disease, such as a viral infection. That theory is false. More accurately, it's a half-truth that misleads people into believing the full lies of Big Pharma and globalists.

How infections really work: In the natural world – absent complete chemical sterilization – we are always surrounded by microorganisms. They are everywhere. Thus, **infectious diseases are caused by microbial exposure (or other agent), exceeding the immune system's ability to contain it.** In other words, infections are caused by a combination of: (1) the quantity of microbes that get inside you and their virulence, relative to (2) the body's ability to keep them from multiplying.

Using simple logic, even people that believe Fake News can agree that the preceding idea is true. But mainstream medical "experts" have brainwashed the masses into believing that *any* exposure to viruses or bacteria will make you sick. This is quite obviously not true. **Your immune system (which you have control over) is the bigger factor in whether you get sick or not.** This seemingly minor omission makes all the difference in what you'll believe… and put up with.

And the result? Their fake stories promote fear and obedience in sheeple due to the fact that invisible microbes are much harder to control than taking personal responsibility to boost your immune system with things like vitamin D and A, eating right, and reducing your wireless radiation exposure. Furthermore, their strategy hides the truth from you and keeps you dependent on them. Now can you see the subtle mind manipulation happening here?

Top: Louis Pasteur.

Bottom: Florence Nightingale, by Henry Lenthall, circa 1850s.

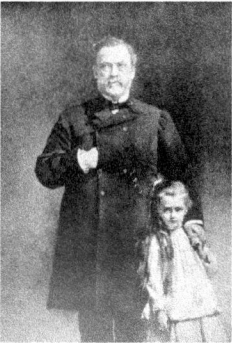

Louis Pasteur's "germ theory" *vs.* Antoine Béchamp and Claude Bernard's "terrain theory"
Louis Pasteur made the germ theory famous starting in the 1850s. He studied the growth and behavior of tiny organisms under a microscope and concluded that germs cause disease. But if germs really cause disease, all we have to do is find something to kill germs and we can wipe out disease… right? Well, not exactly. We have plenty of things to kill germs, yet disease is skyrocketing with no end in sight. Indeed, the harder we try to wipe out microorganisms through antibiotic practices, the more rapidly that drug-resistant pathogens spread.

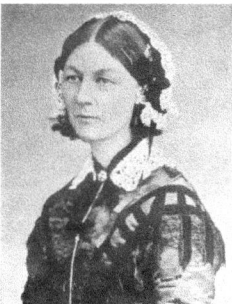

Florence Nightingale puts the terrain theory to the test
Around the time that Pasteur was conducting his research in the 1850s, a natural health pioneer, Florence Nightingale (founder of modern nursing born to wealthy parents), was sent to look after

soldiers injured in the Crimean War. When she arrived, conditions in the hospital were appalling. The plumbing didn't work, raw sewage polluted corridors, rotting food filled the kitchen, soldiers waited days or weeks for treatment, and the mortality rate was 50%. Soldiers had a better chance of surviving the battlefield than that hospital. She wanted to help, but knew it wouldn't be easy.

To get started, she and her cadre of thirty-eight nurses offered to clean the filthy facilities that she believed to be causing the terrible mortality. But the doctors refused her entry into the wards. Instead, they sent nurse Nightingale to the kitchen, so she started there. She scrubbed everything in sight. She telegrammed her father and had him send a shipload of clean linens, clothes, mattresses, bandages, and a cook.

Two and a half weeks later, another ship of wounded arrived that pushed the hospital further over its capacity. Staff was already overworked, so the doctors reluctantly agreed to let Florence and her nurses into the main hospital. The first thing they did was scrub the walls and open the windows to let fresh air in. She made all the doctors wash their hands between operations. She got the plumbing fixed. She put the clean linens into use. She cleaned up every nook and cranny in the hospital where germs can fester and, within six months, the mortality rate was 2%.

When Nightingale returned to England, she was hailed as a hero. But she objected. To her mind, all she did was improve the sanitation, hygiene, and nutrition. Florence Nightingale knew that germs don't cause disease. Germs are the result of unhealthful conditions. She knew what our medical science is just now beginning to accept: pathogens can't thrive in a healthy environment. Whether through cleanliness, a strong immune system, or the presence of good bacteria, harmful germs have no purpose or place in healthful conditions. Pathogens don't thrive in a healthy body.

Example of how an environment attracts its inhabitants

I live in a place filled with trees and shrubs. It's basically a forest. And no matter what anyone in the community does to try and keep bugs out, they will always be around. Naturally, a few of them find their way inside and eat anything edible. So, to no surprise, the summer after I moved in, I found some ants marching around like they owned the place. Now, having learned what I did from Barbara O'Neill, I knew poisonous ant traps are one way to try and get rid of unwanted pests. But a better strategy is to thoroughly clean the place and remove all the food that they like.

I did it. And it worked. I've seen scouts from time to time on what seem to be reconnaissance missions. But they don't come back with reinforcements. So instead of striking back at the ants directly, which is a person's natural instinct, I eliminated their reason for being there: food and provisions. Once the things that attracted them were gone, being there was a waste of resources. So they left and sought sustenance elsewhere.

Summary of the germs *vs.* environment debate

Symptoms of modern diseases – such as mental disorders, autoimmunity, and even weight problems – have no reason to be in the body when conditions are not right for them to exist. They are reactions to, or a product of, problematic conditions in the body. And when you fix those flaws, your fault detection/alert system called *symptoms* tells you by turning off the body's responses to those irregularities. Symptoms cease to exist.

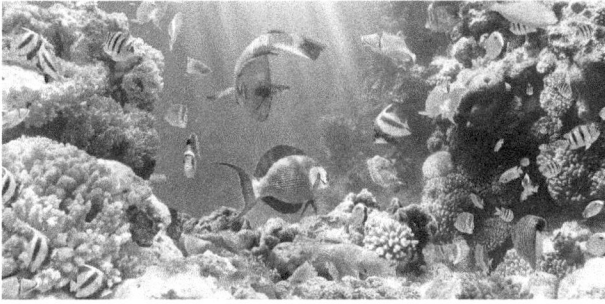

Nature favors life

And life proliferates to the fullest extent that it can, wherever that may be: in the soil, human body, atmosphere, Mariana's Trench, volcanoes, oil wells ten miles deep – even nuclear reactors. Voids don't exist for long in nature, wherever life is capable of growing. That means in both soil and our microbiomes, some sort of biology will fill any space fertile enough to host life. That life will continue to grow, until the space is as full as resources allow.

It's for these reasons that pathogens can only take root when probiotic organisms are absent. You have a certain amount of space available in various bodily compartments. And that terrain is going to be colonized by one life form or another. When beneficial critters are abundant, pathogens will be present, but their numbers limited. On the other hand, when the good guys are weakened, only then can pathogens take over.

Sunlight supports life, while moonlight supports death and decay

Sunlight and moonlight have distinctly different qualities. Sunlight gives us (i.e., used to give us) a golden light that's warming, drying, life-giving, and topically antiseptic (disinfecting). It helps regulate our pineal gland and production of many biochemicals we depend on – including vitamin D, melatonin, serotonin, 5-HTP, and tryptophan. Our sleep cycles, hormone levels, brain function, and mood depend on sunlight.

Yet, plants need sunlight even more than we do. Using chlorophyll, plants capture sunlight to make food for themselves and others. They need the sun's warmth to suppress microbial populations on their surfaces. These foundational processes support life on earth by feeding the entire food chain.

On the flip side of the circle of life, moonlight has the opposite effect of sunlight. It radiates a silvery light that's cold and dampness-forming. In doing so, moonlight increases condensation, microbial activity, and decomposition, thus completing the circle of life. We've all felt it: Clear nights get much colder, much faster, than overcast ones. And although clouds do slow the release of earth's heat like a blanket, I believe the bigger effect is thermal induction.

Consider this: Just as infrared light can make atoms vibrate faster to produce heat, the moon may absorb heating frequencies from the sun, and reflect cooling frequencies to earth. When absorbed by objects on earth at night, these frequencies slow the vibration of atoms in a material, thereby cooling it. In fact, studies have shown that coldness can be induced by EMF radiation, just as heat can. Believe it or not, **moonlight (*vs.* "moon shade") has actually been shown to reduce temperature by 2–10°F.**

Night is when molds, fungi, and some bacteria spring into action

Symbolized (and powered) by the moon, nighttime helps decomposer microbes break down fallen leaves, branches, diseased plants and dead animals. Conversely, daytime is a rebirth from rest. Symbolized (and powered) by the sun, the days are about creation, health and activity. Symbolically, days are life and nights are death.

It's for these reasons the sun and moon have been used for millennia to represent the battle between good and evil. For ages, ancient myths and legends told tales of astrological gods that ruled the sun and moon. Far from mere entertainment, seasonal rituals involving sun and moon have fascinated man from the dawn of time to the present day for good reason.

Yet we tend to view the manner in which ancient peoples worshipped as amusing customs and primitive beliefs peculiar to their group. Little did we know, man's ancient observances had more to do with reality than we ever realized. Their practices were more practical than we thought, while our modern ways are getting more things wrong than right.

Our way of life promotes degeneration and death

Who can deny, we're being pushed into states of sepsis (self-injury through immune hyper-activation), necrosis (cell death), and putrefaction (rotting). Our culture is being driven into breakdown mode by almost everything in our environment: dirty food, water, air, energy, lifestyle choices, medicines and electrosmog. It's plain theft of our life-giving energy and healing capacity. This makes us live in perpetual survival mode, rather than our natural state of thriving.

And humans aren't alone. Look closely at the trees and shrubs in your neighborhood. Do they look like they're thriving? For those old enough to remember the days before cell phones and Wi-Fi, do you see as many insects as you used to (that feed the food chain)? Do you see early morning dew on plants anymore? To top it off, do an image search for "massive fish die off" or "massive dead birds" on your favorite search engine.

I looked into this effect again to confirm my conclusions for the 3rd Edition. I'm now more confident that moonlight does indeed have a cooling effect. Link to YouTube video entitled "Colder in the Moonlight (3:36 in length)": https://youtu.be /cH-M4s7S_7I

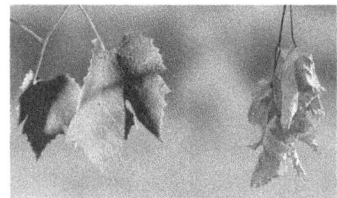

Now think about this: The things that are stressing plants and animals into oblivion are affecting your biochemistry right now too. The human body just has better coping mechanisms than lower life forms, enabling it to resist disease for longer. Taking full advantage of this fact, the elites pacify us with chemical, pharmaceutical, dietary, lifestyle and psychological entertainment, while their products, programs and approaches suck the life out of us. They're killing us slowing but surely.

Birth, growth and life are supposed to be the favored state of Nature. But there's way too much degradation built into our society now, with more being forced upon us with each product update. On a planetary scale, it's quite obvious the entire planet is showing signs of advanced disease. A perpetual state of struggle and survival is the new normal.

Myth: The human body is stupid, fragile, and needs help. Reality: Biology is smarter than we ever imagined

The human body is so exquisitely engineered, yet inconspicuous in its operation, that medical science still thinks of symptoms as defects. Our adaptation systems are so fault-tolerant that the body takes a beating and just keeps on ticking – sometimes weathering decades of punishment before exhausting its resources and sounding the alarm: 'If your choices don't change soon, health crises are going to pay you a visit.'

Unfortunately, we, as a culture, never learned how the body works, why it malfunctions, what symptoms mean, or how to fix glitches. Our institutions have dropped the ball in teaching us the root causes of disease. So we, as consumers, are left to our own devices to find scattered information, know what's right or wrong for us, and fight to get what we need. These are the basics of intentional wellness. But most people are lousy at fending for themselves because they never learned the fundamentals of self-care, such as the following:

Symptoms help you decipher the body's pleas and warnings

Symptoms are not the source of health problems, as organized medicine would have us believe. As expressions of disequilibrium, they are a feedback mechanism designed to make us aware of how stressed or broken the body is. In the early stages of disease, symptoms cause a fuss to warn us about deficits and malfunctions that the body is not able to fix on its own. They warn us about our iffy ways and request that changes be made, while you're still able. Later, when disease is advanced, symptoms tell you that the body is upset beyond its ability to cope.

The meta-example we're all familiar with is pain. Pain isn't the source of what ails us. It's a reaction to disease which motivates us to change. But it's the broken bone, gut dysbiosis, arthritis, or blocked artery that's really causing the pain. So why not fix the source, if/when you can?

Which brings us to a main point of *Gut-Brain Secrets*: The causes of most chronic disease are not a mystery that medical science will one day figure out decades from now. They're already known to those who want to hear the truth and seek it. And alternative healers have already worked out a great many solutions to reverse modern diseases… solutions you've never heard about because they've been suppressed.

Your call to action: If you want be in excellent health for your maximum intended lifespan, find out what's causing symptoms and straighten those out. Learn what your symptoms are trying to tell you and, empowered with that knowledge, you'll be halfway home to fixing them. When you do that, symptoms become an alert system and blessing in disguise. It all comes down to how fluent you are at understanding the body's clues, and in what you do when in possession of accurate information. On the other hand, if mainstream treatments focus all your efforts on symptom relief, disease is sure to persist. Bottom line: We know more about the body than we've ever known. We have more options than we've ever had. And now your family's health depends on you knowing the right information.

How hunger cravings work

The body has complex nutritional needs that change by the moment. One minute you may be stressed at work and need extra vitamins and antioxidants. Twenty minutes later you may be exercising so you need extra potassium and other electrolytes. After working out, you may need extra protein to rebuild muscles. At any given moment, there are thousands of processes happening in the body. And you need hundreds of nutrients to run those processes.

The great mystery within us is how your biology communicates those needs your behavior and reward systems to motivate you to eat what it needs. Think about it: If your body needs X amount of vitamin D, Y amount of protein, and Z amount of magnesium, how is it supposed to tell you *which* nutrients, and *how much*? And then, how would your rational mind figure out which foods contain those nutrients, and how much you need to eat of each, to get exactly what you need?

This is one more instance of the genius of our innate intelligence silently serving you, without your conscious awareness being informed or involved. All the systems in your body – your microbiota, mitochondria, cells of the gut lining, hormones, neurotransmitters, and nervous system – they all work in concert to tell your brain and taste buds what to eat. The end result being hunger cravings.

First, your body senses it's low on certain nutrients. Through innate intelligence and experience, your body knows which vitamins, minerals, enzymes and other nutrients are found in certain plants, animal products, ingredients and seasonings that you've eaten before. In fact, your gut knows better than your conscious mind what's in the food you eat. It knows that oranges give you vitamin C, fish has omega oils that are good for brain function, and steak is abundant in protein.

Your innate biology is keenly aware of which foods it needs to request through your behavior and reward systems to get the nutrients it needs. And that's one reason you may crave a grilled cheese sandwich when you need calcium, spaghetti when you could use more lycopene, or fresh berries when you need antioxidants. That's how hunger cravings work.

Your body is constantly monitoring nutrient levels and adjusting its hunger cravings according to what your body needs at that moment. It even requests any number of over 72 trace minerals by craving sauces, spices or ingredients. Of course, with soil and foods now depleted, the body doesn't always get the nutrients it asked for. So it triggers hunger cravings sooner than it would have, had those nutrients been received.

However, the built-in connection between cravings and nutrition apply mostly to foods that haven't been modified much from their original form. As you may guess, "fake foods" use a different formula to drive consumption. Food companies use flavor-enhancers such as glutamates, salt, sweeteners, artificial flavoring, and lots of processing in order to manipulate our noses and tongues into doing just that: *driving consumption*, thus corrupting the tie between cravings and nutrition.

The immune system can employ pathogens to chelate heavy metals

The human body uses viruses and fungi to do its bidding in fighting toxins. *The enemy of my enemy is my friend.* Buried deep within the infinite intelligence of our biology, the immune system can actually increase or perpetuate pathogen activity as a way to chelate otherwise hard-to-handle heavy metal and chemicals. In some cases, the body will allow an active viral, bacterial or yeast infection to persist longer than usual because that germ is detoxing heavy metals that the innate detox system cannot. While in other cases, it may let an old virus out of storage and revive it in order to combat a particularly dangerous threat. The theory being, each type of microorganism has different attributes. Some of them have special access or ability to chelate heavy metals that normal immune cells and processes don't have. Some of them thrive in the company of heavy metals.

So when you interfere with this counter-intuitive healing process by taking antimicrobial/antifungal drugs, reducing a fever, or otherwise cutting a sickness short, you may be undermining the body's ability to eliminate toxins. In other words, a never-ending illness or overgrowth might be your body's backup strategy to manage an on-going, more destructive, source of heavy metal poisoning that it can't handle conventionally. Likewise, many people believe the immune system can employ less harmful pathogens to fight more destructive ones.

For example, many practitioners suspect the immune system is able to create or prolong a candida infection to help remove mercury – effectively turning candida into an alternative means to detoxify heavy metals. In these cases, a candida infection will be extra hard to extinguish, until you fix the mercury problem first.

Most health problems are present for years, or even decades, before you notice symptoms

Some organs can lose over 75% of their function before giving you symptoms. Before that, you may not even notice when your body is battling adversity. This is how small upsets progress into disease. The body, in its rugged design, doesn't trouble you with every imbalance it's managing, or disorder it's trying to straighten out. It just goes about its business and seldom complains. Only when you are so far in arrears with your obligations such as sleep, nutrition and detoxing does the body give you warning signs that it's in distress. Only after you overtax organs for some time does the body call '911' and force you to problem-solve.

Prior to that, the most your body will ever trouble you with is loose stool, skin problems, recurring tiredness, shortness of breath, or brain fog. These are signs that the body is actively engaged in a healing process or dealing with a deficiency. For instance, you can assault your microbiome every day with chemical and biological assailants and, still, it manages to cope for years, or even generations. Unfortunately, by the time you notice symptoms, your microbiome is likely to be quite corrupted.

The takeaway: When your body is undergoing a healing/rebalancing process, just let it do its thing and don't interfere. Don't suppress symptoms, as conventional medicine is fond of doing. That may give you short-term relief, but your condition may worsen over time. You want to figure out what caused the problem and solve that. In most cases, that is now possible, given our new understandings about how Nature nurtures the body and technology torments it.

"Man's Way" vs. "Nature's Way"... that is the question

To be sure, each approach – medical interventions vs. self-healing – has its advantages and disadvantages. Each has a place in healing. To name a few, Western medicine is great at keeping you alive in life-threatening emergencies. No system is better at trauma care than Western medicine. The downside is, Western medicine sucks at explaining chronic, degenerative disease, preventing it, and treating it. On the other side, Nature's way is far better at helping you heal yourself. But it's nowhere near as good at emergency care. You need to know the strengths and weaknesses of each so you can use them both to your advantage.

4

GOOD FOOD, BAD FOOD
(Sources of Nutrition and Toxins in Food)

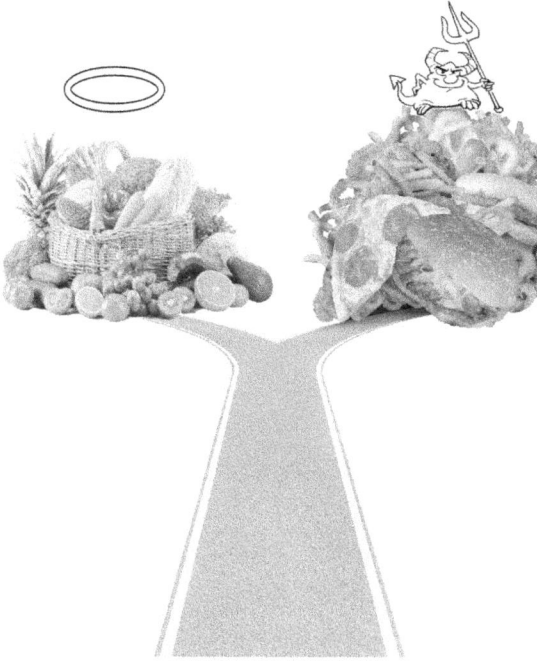

Food is __the__ best medicine, or it can be the most insidious poison

Food is __the__ strongest medicine for reversing modern disease. Not instantly, and not by itself, but by helping the body heal itself – which is a very different way of thinking than what we're taught. In contrast, drugs merely suppress symptoms and do nothing to address root causes.

Good food is instrumental to human health or sickness because quality food feeds our good gut bacteria. It supplies the body with resources it needs to fight toxicity, disease, and epigenetic changes to gene expression. Food grown as Nature intended gives your body what it needs to maintain, protect and heal itself. And bad food does the opposite. It toxifies you. Poor quality food gives you less nutrition and more free radicals per calorie. It feeds pathogenic gut flora, which turns your microbiome against you in terms of barrier function, food sensitivities, autoimmunity, and vitamin production.

The food we eat drives day-to-day operations and adaptive mechanisms. The most important of which is the vitality or fragility of our microbiome, because it's the microbiome that determines the health or sickness of you. All disease – physical or mental – begins in the gut, as you will soon come to appreciate.

The food chain explained

The Sun: Nature had a plan when it designed the food chain. It starts with the life-giving energy of the sun. The sun's energy is the only perceivable resource that is constantly added into our ecosystem. All other matter on earth is recycled.

Plants: The sun shines on plants. And plants, through photosynthesis, harvest the sun's energy, turning it into the solid matter that feeds the entire food chain. No other life form can convert electromagnetic energy into matter quite the same way.

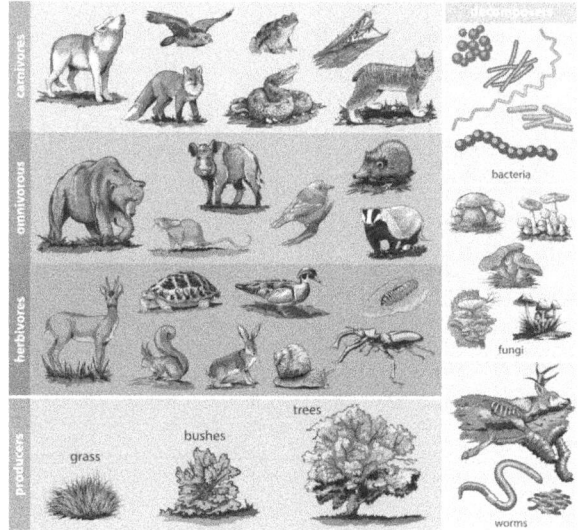

Herbivores: Next rung up the food chain are herbivorous animals – like cows, giraffes and pasture animals. Their entire digestive tract is specially designed to eat grasses, leaves and plants. To access all the nutrients in plant material, they've got grinding teeth, some have stomachs with multiple compartments, and a few regurgitate food multiple times to chew it more than once.

Another interesting feature about the digestive tract of herbivores is their ability to convert plant material into something with completely different properties. Incredibly, the bacteria in a cow's stomach converts grasses – which contain no fat, cholesterol, or fat-soluble vitamins – into short chain fatty acids. So cows, with the help of their gut bacteria, convert fibrous plant roughage into saturated fat, cholesterol, and fat-soluble vitamins. Later, when carnivores and omnivores higher up the food chain eat the cow or its products, they receive a completely different set of nutrients than what the cow itself ate.

Carnivores: Above herbivores in the food chain sit carnivores. Carnivores are designed to eat herbivores. You can tell by the design of their digestive tracts, and by the shape of their teeth. They have sharp canines designed to tear. And you can tell they're meant to eat and run by their speedy physiques, their high metabolism, their highly-acidic single stomachs, and their "swallow it once" style of eating.

Omnivores: At the top of the food chain, we have omnivores such as humans. Everything in our bodies – our teeth, GI tract, microbiome, and biochemical systems – is designed to eat almost anything we can get our hands on. But that doesn't mean the cycle ends with us. We eventually get recycled too. When we die, our bodies decompose and return to the earth to feed the next cycle – just like everything else.

Humans are designed to eat both animal foods and plant foods

You need only look at our multi-purpose teeth and single stomach to see that our digestive systems aren't meant to operate the same as herbivorous animals. Our digestive tracts are not designed to convert plant matter into the fatty acids we need for optimal brain and nervous system function. Instead, we're meant to eat a variety of foods to meet our nutritional needs.

Nature has given us two types of foods for that purpose: plant foods and animal foods. Each group is meant to give us something different. Animal foods nourish us, while plant foods cleanse us. Ideally you get both in your diet to support all of your body's needs. But if you had to

Tomato | Cucumber | White Onion | Purple Onion | Garlic | Carrot | Lettuce

Potato | Red Cabbage | White Cabbage | Radish | Eggplant | Mushroom | Zucchini

Yellow Pepper | Red Pepper | Artichoke | Corn | Beet | Broccoli | Avocado

Spinach | Cauliflower | Celery | Red Chili | Green Chili | Sweet Potato | Green Bean

Kohlrabi | Asparagus | Olives | Pumpkin | Fennel | Spring Onion | Turnip

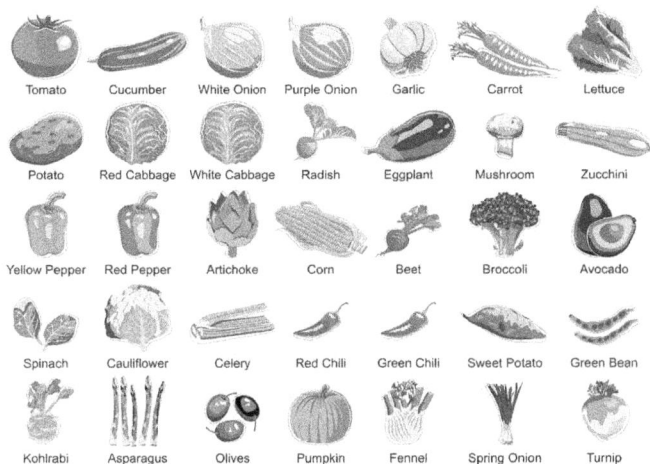

pick only one, you'd be healthier living exclusively on animal foods (naturally-raised, in particular). Conversely, you'd experience a variety of deficiencies and problems living on plant foods alone, as Dr. Natasha Campbell-McBride has seen in her clinic.

Vegetables don't nourish and feed the body as their primary function. Instead, they are cleansers

It's been drilled into our head since we were old enough to shovel food into our own mouth: 'Eat your vegetables; they're good for you.' Turns out, that's partly true. Vegetables are indeed good for you, but not for the reasons that mother and media have told us. You see, vegetables don't do a good job of nourishing the body and sustaining us long-term. Rather, they're good at cleansing our innards. They maintain our inner ecosystem and keep it running smoothly. That's why they're good for you.

Plants are largely indigestible to humans. Their vitamins and minerals are largely inaccessible to us because our digestive systems aren't designed to break down the fibrous material of plants and release the nutrients that are locked inside. Have you ever seen kernels of corn exit you almost the same way they went in? That's what I'm talking about.

On the other hand, cows, goats and other pasture animals *do* have a way to digest plant material properly. But we don't. To illustrate, a cow will chew a mouthful of grass many dozens of times before she swallows it. Her multiple stomachs called rumen then break down the fibrous plant material and ferment it with probiotic bacteria for a while. That "cud" is then regurgitated, chewed some more, and swallowed again, repeatedly. Scientists have estimated a cow will chew a mouthful of grass almost 200 times before she's done with it.

Another reason vegetables alone don't sustain us is that most of them contain no fat. That means you don't get crucial fat-soluble vitamins such as A, D, E and K from them. And that carries major health consequences, as we discuss later. So if you had to rely strictly on plants alone, without special foods to supplement, your mental and physical health deteriorates into disorder over time.

Are vegetables packed with vitamins?

While that may be true, we humans can't absorb and use those nutrients efficiently because only a small percentage of those vitamins are present in a bioavailable

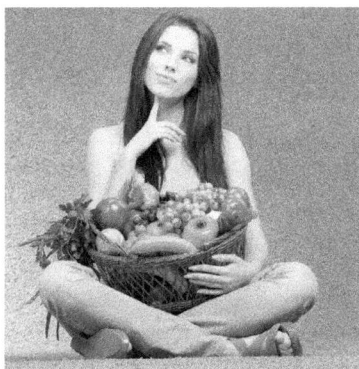

form. The idea that vegetables are packed with nutrients is based on a lot of theory and logical leaps of faith that boil down to this: Nutrition scientists assume their laboratory procedures are an accurate reflection of how the human digestive tract works. But it isn't.

Labs have their procedures for assaying nutrients levels. And the human digestive tract has a very different way of processing foods in real life. Laboratories break down food with mechanical processes and solvents. They then measure vitamin and mineral values with high tech equipment such as atomic spectroscopes and whatnot. Scientists assume the human body metabolizes nutrients the same way – completely ignoring the fact that if nutrients are presented, or digested, into a form that the body can't use it's worthless to us.

So although nutrients may be present in one form or another, they could be going right through you, as they often do. Even if the nutrients are liquefied in a blender, they're still trapped in a fibrous cellular structure that our bacteria don't get much time to process. Contrast that with how a cow's multi-stage fermentation process breaks down fiber.

Now, this is not to say that plants don't have positive benefit. Their most valuable feature is that their fiber acts like a broom. It sweeps the GI tract clean as it passes through. Whole vegetables supply us with small amounts of minerals and vitamins. They give us antioxidants and active enzymes (when eaten raw). They remove toxins. And "prebiotic" fiber in plants, which is indigestible carbohydrates, feeds our gut flora.

Our ancestors knew how to get the most nutrition from vegetables

They learned to cook vegetables before eating them. Contrary to popular belief, **cooking vegetables thoroughly actually raises their vitamin and mineral availability – some nutrients by hundreds of times – by breaking down their fiber and freeing up their nutrients**. Another way to free up a plant's vitamin and mineral content is to do what Nature does and ferment it first – like a cow's stomach does. Traditional cultures prized fermentation for its ability to preserve foods. But what they may not have known is that probiotic bacteria enhance the nutritional value of foods by converting inaccessible minerals and vitamins into bioavailable forms.

Fermenting dramatically increases the nutritional value of foods. Unfortunately, ancient peoples may not have known exactly how fermentation supports our gut bacteria and nutritional needs, so our ancestors of the 20th Century found fermentation easy to abandon. It's only within the past few decades that health teachers have discovered why fermentation enhances human health and started to return to the practice.

Our ancestors knew grains are hard to digest

Every life form is born with an urge to survive and replicate hardwired into its DNA. Animals want to survive and reproduce. Microorganisms want to proliferate. Plants are no different. They want to survive and pass on their genes, so they have defense mechanisms that discourage animals from eating them. Take grains such as wheat and rice, for example. They are actually seeds. They contain all the nutrients that a baby plant needs to sprout and start growing – all in a self-contained package. That makes seeds a nice meal for animals – were it not for their built-in defense mechanisms.

The survival strategy of seeds and grains is to either pass through the GI tract of an animal undigested so the droppings get left behind. Or else substances in the grain make the animal regret eating it, so it learns to eat less the next time – which is exactly what lectins do. Lectins are proteins in a grain that make their carbohydrate complexes sticky, thereby inhibiting their breakdown. This gives animals a tummy ache, which discourages them from over-eating the grain – humans included.

As a result, grains, in their natural state, are difficult for humans to digest. *Ancient* grains cause mild to moderate distress to the gut and the rest of the body – including flatulence and leaky gut. This was not a problem when ancient cultures specially-prepared and consumed breads only occasionally. But it's become a big problem in the last seventy years as breads, pastas and carbs have become part of virtually every meal we eat in the West. Grains also contain anti-nutrients like phytic acid that bind to essential minerals such as iron, zinc, calcium and magnesium, preventing us from absorbing them.

Our ancestors knew grains were a great complement to our diet. Yet they understood there were rules to making grains easier to assimilate. In addition to eating them in moderation, our ancestors helped the digestive process along by soaking the grains in water for a day or more, and/or cooking them thoroughly, before eating. This unfolds their cellular structure and breaks down some of the lectins, thereby easing the workload on the digestive tract in gaining access to their nutrients.

The hazards of veganism/vegetarianism
Dr. Natasha has never seen a healthy long-time vegan in her clinic
This is primarily because most herbivorous humans don't get enough fat-soluble vitamins and cholesterol in their diet to support essential operations. As a result, their body can't manufacture sufficient sex hormones and stress hormones, which are made from cholesterol. They can't produce enough neurotransmitters, causing brain function to suffer. And they have a hard time maintaining cell growth, tissue repair, nerve function, heart function, and other very important biochemical processes.

One of the first things that happens after vegetarians are thoroughly depleted is that their immune system collapses. They get sick and they take antibiotics, which damages their gut flora. This compromises their immune system further, because 85% of the immune system is located in the gut. So they get sick again. This cycle repeats itself until their gut is thoroughly corrupted and they develop psychological problems such as anorexia, anger management issues, and altered perception.

But that's not to say vegetarianism is meritless. Despite posing legit health risks, it is possible to be a healthy vegetarian. You just have to know what you're doing to avoid nutritional deficiencies. You have to know the right foods to eat, or supplements to take, to give your body what it lacks in the absence of animal foods. This usually includes eating animal products such as eggs, butter, and milk products.

Being a healthy vegan is quite a bit harder

The first 6–12 months you're on a strictly vegan diet, you may feel great and be full of energy. But after you cleanse and cleanse and cleanse… and you can't cleanse any more, nutrient deficiencies catch up to you and you start to feel washed out. You start developing serious health disorders because you're not getting enough cholesterol. You may not be getting enough protein. You're not getting vitamins A, D, E and K, which are fat soluble, and are very hard to get in sufficient quantities without animal products.

These deficiencies cause problems in almost every system and process in your body because these vitamins enable other vitamins to do their jobs. Remember, your brain, hormones, nerves, and every cell in your body are made out of fat and cholesterol. And when you don't get enough building blocks to supply these structural and biochemical pathways, things break down and go seriously wrong – particularly your psychology.

Behind closed doors, celebrity vegans and living food gurus suffer from chronic health problems

They don't admit to it publicly, because it would hurt their reputation and income. But many, if not most, of the world's leading promoters of veganism (and some vegetarianism) privately suffer from teeth and bone issues, among other embarrassing health conditions.

It may take many years, or even decades, for nutritional deficiencies to catch up to them. But this goes to show: veganism, fruitarianism, and some vegetarian diets lack the fat, cholesterol, and fat-soluble vitamins that humans need to run crucial bodily processes. These diets often work great short-term, or when you're young. But they're not sustainable over a lifetime, because those diets are far better at cleansing than they are at building and maintaining mind, body, biochemistry, and immunity.

For more information about the downsides to vegan/vegetarian diets, check out Dr. Natasha Campbell-McBride's book Vegetarianism Explained: Making an Informed Decision.

Animal products are best at feeding the body

Animal products – particularly naturally-raised – are much better at building and maintaining the body than plants because they are a more complete food for our physiology. Animal products contain the specific nutrients that the animal needed to build its physical structure, and run its biochemical processes, which is very similar to what we need as well.

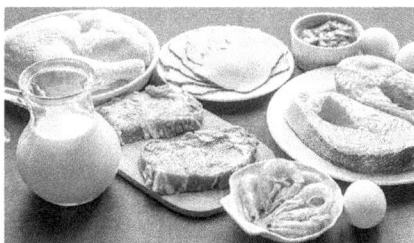

Organs and fat tissue store nutrients. Nature designed animals' systems to concentrate vitamins and minerals in their internal organs and fat stores to even out feast and famine periods. So organ meat and fat are the healthiest for you – not so much lean muscle meat. Organ meat has dozens or hundreds of times the essential nutrients that lean muscle meat has. The most nutritious is liver. Animal livers store and use the same nutrients as our own livers. So eating liver is a shortcut to getting what *your* liver needs to function well.

Saturated fat. Saturated fat, which comes mostly from animals, is the healthiest type of fat for the human body because they're very stable. You can cook with them, and they don't break down under high heat the way other fats do. Saturated animal fats are similar to our own fat. Our ancestors were raised on them, so the body recognizes them and knows exactly how to metabolize them. It also knows how to get rid of them after it's done using them. For these reasons, saturated animal fat should make up the bulk of your fat consumption.

Fat-soluble vitamins. Animal products are far and away the best source of fat-soluble "master vitamins" A, D, E and K_2. The body uses vitamins A and D, for example, to perform a wide variety of digestion, absorption, cell growth, and immune system processes.

Protein. The body needs protein to build muscle and support a whole host of processes. Animal products are our best source. Protein also slows digestion and balances out blood sugar highs and lows.

Cholesterol. Animal products are the only dietary source of the essential nutrient cholesterol. Contrary to what public health officials tell us, the body needs cholesterol because our cell membranes, nerves, and brain tissue are made of cholesterol. It's a raw material used in hormone production. Cholesterol is so important to our physical and mental well-being, the liver and every cell in the body makes it. This is no accident.

The real skinny on fats
The vilification of animal fats is absurd

The food industry has told us for decades that animal products are going to give us cardiovascular problems, and that their fabricated foods such as vegetable oil will save us. That's a laugh. If their made-up stories were even half true, we'd have seen a decline in chronic diseases by now. But what's actually happened in the last few decades? Disease and disorder have skyrocketed, particularly mental health disorders. Just a cursory examination reveals their theories to be extremely suspect in some cases, misleading in others, and downright fraudulent in others.

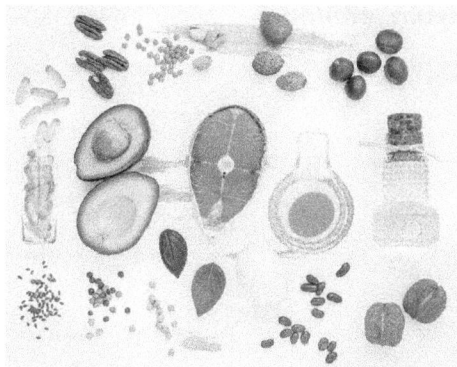

The truth on animal products: When you're deficient in fat, cholesterol, and the all-important fat-soluble vitamins A, D, E and K, things inside you don't work the way they should. Your muscles, bones, vital organs and nervous system starves, because they rely on building blocks and activators to function properly. It's like trying to construct a home without building materials. Without these nutrients, your neurotransmitter and hormone production suffers, which causes your personality to change. You change. You're a different person because your brain isn't getting what it needs to function correctly.

But there are two downsides to saturated animal fats

Animal fats tend to accumulate toxins, just like our own fat tissue does. And fats, by their very nature, are concentrated stores of calories. So they factor into the "calories in *vs.* calories burned" equation in weight loss. Although, contrary to industry propaganda, the body is able to readily burn animal fats, while fabricated fats and refined carbs are problematic for our systems to digest and metabolize.

The net result is that manufactured fats cause inflammation and chronic disease. And refined carbs contribute much more directly to weight gain than do saturated fats. Bottom line: The benefits of eating animal fats greatly outweigh the risks. They're much healthier for you than man-made fats, or no fats at all. So choose naturally-raised animal fats (and cholesterol) over man-made fats at every opportunity.

Vegetable oil manufacturing is similar to petroleum refining

The process of extracting, purifying, stabilizing, and deodorizing vegetable oils looks eerily similar to petroleum refining. They're both produced using high heat and high pressure. They're subjected to light and petroleum solvents. And both are highly profitable for manufacturers.

Fabricated seed oils wreck your health because they're highly processed and far removed from the way they occur in nature. That's harmful to your health because your body can't use them as food, and must remove them as the toxin that they are. In fact, they're so corrupted from their natural state, they have to be deodorized or you couldn't stand the smell.

The reason they're made and promoted so vigorously is because they can be made cheaply in mass quantities. They're ubiquitous throughout the food industry because they keep ingredient, cooking, and spoilage cost down. This turns into

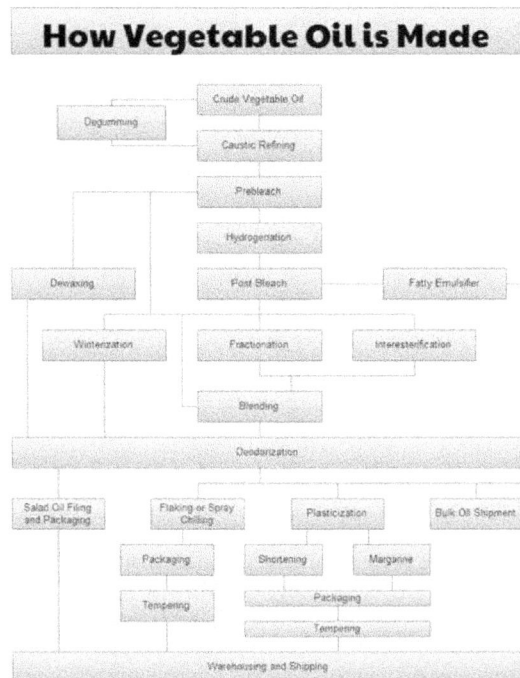

How Vegetable Oil is Made

longer shelf life and greater profit margins. But don't let the PR of Big Food fool you: man-made vegetable oils are not healthier or "a smarter choice," as they're being portrayed. It's a lie.

You can't put man-made vegetable oils in the same category as vegetable oils created by Nature. Natural vegetable oils are fragile. They're damaged by heat, light, and high pressure. So as soon as you do more than cold-press oil out of an olive or avocado, as examples, you start producing an end product that's foreign and unhealthy to the body. Your body doesn't recognize these "industrial" oils and has to work hard to get rid of them.

Everyone now agrees: hydrogenated trans-fats are bad for you

For a variety of reasons, fat needs to be in a solid form for food companies to use it commercially – margarine is one example. So, in 1901, a German chemist, Wilhelm Normann, came up with a process to turn liquid fats into solid ones. The process, called hydrogenation, basically turns a liquid vegetable oil (already harmful to human health) into a solid by adding a hydrogen atom. This makes hydrogenated fats even worse for you by promoting inflammation.

When you eat hydrogenated and partially-hydrogenated vegetable oils, the digestive system doesn't recognize it to be food. So it treats it as a pollutant that it has to detoxify. In fact, margarine is one molecule away from being plastic. Similarly, fabricated vegetable oils harm your health through many of the same mechanisms that trans-fats do. Even though they're liquid at room temperature, they're still foreign to the human body. Like trans fatty acids, the body knows fabricated vegetable oils are not food, and does its best to minimize the damage that they do.

Saturated fats and animal fats are good for you. Trans-fats are horrible for you. And man-made vegetable oils are almost as bad

Big Pharma has misled us through fake nutrition science and the media. They claim saturated fats and animal fats cause heart disease. They claim vegetable oils are healthiest for you. But the facts show otherwise. Many decades' worth of clinical evidence, public health data, and real-world experience have demonstrated those claims to be patently false.

Saturated fats and animal fats are not an enemy to good health. Saturated fats do not clog arteries. In fact, they're more than good for you; they're actually essential to brain, nerve, heart, and immune system activity. Fat, in general, enables the body to use a variety of fat-soluble vitamins. Without fats, you can't solubilize and transport many vitamins where they need to go (in water-based blood). And your liver doesn't work properly. What's more, animals raised on their natural diet store vitamins A, D, E and K_2 in their fat tissue. So when you eat animal fat, you're getting concentrated sources of essential vitamins. And your system is able to utilize other vitamins properly.

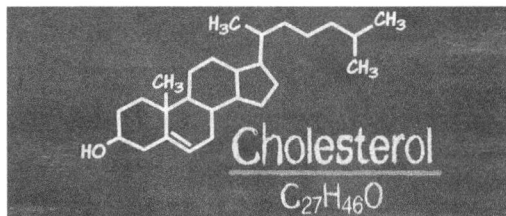

Cholesterol

Cholesterol is not the bad guy. It does not cause heart disease. And the conspiracy to deceive us all has been carefully planned, extremely well-funded, and manipulatively orchestrated.

The truth of the matter: cholesterol is an essential material for

- tissue repair
- development and normal functioning of the brain and nervous system
- hormone production, such as cortisol, testosterone, estrogen
- vitamin and nutrient synthesis (particularly vitamin D and CoQ10)
- production of bile salts (that break down fats)
- many other processes in a healthy body.

Consequently, cholesterol is needed for blood vessel repair, coping with stress, sexual response, heart and muscle function, digestion of fats, and dozens of biochemical processes in the body. For those affected by ADD, cholesterol helps regulate your mood through production of feel-good chemicals, such as serotonin. Cholesterol is also one of the body's most potent antioxidants (bet your sources never told you that).

It's so important to bodily operations that your liver, which makes about 85% of your daily requirements, actually increases or decreases cholesterol production, based on how much of it you need at that moment. Without sufficient cholesterol in the bloodstream, these all-important mechanisms malfunction, causing all sorts of problems – including anger, violent behavior, depression, muscle degeneration, debilitating back pain, infertility, loss of libido, fat-soluble vitamin and mineral deficiency, free radical damage, stroke and heart failure.

Cholesterol is your ally in good health. So not only is it foolish and futile trying to reduce blood-cholesterol levels, it's harmful to the body's maintenance and repair processes. To put it plainly, having abnormally low blood cholesterol hurts your health in many ways. Which means **cholesterol-lowering statins are destructive to your body and can cause catastrophic health crises.** Do not believe people who try to tell you otherwise. They are either misinformed, or they know the truth and are lying to you. True, cholesterol is found "at the scene of the crime." But it is not the cause of heart disease. Rather, it is there helping out. It's like repeatedly finding firemen at the scene of every fire and concluding that firemen must be causing the fires. Don't be fooled.

Dr. Natasha Campbell-McBride tells us the truth about cholesterol

"As I was telling all of my patients for years to eat animal fats, naturally a question would come up: 'What about heart disease? Am I going to die from heart disease on your diet?' Having spent many hours explaining to hundreds of people why animal fats are good for us, and that they have nothing to do with heart disease, I thought I better write a book about this. (*Put Your Heart in Your Mouth* is the result.)

Fats and cholesterol are the essence of life. We are made out of them, to a large degree. Cholesterol is one of those molecules without which we cannot live. It is involved in so many functions in the body. So Mother Nature went to great extent to provide every cell with biochemical machines to produce cholesterol. Every cell in the body produces cholesterol all the time. Blood cholesterol is maintained by our liver. The liver produces it and throws it into the bloodstream.

It has been estimated by physiologists that only about 15% of cholesterol floating in your blood might come from food. The rest – 85% – is produced by your liver. And study after study, all over the world, has confirmed the fact that **diet – what we eat – has no effect on blood cholesterol whatsoever.** You can live on a high cholesterol diet of eggs and butter only, or you can eat no cholesterol at all, and you will have the same levels of cholesterol in your blood either way… because cholesterol is a very important substance in the body. It's fulfilling many, many functions around the body. It's a busy substance. It's doing good work. And the body will maintain that amount of cholesterol in the blood that it needs for all those functions at that particular moment in your life.

There are many things that can increase blood–cholesterol levels. The most common reason is some sort of damage in the body – any kind of damage – particularly chronic inflammation. Why is this? Because cholesterol is essential for healing. We cannot heal any wound, any scratch, any damage in the body without huge amounts of cholesterol. So when there is any damage in the body, inflicted by anything – whether it's an infection, or a toxin, or whether you went to the dentist and there's been damage to your gums, and your root canals, and other things – it's damage.

Or whether you had surgery so your skin has been cut, and other tissues have been cut. So a lot of healing has to happen to heal all those cuts, and heal that bruising and damage… Whether you went through a very stressful period in your life, so there was a lot of free radical damage, and other damage done in the body… Whether you have an ongoing inflammation in your body, for whatever reason, which is inflicting damage to your tissues around your body… In order to heal that damage, you need lots of cholesterol.

So every damaged part of your body sends messengers to the liver immediately. It signals to the liver. The liver gets into gear, and it starts manufacturing cholesterol – in large amounts, and sending it to the site of the damage to heal it and seal it, and to repair it, because the inflammation process, and the repair process, both require large amounts of cholesterol.

So if your cholesterol is high it means your body's doing something. It's repairing something in your body. It's healing something. Don't mess with it. Don't interfere with it, because you will do a lot of damage in other parts of your body. So if your blood cholesterol is high and your doctor says, "Oh, you have to go on statins. This is dangerous," just think to yourself 'My body is healing something.' What might it be? What have I done? What have I damaged recently? Maybe I've got inflammation. Maybe I've had the flu. Maybe I've been to the dentist? Maybe I've had something else happening to me – that's what's happening.

All our steroid hormones in the body are made out of cholesterol. Cholesterol is the building block of steroid hormones – all our sex hormones, our adrenal hormones, and other steroid hormones. That is why our low-cholesterol diets, and our low-cholesterol foods, and our low-fat diets, and our toxic bodies, are to blame for our infertility epidemic.

A lot of people in this world cannot produce enough sex hormones. They haven't got enough cholesterol, or their pathways of production of cholesterol in the body are damaged or blocked, so they cannot produce enough cholesterol. These people have been studied quite extensively by a lot of renowned researchers who found that they've got consistently low blood cholesterol because their bodies are unable to produce enough cholesterol.

The first thing that has been observed in these people is that they have low self-control. They're aggressive. They're reactionary. They're cranky. And they have difficult personalities. These are people difficult to deal with, and difficult to live with. That is why every spouse, pretty much, of a person who is put on statins, which impair production of cholesterol in the body, comments that 'Gosh, overnight, as soon as he started taking statins he became cranky. His personality changed. He became intolerant and impatient and unpleasant. And a very different person'.

One of the hungriest organs for cholesterol is our brain. About 20% of myelin is cholesterol. So that fatty substance that the brain is coated in – every structure in the brain is coated in – 20% of it is cholesterol. And it has to be renewed all the time. So fresh cholesterol has to be delivered there all the time to renew myelin, to rebuild it, to regenerate it. Other structures in the brain require huge amounts of cholesterol for its structure, and for its function. The brain cannot function without cholesterol.

Myelin: Fatty layer of nerve insulation.

That is why people put on statins lose their memory. They're likely to develop dementia. I'm sure a large percent of our dementia epidemic amongst our elderly people is due to statin prescription. I have no doubt about it because every elderly person in Britain (where Dr. Natasha resides and practices) certainly is on statins. They're all popping cholesterol pills, because their doctors put them on cholesterol pills.

And yet research after research has demonstrated when you give elderly people eggs and butter [which contain large amounts of cholesterol] for breakfast their memory improves, and their cognitive ability improves. And that has been proven with psychological/psychometric testing. All people need more cholesterol. All the people with higher levels of cholesterol in their blood are healthier, stronger, and they're 100% "here" – no dementia at all. And they're usually fitter, these people. And cholesterol is so important for older people.

The older we become, the more we need it. So much so that one of the major researchers in this area has posed a question, "We need to take steps to increase blood cholesterol in our elderly population." Which sounds like an anathema, doesn't it, to the mainstream? Because they're doing just the opposite: they're putting everybody on statins, and they're reducing their cholesterol levels in the body. The brain cannot function without cholesterol.

That is why the GAPS diet is very rich in cholesterol, because we need to rebuild the brain. We need to feed it properly. We need to allow it to rebuild its structure, and to function appropriately. There are many other functions of cholesterol in the body. For example, vitamin D is made out of cholesterol, when the skin is exposed to the sun."

Violent offenders are shown to have low cholesterol
Researchers discovered that 4 out 5 violent offenders in prison have very low cholesterol levels. This fits well with what we know about low cholesterol causing deficiency of the stress hormone cortisol. Low cortisol makes people less able to cope with stress, triggering all sorts of anti-social behavior like road rage, anger management issues, and acts of violence. Vicious dogs have also been found to have low cholesterol levels.

Heart attacks were rare before man-made vegetable oils arrived
To illustrate the lunacy of the "cholesterol-heart attack" theory, consider this: Prior to the invention of human-engineered vegetable oils around the year 1900, people cooked in animal fats, and ate mostly animal products. In 1921, the first incidence of heart attack was reported.

Before that, atherosclerosis did not exist. Or, if it did, it wasn't widely reported in the medical literature. So if cholesterol in eggs, bacon and milk products causes heart disease, why were heart attacks unheard of prior to the 1920s, even though plenty of people were eating high-cholesterol foods for breakfast, lunch, and dinner?

Calling HDL "good cholesterol" and LDL "bad cholesterol" = B.S.
When the "cholesterol-heart disease" hypothesis was first proposed, there was no distinction between high-density lipoprotein (HDL), low-density lipoprotein (LDL), and triglycerides. In the decades since, expert opinion and mounting research have forced proponents of the cholesterol-heart disease theory to give their idea a makeover. They now say that cholesterol traveling *to* the damaged blood vessel is bad, and the cholesterol traveling *away* from the repair site is good. How silly is that?

The food industry and the medical profession are claiming the very foods that Nature designed the human digestive tract to eat – the staple foods our ancestors survived on for millennia – are killing us because they're found in blocked arteries. Apparently animal fats and animal products are confusing the body and causing it to malfunction. On the other hand, they want us to believe that foods made by scientists in a lab for commercial gain are ones the body likes and knows how to process.

General news release: American Medical Association, October 12, 1962
"The anti-fat, anti-cholesterol fad is not just foolish and futile. It also carries some risk. Scientific reports linking cholesterol and heart attacks have touched off a new food fad among do-it-yourself Americans. But dieters who believe they can cut down on their blood cholesterol without medical supervision are in for a rude awakening. It can't be done. It could even be dangerous to try."

ADD individuals need to eat lots of cholesterol and saturated fat
ADD children and adults need lots of cholesterol and saturated fats for brain function, in a form as close to Nature as possible. Make sure to eat plenty of animal fat and meats (particularly organ meats), eggs and, if well tolerated, raw or organic milk products because cholesterol in food is virtually the same as that made by the liver. When you eat cholesterol, the liver doesn't have to work as hard making it.

Cholesterol conclusion
This "diet-heart" hypothesis, as it's called, is not harmless profiteering and fear-mongering by food companies and medical companies in collusion with government agencies. It's actually inflicted an incredible amount of suffering on millions of trusting people. Based on what? There is no connection between cholesterol levels in the blood and heart disease … zero (which statin literature freely admits to in fine print). If anything, cholesterol lowers the risk of heart disease. So, word to the wise: You should be thanking cholesterol for all that it does for you, not demonizing it.

To learn more about "the great cholesterol lie" watch Sally Fallon Morell's (President and Co-Founder Weston A. Price Foundation) presentation "The Oiling of America" (youtu.be/fvKdYU CUca8).

Nutrient cycling
What makes fruits, vegetables and water taste good?
You can tell if a plant got the minerals it needed by the way it tastes, because it's *minerals* that make fruits, vegetables and water taste good. Not all minerals, but the *right blend* of minerals that the fruit or vegetable likes. Contrary to Big Ag principles, plants know which nutrients they need. They know a lot better than modern farming does. And they will get it, if they're allowed to grow as they wish.

Exudate: see page 53.

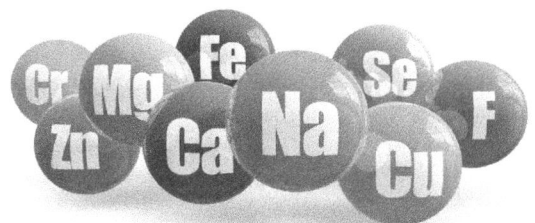

Plants tell microorganisms in the soil to bring them the proper minerals to grow big and tasty. They do this by releasing exudates through their root system that feed the bacteria species that give them the minerals they prefer. The farmer doesn't have to add any inorganic fertilizer or soil amendments when there's good biology in the soil.

Conversely, modern farming pushes chemical fertilizers onto plants in unnatural proportions – basically manipulating their growth mechanisms into growing as big, and as fast, as possible. In addition to killing biology in the soil, this causes the plant to uptake excessive amounts of some minerals, and a deficiency of others. This makes for some gross tasting fruits and vegetables. For instance, too much nitrate is a common culprit in making fruits and vegetables taste bitter. You can usually distinguish these commercially-grown plants from organic ones because conventionally-grown fruits and vegetables are often amazingly consistent in size, shape and appearance.

Whereas organic fruits and vegetables tend to grow in all different sizes and shapes. You need only bite into ripe fruit that was grown as Nature intended to prove to yourself that Nature knows what it's doing. Even vegetables not known for their sugar content have a sweetness to them, such as vine-ripened tomatoes, bell peppers, and even lettuce. Conversely, substances that harm your health taste bad. But the interesting point here is that the body knows what's in the food that you're eating. And it knows if it's good for you or not.

Case in point: I've always thought Portland, Oregon has some of the best tap water in the country. It tastes as good as bottled water with minerals added for flavor. I believe it's because of the relatively uncontaminated, mineral-rich, and non-fluoridated water that travels only a short distance from where it fell as rain or snow. The Bull Run water shed, as it's called, is so clean, it almost doesn't need to be decontaminated before it's drinkable.

The nutritional value of a plant drops quickly after it's picked

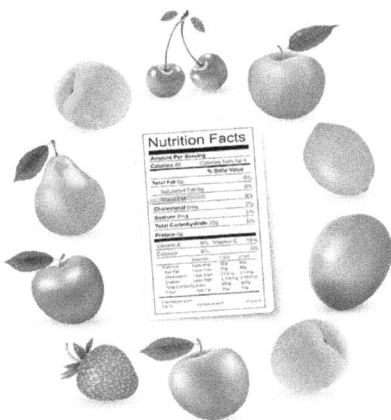

The moment you pick a fruit, vegetable, nut or grain its nutritional value starts to decline. It drops quickly because nutrients stop being added to its creation, and instead start being consumed by microorganisms inside and outside in order to return its nutrients back to earth. In fact, fruits and vegetables lose anywhere from 15–90% of their *vitamin* content in 7–10 days after picking. *Minerals* leave a little slower as the fruit/vegetable "breathes" and dries out. *Proteins, enzymes and other nutrients* will also degrade as the fruit/vegetable ripens.

On average, fruits and vegetables will lose about a third to one-half of their nutritional content 3–5 days after being picked, as it literally consumes itself from within. But, oddly enough, when a fruit or veggie is picked, it doesn't "die" right away. Rather, it continues to live and grow for a few days to a couple weeks, albeit without its old supply line: its roots. For instance, green onion lovers are quite familiar with the way they continue to grow for weeks after being pulled from the ground. This goes to show you, produce has a life force that expands as the plant takes up nutrients from the soil. It plateaus for a short while after being picked. And then its life force leaves rapidly, when the time comes.

Sprouting dramatically increases a seed's life force that it gives you

Due to their concentrated and balanced set of nutrients, seeds, grains, nuts and legumes offer good health benefits. But sprouting them prior to eating takes their life force benefits to another level. The very act of germinating a bean before eating maximizes the life force it gives to you because, as it begins to sprout, the bean draws in a burst of extra-dimensional energy to give it the best start in life. Tip to remember: Newly sprouted seeds, growing full-tilt, are among the healthiest ways to eat plant foods.

Becoming bioavailable

"Bioavailable" means *in a form that the body can use.* Prior to that, many nutrients in food and supplements need to be broken down or rearranged on a molecular level – usually with the help of enzymes – to be recognizable to the body and usable. Particle sizes can also be too big to fit into cells, for example, or be incorporated into biochemical processes.

Not surprisingly, bacteria and fungi, whether in soil or your gut, do a lot of that work. Microbes eat inorganic minerals from the earth and break down or rearrange larger, un-usable molecules into microclusters of very few atoms, which are easy to assimilate, thereby making minerals bio-available. Our own digestive system can also break a limited amount of inorganic minerals on its own – provided you have sufficient enzymes from live, uncooked foods, such as raw vegetables, fruits, and even meat.

Absent this type of probiotic/enzymatic, external/internal activity, minerals can't get into cells and do you any good. Instead, they just clog up your system and need to be dealt with as a waste product. So minerals are either a benefit or a hazard – depending on the form in which they are present, and the resources you have to break them down, such as enzymes and microorganisms.

Soil science

Before Dr. Elaine Ingham came along, most scientists, growers and agriculture companies thought of raising plants as basically a "minerals applied, minerals uptaken" sort of thing. Whatever is in the soil gets taken up by the plant to feed itself, and ultimately goes to the animal that eats that plant. Minerals in the earth basically get consumed and depleted over the course of several growing seasons and that's it. You don't get any more until: (a) the next volcanic eruption, (b) a biblical-scale flood deposits minerals in the area, or (c) you put "it" in the ground yourself.

Thus, most members of the grower community thought of farming as a chemical equation that Big Ag companies could solve with technology and chemical crop amendments. But that's not how agriculture works in Nature (is supposed to work) – from a nutritional standpoint, sustainability standpoint and, often, yield standpoint. In the ways that really matter to the health of people and the planet, modern farming works very much in opposition to Nature. Like drugs and modern medicine, modern farming basically forces Nature to do things against its will, or at least out of its comfort zone.

Soil is the foundation of life and health for the entire food chain

Over the past several decades, soil science has focused primarily on the chemical and physical properties of soil – particularly mineral levels that plants need to grow big and fast. But science is rapidly waking up to the fact that the *biology* in the soil – the life in the soil – has a bigger influence on its productivity than its mineral and structural composition. To put it more potently, soil must contain life.

Without a complex hierarchy of life forms living in and around it, *soil* isn't soil; it's just dirt. *And dirt don't grow much* (at least not without a lot of help). For us landlubbers, soil is where the food chain starts (and begins again). Soil feeds the plants. Plants feed the animals. Animals feed people. And everything returns to the earth when it dies to be recycled. So, naturally, if you want healthy bodies and healthy minds, you need to start with what's happening in the soil.

Organisms in soil are a tiny ecosystem, not unlike that of the gut

In the mid-1980s, soil microbiologist Dr. Elaine Ingham, and her husband Dr. Russ Ingham, started doing groundbreaking research into what lives in the soil that ultimately feeds the entire food chain. What they discovered shocked farmers, educators and agricultural scientists alike, because even industry veterans had no idea how destructive modern farming practices were until they learned how microorganisms in the soil govern plant health.

They didn't realize that microorganisms in soil enhance nutritional content for plants and the food chain, let alone the extent to which they make it happen. No one knew precisely how tiny creatures in the soil cooperate with plants to form a complex and interdependent community where each type of organism has a job to do, and is there for a reason.

A few inquiring minds knew something about how soil structure helps its inhabitants get their basic needs met, prevents erosion, and protects the environment from contamination. People had their suspicions. But no one could really say specifically why life in the soil means so much to so many. It's a remarkable story that's vital to the health of every organism on earth, as well as the planet itself, because the wellness of perhaps 99% of all life on earth comes from the soil. Like the gut, small but inconceivably intelligent microbiota make magic happen in the soil for every living being's benefit.

Or the opposite is true: toxicity, weakness, poor nutrient profile, and abnormal genetic expression emanate from a corrupted growing medium that many people wrongly call "soil." And it happens when a thriving community of microlife in the soil is lacking. What's more, much of the information that follows is virtually unknown outside of the "bio-friendly farming" community. Hopefully, we can change that.

The soil food web

While doing research at Colorado State University, Dr. Elaine Ingham examined what the different groups of organisms in and around soil do for that ecosystem. She coined the ecosystem the "soil food web."

The Soil Food Web (Source: USDA.gov)

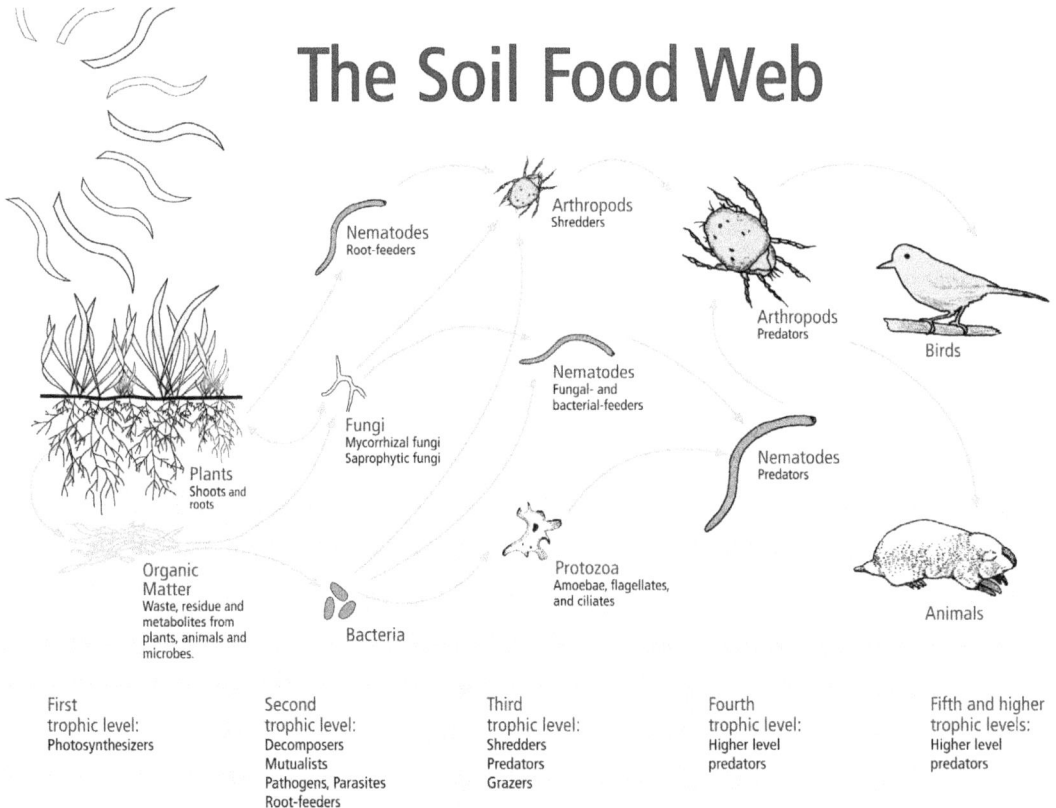

The Soil Food Web

| First trophic level: Photosynthesizers | Second trophic level: Decomposers Mutualists Pathogens, Parasites Root-feeders | Third trophic level: Shredders Predators Grazers | Fourth trophic level: Higher level predators | Fifth and higher trophic levels: Higher level predators |

The 5 trophic levels (groups of organisms) of a healthy *soil food web*:

1. **Photosynthesizers.** Plants. Other important components: waste matter, residue and metabolites from plants, animals and microbes.
2. **Micro-decomposers.** Bacteria, fungi and tiny nematodes (worms).
3. **Shredders.** Protozoa, slightly bigger fungal- and bacterial-feeding nematodes and microarthropods.
4. **Higher level predators.** Macroscopic predatory nematodes and arthropods (e.g., spiders, ants, centipedes).
5. **Higher level predators.** Birds, rodents, etc.

Soil must have most of these groups of critters to be considered true soil. Otherwise, call it what it is: dirt. **Any growing medium that's lacking the basic life forms needed to cycle nutrients and create space for its inhabitants is not soil, it's just dirt, clay, or what have you.** And dirt won't grow things very well, nor for very long, without regular applications of chemical fertilizers. Moreover, you get a fraction of a plant's potential nutrient content when you grow using "conventional" methods.

Each class of organism in the *soil food web* plays a role in
- nutrient cycling
- soil structure
- water retention
- nutrient density
- yield
- disease resistance
- decomposition
- erosion control
- population control of the others.

Each micro- and macro-organism group supports the health and productivity of the community, in an ecosystem more dynamic and dependent than previously thought. Each organism is doing something that needs to be done in the soil to grow the healthiest, most nutritious plants possible, and sustain the group. So, as Nature would have it, organisms in the soil food web form a community much like microbes in the gut. Yet no one had ever studied exactly what each of these groups is doing in the soil. Experts had just observed microorganisms like bacteria and amoeba living in soil and figured they were opportunists, just looking for a place to stay.

Dr. Russ Ingham did an experiment that changed everything we know about soil composition and plant health
He tried growing a wheat seedling in soil that had been sterilized – adding back each type of organism, one at a time, to gauge each one's

contribution. He started with just bacteria. It didn't go well. The plant died. Same thing with just fungi; the seedling just died faster. Then he added bacteria and fungi together, and the plant still died. Then Dr. Russ added bacteria and protozoa. And the plant grew, but it wasn't happy. The difference was, protozoa and bacteria together made more minerals available for the plants to use.

Next, he put (1) bacteria, (2) bacteria-eating protozoa, and (3) bacteria-eating nematodes in at the same time, and the plant grew even better because there was even more nutrient cycling (exchange) going on. He proceeded to try every combination to determine each group's specific effect on the rest of the ecosystem. With each successive experiment, it became more and more clear that each group of organism does something important for the community of critters in the soil and beyond.

Bacteria and fungi have a superpower that fuels the food chain

As valuable as those discoveries were, there was one biologic activity more profound than any other. The Inghams came to the stunning realization that there's one essential mechanism that initiates everything... something Big Ag lacks in both principle and practice. This mechanism lays the groundwork for all life on earth (dry land, that is). It starts the entire food chain. Without it, life on terra firma would not exist.

Bacteria and fungi secrete enzymes and acids that solubilize (dissolve) minerals locked up in sand, silt, rock and clay – converting them into a plant-available form. These microorganisms get the whole food chain started by releasing minerals from the earth so they can be absorbed and used by plants as their food. It's an indispensable step in the cycle of life – as important as sunlight itself, because minerals are present in inexhaustible quantities almost anywhere on dry land that you choose to look. But you need bacteria and fungi to unlock them.

> *"There is no soil on the face of the earth that lacks the nutrients to grow healthy plants."* —Dr. Elaine Ingham.

In fact, Dr. Elaine says one grain of sand contains enough trace minerals to supply an acre of crop for a year!

The problem is, those minerals are usually not abundant in a bio-available form because minerals in rock, sand, silt and clay are bound in the crystalline structure of the silica layers that comprise rocks. Thus, they're unusable. In order to be released, the minerals first need bacteria and fungi to gobble them up and convert them into an organic form by metabolizing them. These newly solubilized minerals then get stored in the physical structure of bacteria and fungi as organic compounds. However, they're still not accessible to others.

The next step is bacteria-eating protozoa (single-celled organisms with animal-like behaviors such as amoeba), microarthropods and earthworms will eat the bacteria that have collected extremely high concentrations of minerals in their cells from all the minerals they consumed. Now loaded with more minerals than they can possibly use, and harmful if retained, these little predators move around and deposit mineral-rich feces near the plant's root surface, which the plant can then absorb. That's how minerals become accessible to the food chain.

The net result of Nature's growing process is that plants receive the maximum amount of nutrition that they need, which produces the most nutrient-dense plants possible. And, contrary to the way our ancestors farmed, crops never need to be "rotated" when grown in this bio-friendly way. When you have a healthy ecosystem of microcritters in the soil – that is, when they're in balance – you don't have to add anything to the soil. Nature figured out this nutrient exchange thing in the food chain long ago. She's many steps ahead of us (and is likely to be for some time).

Mycorrhizal fungi form a smaller, finer root system around a plant's own roots, thereby increasing its nutrient absorption

Plant roots have limited ability to extract nutrients directly from soil, due to their limited surface area. So many kinds of plant partner with a beneficial fungus called "mycorrhizal fungi" to absorb the nutrients that bacteria unlock through the process described above. Mycorrhizal fungi grow around the root system of these plants, forming a more complex pseudo-root system that envelope the plant's own roots with finer branches. In doing so, mycorrhizal fungi do most of the nutrient gathering work for the plant by multiplying its absorption capacity.

The mycorrhizae attach itself to the plant's roots, and with its super-fine web of filaments, supply the plant with minerals pulled from the soil. In return, the plant feeds sugars and proteins to the mycorrhizae through its root exudates. This symbiotic relationship gives plants maximum absorption capability and nutrient density – much of which is missing in modern farming practices because beneficial fungi is not supported (to put it kindly) in commercial agriculture. **Net result: With most crops, natural farming techniques easily outproduce conventionally-grown ones.**

The importance of soil structure

Microbial life at the bottom of the food chain – bacteria and fungi – have another skillset that's sorely missing from mechanical farming. And that is, they create "soil structure" – like a tiny cave system. Without this active community of microlife underneath the surface, the sand, silt, clay and rock of the earth get more and more compressed over time. Eventually, most material without organic life in it gets so compacted that natural geologic processes turn it into rock. Indeed, that's how rock is made.

Conversely, when you have biology in the soil, it creates *structure* consisting of clumps and voids held in place by the cross-linking fibers from fungi. These open spaces allow water to penetrate much more easily into soil, move through it, and stay in the soil like a sponge. In fact, biologically-structured soil absorbs and retains moisture up to 70% better than conventional farming techniques – which means you don't have to water nearly as much. In some cases, you never need to water your crop – even going many months without rainfall. In fact, some crops can survive on the moisture absorbed from morning dew alone!

Good structure also keeps nutrients in the soil, and prevents toxic run-off such as inorganic fertilizers, herbicides and fungicides from contaminating waterways downstream from these factory farms. In addition, soil structure allows air and oxygen to move through the soil, allowing microorganisms deep below the surface to breathe.

Soil structure gives microorganisms a place to live, and protection from being displaced

Soil microbiota is housed and fed with the help of cross-linking fibers produced by fungi, called "hyphae." You can think of fungal hyphae as an underground network of structural support cables – like that of a pop-up tent. After microcritters break up the dirt/clay hardpan into little clumps called "aggregates," the fungal hyphae interconnect the clumps so they and the gang don't move around.

This gives microorganisms something stable to hold on to so they don't get washed away with the first rainfall. As you might suspect, the spaces between the clumps are the most important feature of soil structure. The spaces create living quarters, short-term storage facilities, transportation tunnels, and ventilation shafts for all the members of the soil food web to live in. And the fungal hyphae keep everything in place.

Soil structure and microlife form an active, living filter that traps and neutralizes toxins

Another secret skill of soil bacteria, like their intestinal counterparts, is that they're good at detoxifying harmful substances in the soil, such as heavy metals, industrial chemicals and petroleum pollution. Bacteria have a knack for either altering the chemical properties of pollutants to neutralize them of toxicity, or grabbing hold of them until they can be washed away. Plus, bacteria are always reproducing, so their detoxification capacity grows or continues without re-applying chemical "detoxifying" agents.

However, because each toxin has a different molecular structure, and differing effects on the body, you may need several strains of bacteria to deal with the toxins at-hand. Unfortunately, we're losing microbial diversity due to modern growing practices and, along with it, go the planet's natural toxin filtration capacity.

Healthy plants can protect themselves

When indigenous soil bacteria are present and productive, chemical pesticides and herbicides are generally not needed, because beneficial bacteria coat the plant's above-ground foliage with a protective layer that acts as a physical barrier against pests and disease. Below the surface, plants in robust health produce herbicidal compounds that keep competitor plants (particularly weeds) from growing in their immediate ground-space. It's only when the natural balance of the ecosystem is upset by tilling and inorganic fertilizers that man needs to step in and "help" a crop by adding herbicides, fungicides and pesticides.

Plants are smarter than we think

Plants are actively orchestrating the show the whole time. They know what they need. And they know how to get it, because they are the ones controlling the microorganism populations that help them grow. They do this by secreting sugar, protein and carbohydrate "exudates" – basically cakes and cookies – through their root system.

The plant releases exudates through its root structure that selectively feed those exact strains of bacteria that are good at providing the plant with the specific mineral combination it needs at that moment. You see, each strain of bacteria has a particular talent for converting a certain set of minerals through their normal metabolism.

Through this process, the plant partners with bacteria and fungi as a home delivery service to bring it whatever food it wants, when it wants it, which may change nearly minute-to-minute. The plant actively adjusts bacterial populations around it to get the exact nutrients it wants. By maximizing the nutrients it gets from the soil, the plant optimizes: (1) its health, (2) its resistance to pests and disease and, of course, (3) its nutritional value to those that eat it.

The difference is, plants grown as Nature designed them to grow are better at fighting off pests and disease. It's only when modern farming corrupts the growing process that they grow vulnerable to attack. It is then that they need to be watered and fed like dependents. Extrapolated out, when any life form is nutrient deficient – people, plants or animals – its resistance suffers, and its health diminishes – even if it looks well-fed.

Commercial farming fights Nature every step of the way

- It lowers nutritional content
- reduces the disease-resistance of plants
- uses more water than natural growing techniques
- increases erosion
- produces runoff that poisons everything downstream
- creates dependence on chemical fertilizers, pesticides and herbicides.

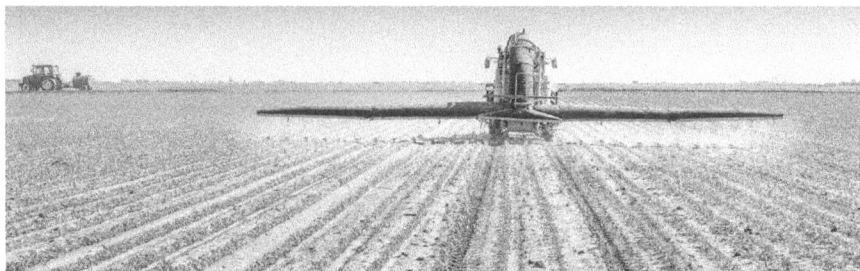

About the only beneficial things that modern farming does much better than Nature are commercially-oriented. That is, it's great at producing volume and consistency, raw tonnage and profit potential. Everything else that benefits people, animals and planet decreases with factory farming.

What makes commercial agriculture so destructive? Let's count the ways

1. Tilling destroys beneficial fungi, fungal hyphae and more. Without microorganisms creating structure in the soil, farmers have to till the soil to break it up and make it breathable for inhabitants. The problem is, tilling the soil kills beneficial fungi, along with its consumers. Tilling compresses the ground beneath it into a layer of earth that's hard for roots, oxygen and water to permeate. Roots may then run into this "compaction layer" that can sometimes be denser and harder to penetrate than solid concrete. When soil is compacted, oxygen can't reach oxygen-breathing microbiota, leading to anaerobic conditions. Water can also accumulate at compaction zones, causing root rot.

Aerobic: with oxygen. Anaerobic: without oxygen. Hypoxic: low oxygen.

2. You get weeds, and need to use herbicides such as glyphosate, which causes leaky membranes in people. Tilling encourages the growth of undesirable plants, because bacteria-dominated soil is a magnet for weeds. Weeds compel herbicide use such as glyphosate that cause leaky gut, leaky brain and GAPS conditions.

3. Inorganic (chemical) fertilizers kill beneficial life in the soil. Fertilizers kill probiotic populations that release nutrients from the soil so plants can use them. Without bacteria present to make nutrients available to plants, you have to apply chemical fertilizers to "spoon-feed" plants the minerals they need. This kills more bacteria. You then have to add more fertilizer to feed the plants. And so on, and so on. It's a vicious cycle of addiction and dependency that depletes plants, land and people of nutrients.

4. Glyphosate steals minerals and is a potent antibiotic. The most widely used weed killer in the world, glyphosate, binds to beneficial minerals such as zinc, iron, magnesium, manganese, nickel, cobalt and copper – thus preventing the plant from absorbing them and passing them up the food chain. In fact, glyphosate was originally developed and patented as a chelator to descale mineral deposits from boilers before it was made into an herbicide. Glyphosate is also known to kill microbes due to its mineral-stealing effects, so it was patented as an antibiotic.

In simplest terms, glyphosate corrupts soil like antibiotics corrupt the gut. These two effects – mineral chelation and antimicrobial – interfere with our production and usage of enzymes, B vitamins, hormones and neurotransmitters through mineral deprivation. Which means glyphosate is a big contributor to diseases precipitated by nutrient deficiency – including GAPS conditions, autoimmune diseases, metabolic diseases, depression, sleep disorders and cancer.

In summary, glyphosate is a potent antibiotic that kills beneficial microorganisms by tying up trace minerals used in enzymatic activities. That robs the soil of fertility and deprives plants of the minerals they need for growth and disease resistance. Growers then have to add chemical herbicides and fertilizers to put back some of what was lost.

5. Less bacteria in the soil means more toxins for us. When you wipe out the biology in the soil, and destroy its structure, toxins linger because bacteria are Nature's cleanup crew.

6. Water consumption, runoff, erosion, and downstream contamination. When soil lacks structure, water does not penetrate deeply into the ground. It is poorly retained, so it runs off or seeps through, carrying both top soil and a toxic crop amendments with it. If city aquifers or family wells are exposed, drinking water can become contaminated. As a result, Big Ag practices use far more water than bio-friendly farming. They deplete the land of minerals. They contaminate waterways. And they harm plants and animals living in its wake. Not to mention, destroying the ecology where the minerals were mined to make the fertilizer.

7. "Monocrops" diminish biodiversity, resiliency, yield and nutrients. When you grow large tracts of a single crop (called a "monocrop"), you weaken that ecosystem's health and resiliency. Lack of diversity in the ecosystem decreases: nutrient exchange, strength of the gene pool, and ability to weather adversity. When fewer plants populate the soil surface, fewer microorganisms live beneath it. And the opposite is true: having other plants living alongside your primary crop, or as a "cover crop" between harvests

- cuts erosion
- increases soil fertility
- retains water better
- controls weeds and pests
- and avoids diseases.

Everyone is happy and productive when there's excellent biodiversity above and below ground, because the entire community is supported.

8. Farmers are paid primarily by weight, then size, appearance, consistency, taste, and shelf life... not by nutritional content. It seems utterly ridiculous, but the single most important quality of a plant – its nutritional value – is virtually last on the list of what we pay for when buying fruits and vegetables in a store. Many assume that buying organic ensures them a better nutrient profile, but that belief is unreliable at best.

Is buying organic any better?

The term "organic" is controlled by the USDA. More and more people are buying organically-grown food in order to eat healthier. But really, *organic* primarily means the absence of certain disallowed pesticides, herbicides and fungicides in the latter portion of a plant's growing cycle. *Organic* also requires that plants be GMO-free, which is a "win" for health-minded people. However, calling a piece of produce *organic*

- does not mean the plant was grown in fertile soil;
- that the plant was healthy;
- is more nutritious for you (it was probably still picked early);
- that it's freer of contaminants.

People just assume these things to be true. And, most of the time, they are. But, just as frequently, you should put a big 'question mark' next to these attributes, rather than a 'check mark,' as more and more farmers choose to grow organically for monetary reasons, rather than human benefit.

Part of the reason that there is no ultimate, best choice in produce is that food production and consumer preferences are following in the footsteps of mass production, in that variation is scorned like a manufacturing defect. Consumers and industry now demand that fruits and vegetables be perfectly consistent – even if that means it isn't as good for you. We're so spoiled that we want everything to be big, pretty, similarly-shaped, long-lasting, and decent tasting (not necessarily great). Unfortunately, that often lessens plant health, our health, and sustainability of our farming because Nature prefers variation. Nature doesn't like to grow apples exactly the same size, shape, color and weight when left to her own devices. But we've grown so accustomed to certainty in purchasing mass-produced products that we expect it, and object when we don't get it.

The trouble with soy

Beginning over three decades ago, the food industry conspired with public health agencies to brainwash people into believing that soy is a quintessential health food, of great benefit in a plethora of foods. They made soy out to be a near superfood that should be in every health-conscious consumer's diet. But that argument does not hold water when you know the real truth of the matter.

Well-informed healers now agree the that modern soy plant (not the soy bean Nature created) devastates hormonal systems with its "phytoestrogen" hormone mimics. This screws up hormone function, causing all sorts of problems ranging from gender issues to personality changes to thyroid problems and weight gain. Modern soy also impairs digestion with its genetically-modified DNA.

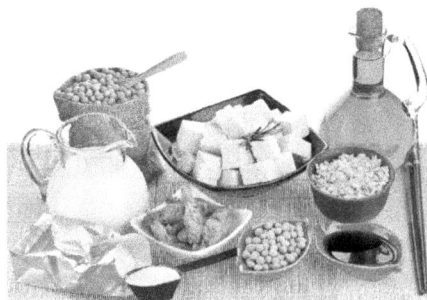

The traditional soy of Asian cultures is not the same as modern soy
Traditional Asian cultures prized their soy-based foods. For hundreds of years (at least), Japanese cultures, like that on the island of Okinawa, enjoyed natto, miso and tempeh in their diet. Whether these played a role or not, Okinawans were famous for their longevity, with many living well over a hundred. Meanwhile, Asian cultures in general made soy sauce and tofu staples of their diets.

To leverage this tradition into sales, food conglomerates and the health field began advertising soy as a blessing to health and longevity – forgetting the fact that traditional soy products are fermented before they can be eaten safely. You see, ancient Japanese and Chinese people knew soy in its natural form upsets hormonal balance with its estrogen-like elements. For instance, tofu has been used in monks' diets to help them maintain their vows of celibacy, as phytoestrogens reduce testosterone and sex drive.

Asian people knew these things from observation and experience, not chemistry and experimentation. So what did they do? Out of necessity, ancient peoples fermented their soy with probiotic bacteria before eating it. That neutralized the harmful effects of soy's phytoestrogens and phytic acid (which inhibits absorption of minerals) so they could eat it in bulk without side effects. Good bacteria made this possible.

In contrast, food producers developed cheaper methods of growing soy, while broadening its usage into thousands of products... without fermenting it first. Now mature, that push to get soy more widely used in food production is feminizing men physically and mentally by raising estrogen levels and lowering testosterone levels.

Soy feminizes men – contributing to homosexuality, early puberty in girls, and gender confusion in both sexes
Phytoestrogens in soy contribute to infertility in men, reduced muscle mass and bone density, lower energy level, and sexual dysfunction, along with a variety of symptoms brought about by low testosterone. Unfermented soy in our diet today is causing men to develop abnormally pronounced pectorals (male breasts) – especially those that consume soy as a way of life (e.g., protein bars, milk substitutes, and protein powder shakes).

Western medicine even had to invent a new name for low hormone in men because it's so common: Big Pharma calls low testosterone "Low T." Soy is even strongly suspected to play a role in the substantial rise of homosexuality in men because it continually subjects the male brain, in its formative and highly-impressionable years, to female hormones at dozens to hundreds of times their normal levels. This is thought to bias the delicate anatomy and function of the brain away from male tendencies, toward a female way of thinking.

Soy increases estrogen in women, causing obesity and disease

In the female population, soy products are the biggest reason puberty occurs 4–8 years earlier than at the start of the 20th Century. Soy also increases women's risk for breast and cervical cancer, polycystic ovarian syndrome, hypothyroidism, and hormone imbalances from chronically high estrogen. Contrary to what the soy contingent tells dieters, soy does not help you lose weight. Sometimes it can short-term. But over time, soy consumption slows your metabolism and causes weight gain through the same mechanism as that of hormonal birth control pills: elevated estrogen interferes with iodine's ability to make the thyroid hormones that regulate metabolic rate.

For babies, soy in infant formula is just plain wrong. Avoid it at all costs. Never forget, when you concentrate soy proteins into "isolates," and put them in foods to cheaply bulk up their volume, that food then gives you phytoestrogen levels 20,000 times higher than birth control pills. That doesn't bode well for the biochemical balance of any human, animal or plant living on this planet. Not to mention the fact that some 95% of soy grown in America is made from genetically modified seed developed by Monsanto to withstand glyphosate use. That corrupts the gut in ways that science is still coming to terms with.

Conclusion: Avoid proclaimed soy products, such as protein bars, weight loss shakes, muscle-building powders, and milk substitutes. And minimize your intake of foods that use unfermented soy ingredients as fillers (admittedly a tall task because soy is being added to everything it seems). They mess with your biochemistry on so many levels you'll never know. If you can find them, get organic (non-GMO) soy foods. Endeavor to try the more elusive fermented soy foods. Those that eat plant-based diets need to consider these words carefully, because soy is a preferred ways for vegans and vegetarians to get their protein.

Monosodium glutamate (MSG)

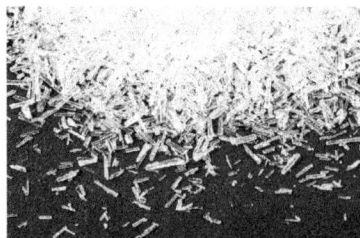

Monosodium glutamate is the refined version of glutamic acid. It's added to thousands of foods on store shelves. The food business calls MSG a "flavor enhancer." But its effects go well beyond that.

The insidiousness of MSG is that it makes food taste so good that it amplifies cravings. It erodes the sensitivity of taste buds, which makes you demand saltier, sweeter, spicier, and more concentrated flavors. It causes you to over-eat. And it's habit-forming. MSG is like a narcotic drug in that it stimulates the reward center of the brain, and contributes to tolerance, dependency and addiction – not just for glutamate-enhanced foods, but more intensely-flavored foods, as well as food in general. And this creates repeat customers for food companies.

Freaky things can happen when you eat too much MSG

MSG (and all the other names it goes by) cause a host of bizarre side effects. Here are a few of the weirder ones, among more than a dozen:

- tiny and dull headaches, to piercing and temporarily debilitating;
- taste buds over-salivating;
- excess phlegm in the throat;
- glutamic acid makes food taste unnaturally good and disrupts the "I'm full" signal, so you continue to eat after you're full.

But weirdest of all, considering MSG's excitotoxicity: **Excess glutamate consumption can cause minor muscle spasms to occur in a random area of your body.** It's an intermittent twitching that's slightly annoying, but subsides in a few minutes. I got these from time to time but never understood what was causing them. I found out these twitches are not a result of MSG accumulating in a random muscle and creating a short circuit. Rather, MSG is actually over-stimulating cells in the brain, partially frying that circuit for a while and causing a "brownout" – like a blinking light bulb that's on the verge of burning out. This is what causes those random muscle spasms that seem to come out of nowhere.

It could be your eyelid twitching. It could happen in your upper lip, your arm, or your back. It could show up as hiccups. But, contrary to what you may think at the time, the malfunction is not happening in that muscle. It's actually a mini-seizure happening in your brain from eating any high glutamate food, such as soy sauce, ketchup, salad dressing, taco sauce or barbeque sauce. Trippy, huh?

It's safe to assume purified MSG is the worst for you, because it's concentrated and unmoderated. Whereas, naturally-occurring glutamates from whole foods are probably a little easier on brain cells – being accompanied by substances that help you metabolize them.

MSG has been used in over 500 scientific studies to fatten mice

When scientists need obese mice to experiment on, they actually have a hard time getting mice to overeat on their own. So, decades ago, scientists discovered that they can feed mice MSG (or inject it) to disable the feeling of being full in their brain (among other mechanisms). This causes mice to eat nonstop, until they become morbidly obese (and diabetic).

MSG spikes insulin levels

You have glutamate receptors all throughout your body – especially in the nervous system. When you eat MSG-laden foods, the glutamate receptors in your pancreas get excited, causing more insulin to be released than you actually need. This causes your blood-sugar level to tank thirty minutes to one-and-a-half hours after eating glutamate-flavored foods. As a result, you get hungry, cranky, tired, sleepy, foggy, and prone to anger and violence. Low blood sugar makes you hungry prematurely.

Insulin also causes your body to store food intake as fat – particularly around the belly. Both of these effects make MSG "enemy #2" (behind sugar) in your effort to lose weight. From the food companies' perspective, it's the ideal additive to get you hooked – despite your intentions and willpower. It's cheap. It's seductive. And it operates so stealthfully that you'd never know you're under its spell.

But the side effect that MSG is notorious for among wellness coaches is that it's an "excitotoxin." Wikipedia: "Excitotoxicity is the pathological process by which nerve cells are damaged or killed by excessive stimulation by neurotransmitters such as glutamate and similar substances." In other words, over-indulging in glutamate-flavored foods literally excites brain cells to death. Thankfully, for most people, the damage is not as immediately crippling as it sounds. The majority of the population can eat MSG in most of their meals and not suffer side effects severe enough, or rapidly enough, to feel any loss of brain cells. But who knows about long-term effects to heavy consumers? The only thing we know for certain is that not a lot of organizations are anxious to fund that research to find out.

Think you can avoid MSG by reading labels? Think again

To disguise MSG from label readers, the food business has come up with more than forty different names for MSG. The way they get away with it is that MSG occurs naturally in foods like meats, cheeses and soy sauce. Since they're not required to list what's in a whole food, they don't have to specify it in their ingredients. Therefore, only the refined form of MSG has to be labeled as MSG. When it's included as an extract, or a concentrate of some other food, it can be called something else.

Here are a few of the most common names used to hide its presence from consumers (called "cleaning up your label" in the biz):

- yeast extract and anything with the word "autolyzed" in it
- seasoning
- anything with the word "flavoring" is suspect
- soy protein and anything with the word "hydrolyzed" in it
- whey protein, whey protein concentrate, and whey protein isolate
- anything with "caseinate" in the name
- malted barley and its derivations
- maltodextrin
- brewer's yeast
- virtually all stocks, broths and bouillons contain some form of MSG.

Companies only label MSG as such when consumers aren't too picky about what they're eating. In other words, when it won't hurt sales, they go ahead and call it MSG – like in Doritos, dips and some salad dressings. Otherwise, most processed foods contain MSG by another name. Indeed, most packaged foods contain more than one form of MSG to hide it.

But who's to blame? Well, we all are. Companies make the stuff, and consumers buy it. Most people know junk food is bad for you, yet it continues to sell – even when its wrongs are pointed out to consumers. So neither side is any more guilty than the other. As a result, our society has become increasingly indulgent and addicted to stronger and stronger flavors.

The flavor "arms race"

If you're old enough to remember the 1980s and '90s, Doritos used to have a nice punchy flavor – but nothing like they are today. Now, when the seasoning of a chip hits your tongue, the taste is so strong it's practically overwhelming if you're not used to it. But the thing that's messed up is, that's your *normal* if you eat stuff like this all the time.

The sad truth is, food companies have had to continually ratchet up the intensity of their flavors, with ever-more powerful seasoning, because the palate of the average consumer has become so corrupted that the most heavily affected say things like, "I don't like drinking water because it has no taste." It's like we're escalating the flavor of everything we eat in an arms race of taste affecting all processed food categories. Consumers are unwittingly demanding hotter, spicier, sweeter, saltier, and more MSG-intensified foods. How can natural foods compete with that? Stay tuned for help overcoming this addiction later in the program.

An analogy we can all relate to: Think of MSG like sugar. The food industry has extracted and purified cane sugar into table sugar to intensify the sweetness. Refined sugar gives the taste buds a massive blast of stimulation when it hits the tongue. Well, same thing with MSG – only the gap between unflavored food and MSG-spiked food is startling.

For instance, have you ever tasted real chicken stock (water that comes from boiling a chicken)? It hardly has any taste at all. But when store-bought broths, stocks and soups hit your tongue, they set off an explosion of taste sensations – as if they're lighting up all the neurons in your brain devoted to taste and pleasure. Same thing with unflavored refried beans *vs.* beans flavored with yeast extract, etc. **In fact, you can add MSG to dirt and people would think it tastes good.**

It's a little hard to tell, but if you pay close attention to flavor, you can identify what MSG makes a food product taste like. Unadulterated food tastes one way: pure, while MSG "supes up" a flavor – like a more intense, slightly unnatural clone of the original. Glutamates are an artificial kind of taste that's like a cousin to the taste of salt. Unfortunately, many people don't even know what real food is supposed to taste like anymore :-(

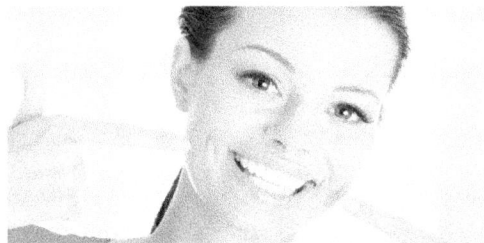

Mythbusting
Myth: Calcium builds strong bones and teeth

Not true… at least not by itself. Calcium is only a building material. Think of bone building and tooth building like this:

- Calcium and minerals are the bricks in the wall that are your bones.
- Collagen, fat and protein are the mortar that holds the wall together.
- And fat-soluble vitamins coordinate the construction by telling the materials where they need to go.

So consuming more calcium is not what you need to build stronger bones and teeth, as the dairy industry would have us believe. Most Westerners don't lack calcium in their diet. We get plenty of it in milk and milk products such as cheese, yogurt and ice cream. In fact, most of us get too much calcium – especially in relation to magnesium.

What we lack is the mineral phosphorus as a building block, "glue" factors in the form of collagen and protein, and vitamins such as vitamins A, D, E and K_2 that come mostly from animal products to facilitate the process. These vitamins, K_2 in particular, make calcium go where it's supposed to – bones and teeth – and not into soft tissues where they're not supposed to be, like blood vessels, kidneys, bile ducts, pineal gland and eyes.

Unfortunately, a shortage of fat-soluble vitamins and binding agents can be a serious problem for vegans and vegetarians. Lack of protein and fat in their diet can cause a deficiency – not only of fat-soluble vitamins, but also collagen deficiency. Thus, they lack the glue that holds things together.

Weight management is more than calorie counting

Calories are a measurement of how much heat is generated when you literally burn a food – as if humans were nothing more than Bunsen burners. The more heat generated when you burn a substance, the greater its calorie count. But this neglects a great many bodily processes, such as how well, or how poorly, a food or ingredient is digested, metabolized and eliminated. It fails to take into account the way residual antibiotics in poultry, for example, can damage gut flora and the pituitary gland, causing weight gain.

It loses site of the fact that pesticides, herbicides, GMOs and preservatives make their way into food production and disrupt our biochemical processes, triggering a cascade of side effects – notably leaky membranes, nutrient deficiencies, overactive immune system and hormonal issues. All the while, Big Food and government agencies want us to obsess over calories, calories, calories in an effort to lose weight. They pretend that's the only diet-related thing we need to worry about if we want to get thin and stay thin. It's classic one-dimensional thinking.

When really, it's everything else besides calories we should be concerned about – e.g., crop amendments, GMOs, heavy metals, artificial ingredients, preservatives, toxins, additives, and the form in which those calories are presented… in addition to how well the body metabolizes and eliminates that food. Take sodium benzoate, a preservative found in some diet sodas, for example. It, and its chemical cousin, potassium benzoate, have been known to damage DNA and mess up your metabolism, leading to kidney problems and weight gain – even when calorie count is negligible.

JAMA agrees: A study published January 2018 in the Journal of the American Medical Association (JAMA), "Effect of Low-Fat *vs.* Low-Carbohydrate Diet on 12-Month Weight Loss in Overweight Adults and the Association With Genotype Pattern or Insulin Secretion," supports the idea that cutting calories is not what you should be focusing on if you want to lose weight. Nor should you focus on cutting fat from your diet. Both of those approaches either don't work very well, or are problematic to implement and sustain (my interpretation, not the study's).

Rather, the quality of your food is more important in achieving your ideal weight – meaning, reduce your intake of refined/processed food, particularly sugar and carbs. And, instead, eat more whole, unprocessed foods grown naturally, with no restriction on quantity, fat intake or calories. In other words, eat as much high quality, nutrient-dense food as you like – the more the better – and your weight tends to normalize. That's the way to lose weight if you're overweight, gain weight if you're underweight, and gain health in the process.

Diet soda drinkers: Its zero calories does not help you lose weight

Calories are not what you should worry about if you want to lose weight and get healthy. Chemicals, toxins and denatured ingredients are the real enemies to ideal health because of the way they wreak havoc on the body's biochemistry. The whole idea of calories is misleading because humans don't burn food just to produce heat.

Rather, our digestive systems break down food into fat or glucose. Our mitochondria then turn those two fuels into an energy source that our cells can use: ATP. Just as important, our mitochondria produce other vital resources in the process, such as water, magnetism and electrical charge. So measuring calories is misleading. Instead, the chemicals, contaminants, additives, fillers, colorings, preservatives, and antibiotic ingredients added to foods – they're the constituents that should concern you, because they may not add any calories per se. But they sure as heck disrupt bodily processes and trigger side effects.

For example, when the tongue tastes an artificial sweetener in the food you're eating, it prepares the body for an influx of energy. After digesting that food for a bit, and finding no sugar present, it goes into a panic mode. It creates hunger cravings to make up for the shortfall. You then end up eating even more than you would have. It's a vicious cycle.

Therefore, calories should be one of the last things you think about when you want to lose weight. Instead, focus your attention on nutrition and purity (meaning, lack of harmful ingredients). That creates optimal health throughout your body. And optimal weight follows.

Salt isn't bad for you... *processed* salt is nutritionally imbalanced

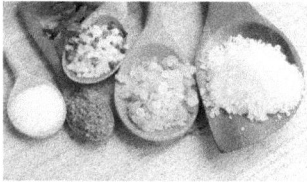

Salt is a vital nutrient. You need a certain amount of it in your diet to maintain good health. For example, the body needs salt to make hydrochloric acid, or else your stomach can't break down food properly and digestion suffers. You need salt for energy, because sodium transports glucose across the gut wall and into the blood. In addition, the adrenals need salt just to function. However, all salt is not created equal. There's good salt and bad.

The thing that makes refined sodium chloride (table salt) so detrimental to human health is it's been stripped of trace minerals in the manufacturing process so it passes those imbalances on to you. You need trace minerals for many bodily processes to occur. On the other hand, pure, unrefined sea salt is good for you. It contains otherwise hard-to-get trace minerals in the exact proportions that our biology needs. Some sea salts have as many as 92 trace minerals. And every one of them is used by the human body to accomplish something. Best of all, you don't need to sacrifice a thing using sea salt, apart from iodine.

Two varieties of salt praised for their nutritional value, purity and cooking qualities are Celtic sea salt and Himalayan pink salt, while dozens of other varieties offer different colors, geologic origins, flavor nuances, and mineral proportions. So salt is like most other foods: It's available as a whole food that supports the body in worry-free ways. Or you can find it in processed, adulterated forms that undermine the biochemical balance of the body in sneaky ways over time.

More evidence there are no coincidences in nature: The mineral profile of sea salt is virtually identical to that of human blood. During World War II, when a soldier was injured in the Pacific theatre and needed surgery, but there was no blood available for transfusions, medics would substitute sea water for blood. Sea salt is not quite as good as human blood, but this emergency hack has been known to save a life or two in a pinch. This shows the extent to which Nature and the human body are on the same page.

On the other hand, refined salt is made the way that it is primarily because industry needs salt to be in its pure form for use in commercial products such as soaps, detergents, plastics and agricultural chemicals. That's why refined salt must be stripped of its minerals.

All sugars are not created equal

Sugars are another area where calorie-centric thinking tricks people into making bad dietary choices. Even though many sweeteners have similar calorie counts, refined white sugar is more likely to cause weight gain because it assaults the pancreas with insulin demand. Over time, this contributes to insulin resistance and increased fat storage. But, even worse for you, high fructose corn syrup (HFCS) is partially man-made. It needs to be converted by the liver into glucose, glycogen or fat before it can be used. HFCS contributes to type 2 diabetes, obesity (particularly around the abdomen), inflammation, fatty liver disease and leaky gut.

In contrast, sugars made by Nature, such as honey, maple syrup and molasses are whole foods that the body knows how to metabolize. Honey, in particular, contains nutrients and active enzymes that help you digest it properly. The lesson to learn: Use sweeteners that are as close to a whole food as possible and you won't need to worry half as much about sugar-related metabolic problems and weight gain.

Don't trust numbers on multi-vitamin/multi-mineral supplements

Just like food labels, multi-vitamin/mineral numbers can be misleading because most brands use synthetic, refined, or otherwise processed ingredients. Unfortunately, these supplements may be doing far less good for you than their naturally-sourced counterparts because they are produced from inferior materials. Most people would never know the difference between quantity and quality, so who cares?

To illustrate how backwards the labeling system is, it's hard for supplement companies to tell you how much vitamin A or D is in a natural fish oil because each batch is different. But, to our disservice, it's easy to give you exact numbers when you use synthetic or processed ingredients – often supplied in powder form – because they're standardized. That's a major reason supplement makers and food companies like using refined sources of vitamins and minerals: they can put exact numbers on nutrition labels.

The problem is, the synthetic versions are far removed from whole foods. They lack the co-factors your body needs to fully utilize the nutrient. They may give you some benefit, but not nearly enough when you need all the nutrients you can get in order to reverse vitamin deficiencies, disease conditions, or a transgenerational-epigenetic defects. On the other hand, vitamins and minerals derived from natural sources are generally much more useable for the human body because Nature packages them with everything the body needs to break the nutrients down and present them in a form in which cells prosper.

Moreover, the supplement market is largely self-regulated, which means it isn't regulated at all unless something seriously abnormal occurs. Hence, many supplements don't meet the content and potency claims. And, even when they do, the vitamins and minerals reported on the label may be in a different form than what the body needs, so their unusable molecules need to be converted into bio-available ones. Otherwise, that particular vitamin/ mineral can't be absorbed and does you almost no good at all, which tends to be the case with all but the best, most expensive supplements.

Even when things are working perfectly, your microbiome, digestive system, and cells expend resources to perform the conversion – ultimately sacrificing a significant percentage of nutrients going from bottle to cell function. Not to mention the fact that the USDA's "recommended dietary allowances" are largely based on opinion, not scientific fact. So, as you can see, there are a number of opportunities for blunders and breakdowns to occur in supplementation.

Food preservation

We forget about the role that food preservation plays in our health, and our food supply, because taste and price are priorities #1 and 2 for most people. We don't stop to consider the virtues and vices of different food preservation techniques because, having lived with shelf-stable foods our entire lives, and having left most of those decisions up to Big Food, we take a certain amount of food stability for granted.

Processed food purposely depletes nutrients to extend shelf life

Have you ever thought it strange that some foods never spoil – Twinkies, for example? Urban legend says they'll sit for 100 years and never go bad. Whether that's true or not, there's a reason some modern packaged foods take forever to spoil or, in fact, never do. And it's not necessarily the preservatives. Rather, heavily refining a food strips it of nutrients that the microscopic recyclers of the world consume – including bacteria, molds, yeast and enzymes. When there's nothing nutritious for microorganisms to eat, the "food" takes forever to spoil, if at all, because that's largely what spoilage is: microbes consuming the food's nutrients to decompose it.

Simply put, when processed and refined foods don't support life on a microscopic level, they also lack the vitamins and minerals to support the nutritional needs of multi-celled organisms higher up the food chain. So, if a food keeps for an unnaturally long time, you better bet the vitamins, minerals and other nutrients have vacated that foodstuff in the refining process. And, in many cases, the nutrient depletion is done intentionally.

The idea of processed food came from the US military

Early in the 20th Century, the US military needed ready-to-eat meals that didn't spoil for their overseas war efforts. Through their research, food scientists discovered that removing nutrients greatly extended their shelf life because the microorganisms that cause spoilage had nothing to eat.

The packaged food industry caught on to this and developed their own methods to remove certain nutrients by refining and purifying the ingredients. Through a process of "enrichment," they then add back select vitamins and nutrients (usually synthetic) to ingredients such as flour to avoid causing more malnourishment than it already does… and to make the nutrition label look more appealing to conscientious moms and dads.

Through this intentional process of nutrient depletion, they dramatically increase their profit potential by keeping food from spoiling before you buy it, which has always been one of the food industry's biggest expenses – hidden in the food that you do eat. That's the dirty secret Big Food would rather you didn't know. It's not nefarious by any means, because the process benefits consumers in many ways. But, being better informed, you now have decisions to make in how you feed your family.

Our society demands more from our food preservation techniques than current methods can deliver

Beginning in the first half of the 20th Century, the food industry sought more ways to stabilize food's color, taste, texture, appearance and nutritional value. Food scientists started developing additives to leave in food products to prevent undesirable microbial activity, chemical reactions such as oxidation, and other changes from degrading the integrity and appeal of the end product.

Today, the food industry uses a wide variety of natural and synthetic agents (and a few processes) to extend the shelf life of foods sold commercially. Their ultimate goal being to create "shelf stable" foods, which means it doesn't require refrigeration and takes a long time to discolor, separate, go rancid or otherwise deteriorate.

Common food preservation methods
- cooking
- canning/vacuum sealing
- freezing and refrigeration
- curing/salting
- dehydration
- smoking
- fermenting/culturing.

With each method listed above, "what you see is what you get," in that each works fairly well protecting food quality, and its benefits *vs.* risks are well-understood. But we should take a moment to appreciate what each of them aims to do as its principal method of action: they inhibit the growth of microorganisms that would otherwise make food go rotten. Once again, microorganisms are a fundamental part of so many natural processes that we routinely take for granted.

To illustrate, here's one antimicrobial phenomenon that benefits us all, yet few are aware of it: A number of food preservation techniques rely on salt to inhibit microbial growth. Thankfully, salt doesn't proactively go around and kill microorganisms the way that antimicrobial agents do. Instead, it grabs hold of moisture so water is unavailable for microbes to proliferate. Unfortunately, salting, dehydration and smoking foods can concentrate salt to unhealthy levels, so it's not a good idea to eat foods preserved primarily with salt all the time.

Food preserving additives can be divided into three categories:

1. **Antimicrobials** inhibit growth of microbes that cause spoilage.
2. **Antioxidants** slow the oxidation of fats that make food go rancid.
3. **Chelators** decrease enzyme activity that causes fruits and veggies to ripen and discolor.

Antimicrobial preservatives. Generally speaking, antimicrobial agents and actions are the least healthy way to preserve food because they wipe out microbial life in food – including bacteria, yeasts and molds. And they don't discriminate between good bugs and bad. Of course, this slows pathogen growth. But it also reduces the benefits you get from friendly flora, enzymes and other nutrient factors, such as phytonutrients often accompanying probiotics. Sodium benzoate, nitrites, sorbates and irradiation are examples of antimicrobial preservation.

When we think "preservatives are bad," the antimicrobial class deserves the majority of that fear and loathing – and for good reason: **Antimicrobials can't help but kill probiotic bacteria, and damage your own cells, in your gut microbiome.** And, even before you eat it, antimicrobials can't help but kill the naturally-occurring probiotic organisms in a food that break it down into nutrients, and neutralize toxins that we can't. In short, we sacrifice nutritional value and detoxification to gain convenience and longer shelf life.

Chelating preservatives. Although they sound worse than they are, chelating agents that block enzyme activity fall somewhere in between antimicrobials and antioxidants, in terms of risk-to-benefit ratio. Chelating preservatives work by binding metallic minerals needed in chemical reactions that cause food to transition from *alive* to *dead and decaying*. That is, fruits and vegetables need enzyme activity in fungi and other microorganisms to ripen, then rot. Without minerals and enzymes, fruit won't ripen at all. This process is helped along by metal ions like magnesium acting as co-factors in the ripening process.

Chelators such as EDTA, for example, preserve canned foods by grabbing hold of their minerals/metals, thus disabling enzyme processes that degrade their color, flavor and texture. Citric acid is one of the gentler chelators in this class. EDTA is potentially more detrimental because it depletes beneficial minerals. And then there are chelating preservatives like polyphosphates that should be avoided, whenever possible.

Antioxidant preservatives. Antioxidant preservation operates through more bio-friendly means than do antimicrobials and chelators. They may not be as potently protective as cooking, salting, freezing or chemical preservatives. But many have little downside, to go along with decent upside. Antioxidant preservatives work by counteracting the oxidation process. As a food sits – particularly when uncovered – oxygen steals electrons from its fats and oils, denaturing their chemical structure. When oxidized, the fat/oil in the food goes rancid, and the food along with it.

Antioxidant preservatives block this process by donating electrons lost through oxidation. This neutralizes oxidation and maintains the food's original freshness longer than it would un-preserved. Vitamins E and C preserve food through their antioxidant activities, while sulfites act as both antioxidants and antimicrobials, so they're potentially more harmful.

A bizarre consequence of eating highly processed and preserved foods

In the Vietnam war, Vietcong soldiers were shocked that American G.I.s killed in combat took weeks longer to decompose than did their soldiers. Their thinking was: Americans consumed so many preservatives that they basically turned into Twinkies on the inside in terms of decomposition rate (my description of their belief). On the other hand, native Vietcong still ate their traditional diet, containing little to no processed foods.

Food preservation method is instrumental to its nutritional value... or its contribution to disease

Indeed, it's not uncommon for preservation method to be the single biggest factor in nutrient availability, toxin exposure, and influence on the microbiome. The way food is preserved often makes the difference between: (1) it being good for you and prized, (2) best left for special occasions, or (3) avoided at all costs. Preservation technique is just as important as which types of foods you choose to eat, how they're grown/produced, and how they're prepared. Note to self: Decrease consumption of preservation techniques that denature food. And increase your intake of foods that are not devitalized through the manner in which they're preserved. Heck, maybe even seek out foods preserved in a way that increases nutritional value and gut health, such as fermentation.

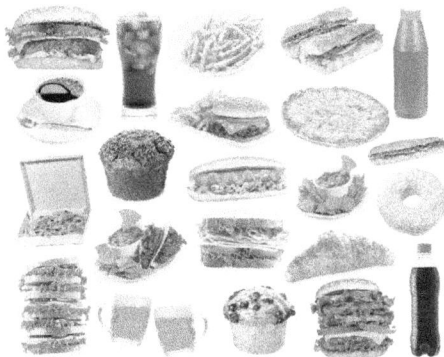

Processed foods
Processed food stresses the body with refined carbs

Refined sugar and carbs spike insulin levels, which overwork the pancreas, contributing to insulin resistance, metabolic syndrome, obesity and diabetes over time. Sugars and carbs also feed bad gut microbes disproportionately more than good because most disease-causing bacteria love sugars. In fact, refined carbs/sugar are their favorite type of food. One of insulin's more surprising effects is that it makes the body store most food types as fat – even seemingly harmless foods like lettuce. Odd as it may seem, insulin can help turn a vegetable that is not much more than fiber and water into fat.

Refining a fruit, vegetable, nut or grain throws it out of nutritional balance, causing vitamin and mineral deficiencies

Most plants and animals – when grown and eaten as close to their natural state as possible – are perfectly balanced for human physiology. Every vitamin, mineral, enzyme, or co-factor we need is included in the whole food so that no nutritional imbalances are created in you. For this reason, it's hard to overdose on whole foods because the body absorbs the nutrients it needs and eliminates the rest.

On the other hand, refining and processing concentrates the sugar and carbs, while it strips the vitamins, minerals and co-factors Nature put in the package so humans and animals can assimilate it properly. For example, one molecule of sugar requires 56 molecules of magnesium to metabolize. Wisely enough, whole fruits, grown naturally, have the same 1:56 ratio so you can eat as much as you want and never develop nutrient deficiencies.

Conversely, when you eat foods with sugar concentrated or added, your body has to steal magnesium that's needed elsewhere, just to digest that sugar. It diverts magnesium used in neurotransmitter or hormone production, for example, to meet the more urgent demand of getting sugar out of the bloodstream as quick as possible. Magnesium deficiency then impairs neurotransmitter production, because neurotransmitters require an array of metabolites, co-factors and building blocks in their construction. Your brain is then forced to run on emergency reserves of neurochemicals.

Most modern humans are starving for minerals because damaged enterocytes aren't transporting minerals through the gut wall. And then refined carbohydrates come along and further sap you of minerals needed to produce both neurotransmitters and brain function. Another process that suffers in a state of mineral deficiency is detoxification. It requires large amounts of vitamins and minerals to bind up toxins and expel them through detox channels.

The ingredients in man-made foods can damage gene expression

Epigenetics: Study of how environmental factors turn your genes on or off

Through the relatively new science of epigenetics, we now know that man-made "foods" damage the way your DNA is transcribed into physical, mental and behavioral characteristics. Processed vegetable oils, man-made sweeteners, preservatives, agricultural chemicals and toxins can switch on genes that cause the body to become insulin resistant and obese, as two examples. Or contaminants like these can contribute to cancer, heart disease and most chronic, degenerative diseases. On the flip side, unprocessed, nutrient-dense food can turn those genes off (a long time after the threats are removed).

So when a morbidly obese family all seem to have the same body type, remember that genetics only "loads the gun" for gene expression to occur. It's the environment – particularly what you eat, and your chemical exposure – that "pulls the trigger" in manifesting those traits. Without those exposures, the genetic potential for those traits remains dormant in your genetic code. But in their presence, you not only trigger those traits to appear in yourself, but you may also pass them on to your children. And, once triggered, those traits often become characteristic of your family tree that is difficult, but not impossible, to reverse.

It can take a long time to cause the damage – sometimes decades in one person, or that long in multiple generations. And it can take even longer to reverse it. In his research with cats, Francis M. Pottenger, Jr., MD, discovered epigenetic changes to gene expression took four generations to repair after being triggered by nutrient deficiencies.

To reverse epigenetic changes, you basically have to remove the offending influences and supply the body with copious nutrition (bio-available nutrition, not just nutrition label numbers). That gives the body the resources it needs to shut down emergency coping mechanisms, jumpstart dormant detox processes, and launch epigenetic repairs to processes such as methylation. Do that and you can switch off undesirable gene expression long-term and seemingly remove it from your family tree.

Underappreciated health protectors

Harmful ingredients and lack of vitamins aren't the only reasons that processed foods are bad for you. It's also the following unsung heroes of health that are knowingly or unknowingly removed in commercial food production that add insult to injury. That's the "secret-within-a-secret" as to why processed foods are bad for you. The absence of these lesser-known, but equally important, nutrients degrade your health when whole foods are turned into processed foods.

- minerals needed for metabolism and detoxification
- beneficial bacteria and other microorganisms (e.g., fermented foods)
- digestive enzymes (particularly in meat)

UNSUNG NUTRIENT HEROES

MINERALS/ MONOATOMICS

GOOD BACTERIA

ANTIOXIDANTS

FIBER

DIGESTIVE ENZYMES

ESSENTIAL FATS

PHYTONUTRIENTS/ CO-FACTORS

MOISTURE CONTENT

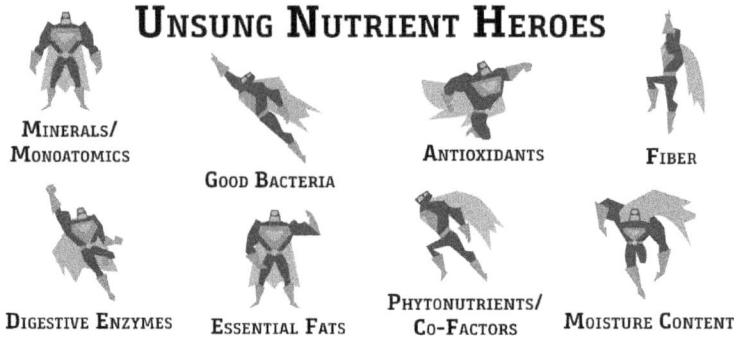

- antioxidants (particularly in raw fruits)
- phytonutrients and co-factors (which we still have a lot to learn about)
- fiber in fruits/vegetables/grains that slows digestion of sugars, cleans the colon, and feeds gut flora
- moisture content (with good stuff in that moisture)
- healthy fats that slow the rise in blood-sugar level.

There are hidden costs to eating processed foods, and foods that resist spoilage

Call this a "withdrawal" from your health "bank account." There's a reason some foods have to be consumed in a few days or they go bad, while other foods last weeks, months or even years without refrigeration. It all comes down to the nutrient value that the food provides to the microbes outside and inside your body, how many of the unsung heroes of health that remain in the food, and how much life-force the food still has left when you eat it.

Conclusion

Optimal brain and organ function require you to assimilate the right nutritional factors, and stay away from those that empty your bucket of wellness. You can't simply eat more vegetables to get healthier. You can't just consume mass quantities of probiotic supplements and expect your health to ascend forever. Instead, you need to limit your intake of secret health saboteurs. And you have to learn a few new concepts to live by, such as replacing processed salt with sea salt, and daily detoxing. It's little adjustments like these that go a long way toward fixing nagging problems, restoring gut health, and optimizing brain function.

Start your wellness journey by unlearning the propaganda that Big Food and Big Pharma have spread about how health is created in a body. Don't believe the lies that they've told about fat, cholesterol, calories, vegetable oils, salt, and the Food Pyramid. Don't listen to what "they" say you should eat, and what you shouldn't, because virtually everything they tell you is wrong. And don't blindly believe the marketing hype you read on labels, because most of what they have be teaching us for decades is the exact opposite of the truth. Learn for yourself and be your own health boss. The truth is close at-hand.

———— ❧ ————

5

GENETICALLY MODIFIED ORGANISMS (GMOs) AND GLYPHOSATE

Starting in the 1950s, agriculture companies went from an approach of working with Nature to a compulsion for controlling and dominating it

Prior to the 1940s, man worked more or less in harmony with Nature to grow enough food for everyone to eat. But, after World War II, industry had so much: (1) extra petroleum-making capacity, (2) unused chemical weapons, and (3) technology momentum from the war that they decided to find new uses for chemicals, instead of going back to the way things were.

Chemical companies shifted their efforts away from feeding the war machine, toward the development of nitrogen-based fertilizers derived from crude oil. In tandem with fertilizers, they turned chemical weapons into herbicides and pesticides. More efficient machinery and processes also made it possible for farms to increase in size. Together, they called these agricultural advancements the "Green Revolution" because of their ability to surpass Nature's limitations and industrialize the growing process.

On the surface, the new technologies and techniques were a smashing success. Efficiencies and yield multiplied. Economies of scale were enjoyed by all. And America became the breadbasket for the world. However, underneath it all, a storm started brewing that would take decades to heat up and boil over. That's because chemical companies basically decided to commercialize agriculture and treat it like any other business with a "no-holds-barred" approach to making money feeding the masses. From that point on, food stopped being mere sustenance and, instead, became a commercial product, just like any other on a store shelf. It was

- to be made as cheaply as possible,
- reduced in quantity and quality as much as consumers would tolerate,
- marketed as aggressively as the law would allow (and then some),
- and supplied by as few corporations as could be.

… Not necessarily sinister, just the way it is. But the most important change brought about by the Green Revolution was in man's new approach to agriculture – as well as his place in the universe – compared to Nature itself. That is, man, in his hubris, started looking for shortcuts and "cheat codes." Today, we call them "hacks" to overcome every inefficiency that

Nature presented in raising plants and animals. The effort (1) started with mechanization; (2) incorporated inorganic chemical fertilizers; (3) made extensive use of herbicides and pesticides; and (4) grew in scale through consolidation and organization of producers, distributors and sellers.

Then, in the 1970s and '80s, Big Ag sought to remove Nature's limitations entirely through genetic engineering. Man thought he was clever enough to call the shots in food production from then on. Technology and mechanization were his keys. And, for a while, it all seemed to work out.

The Green Revolution industrialized agriculture and brought us a plethora of problems to go along with seductive benefits

Our science and industry thought it could do better than Nature. So man basically said to Nature, 'You've done a good job getting us to where we are. But we'll take it from here. Man's science and industry will do the driving from now on.' From that point on, Big Agriculture and Big Food has thought and acted as if it needs to subdue and control Nature, rather than work in harmony with her principles and processes. Little did we know, those early successes signed us up for deferred consequences we'd soon have to repay... and with interest.

You see, Nature has such vast and resilient coping mechanisms that it takes many decades to wear them down and show us the consequences of what we created. Imbalances in nature take longer to turn into disease than in the human body, because Nature operates on a much grander scale and longer timeline. So the 70+ years that we've been abusing the planet with agricultural and industrial poisons is like a few months in "human years."

Big Ag and Big Food have gladly taken the wins, while they've dismissed, denied, displaced or deferred the losses onto the planet and future generations in the form of pollution, disease and environmental destruction. However, it's only within the last three or four decades that we've woken up to the fact that we've been accumulating debts – biological, environmental and humanitarian – that have to be repaid... the worst of which are caused by (1) broad-spectrum herbicides such as glyphosate, (2) genetic engineering (as it's being practiced today) and, to a lesser extent, the (3) Green Revolution itself.

For 50+ years, genetic engineering has been promoted as the solution to

- world hunger (i.e., yield)
- malnutrition (i.e., nutrient content)
- herbicide and pesticide use
- disease and pest resistance
- environmental degradation
- economic prosperity (through sales and exports).

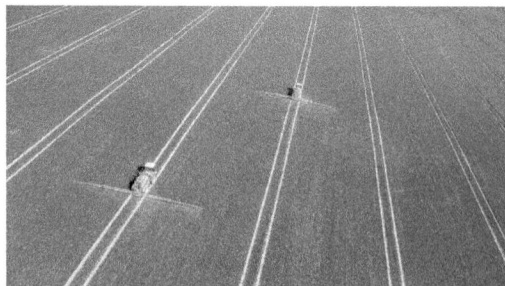

They said we needed GMOs to feed the world's expanding population. The implication being, GMOs would end world hunger. Unfortunately, none of their promises have come true. In fact, we're seeing the exact opposite take place… and it's getting worse.

- **Yield.** No GMO crop has ever outperformed its ancestral/heirloom (isogenic) variety in yield (as court rulings have prohibited Monsanto from claiming). And yields are dropping. Yield is a complex synergy of many genes interacting, not one gene acting alone.
- **Nutrient content.** The nutritional value of GMO and glyphosate-sprayed plants has plummeted. That lowers nutritional content for both humans and farm animals feeding on those plants.
- **Herbicide/pesticide use.** Weeds are developing resistance to the herbicide most GMOs are engineered to tolerate: glyphosate, which requires more and more of it to get the same effect. So the transition is now underway to even more powerful and toxic herbicides such as "2,4-D," atrazine and dicamba.
- **Plant immunity.** In most cases, genetic engineering weakens a plant's ability to cope with stresses and threats. As a result, dozens of once-minor plant diseases are starting to pose major problems for the agricultural industry due to herbicide and insecticide resistance.
- **Environmental contamination.** GMOs, and the herbicides they're engineered to tolerate, are contaminating the planet more than any toxin in history.
- **Farmer income.** Independent farmers around the world despise GMO crops and their makers, because of all the damage they do to everything they touch.

It hasn't worked out the way that they promised

Everything that Big Ag companies have done with genetic engineering prior to non-browning apples and faster-growing salmon has been done for their own benefit – not that of consumers, hungry/impoverished, genetic strength of plants, animal welfare, or planetary health. As for the farmers themselves, they're now being treated like cogs in a big machine.

In other words, GMO crops don't save the consumer any money. They aren't more nutrition (with the exception of beta-carotene in golden rice). They don't taste better. Most don't stay fresh longer. They don't lower herbicide and pesticide use. They don't give plants any better resistance to stress or disease. And they haven't been used to end world hunger, environmental degradation, or climate change. On top of that, they're wiping out US exports to other countries because foreign nations are banning the import of GMOs left and right.

Furthermore, if you ask any farmer who's used GMOs and their chemical companions, most of them say the combination gives them two big benefits: simplifying weed control and increased insect resistance (of certain crops). But, along with that, they're forced to endure miserable drawbacks. For example, agrochemical companies have consistently and aggressively raised GMO seed prices since they gained near monopoly control over most varieties and sellers, leaving growers fewer and fewer options. As a result, most growers have serious reservations about using GMOs and Roundup. And that's only the growers it works reasonably well for. A large percentage would switch to bio-friendly farming if they could. However, that's easier said than done. They feel trapped.

Bottom line: Genetically modified organisms have very little to do with anything except selling more chemicals and monopolizing control over the growing process. Those are the real motivations behind the world-wide proliferation of GMOs and glyphosate.

Did the GMO companies knowingly lie to us, or did they honestly believe what they were saying?

It doesn't really matter. Whether they overpromised or under-delivered, whether sincere or willingly deceitful, the end result is the same: **they can't be trusted.** The ringleader, Monsanto (among half a dozen major players) is a perfect example of what happens when compulsive lying and calculated maleficence are woven into the DNA of a company. This is the company that told us DDT was safe. They said Agent Orange was safe. They said recombinant growth hormone (for cows) was safe. They said PCBs were safe. And now they're telling the world both GMOs and glyphosate are safe. Do you see a pattern of deceit going on here?

GMO crops benefit agrochemical companies the most, growers some, food companies a little, and consumers only in limited ways

For growers, Roundup-ready GMO crops greatly simplify weed control, which is farming's greatest challenge and concern. So it's a convenience factor that permits more mechanization, larger farm size, greater economies of scale, and more predictable outcomes the first few years of use – after which productivity, predictability and profitability decline.

On the surface of it, growers seem to be the ones benefitting from GMOs. But, as we'll soon discuss, Big Ag companies, not the growers, actually end up pocketing most of the benefits in the long-run. Industry experts such as Dr. Don Huber have reported the use of GMOs and glyphosate does not save growers any money in the long run. It's pretty much a wash, because the benefits are negated by the increased costs of buying more herbicide, fungicide, insecticide and GMO seed.

Meanwhile, food companies benefit from GMOs because they reduce ingredient costs and are better for mass production – particularly in packaged and processed foods. It's fair to say some of that cost savings is passed on to consumers – mostly because the US government subsidizes GMO crops. But you may end up paying higher medical bills as a hidden cost.

To many people's surprise, non-GMO food does not inherently mean higher prices, as GMO advocates have suggested. Food prices in the US for decent quality non-GMO food products are comparable to those in countries where GMOs are prohibited. Low GMO food prices just make conventionally grown ones seem expensive by comparison. As for the foods themselves, the newest products of genetic engineering, on the surface of it, seem to offer desirable benefits such as non-browning apples and faster growing salmon. But one has to ask, 'At what cost'?

Image used courtesy of OrganicLifestyle Magazine.com

The price we pay for GMOs

Just think: Pharmaceutical companies study a new drug's effects and side effects in humans before releasing it to the public. On the other hand, new GMOs are put on the market with a bare minimum of: short-term, internally-funded, highly-biased, and usually secret testing on animals… if any testing is done at all. Which is to say, GMOs are hardly studied at all prior to being declared fit for human or animal consumption. That means you and I are the human guinea pigs in the great GMO experiment. In addition, Nature and traditional selective breeding are better at producing the benefits that GMOs claim to offer. For example, selective breeding can do a much better job of improving nutrient density than genetic engineering, and with far fewer side effects.

The downsides to genetic engineering

- **Nutrient loss.** The genetic engineering process obstructs nutrient absorption in plants. Glyphosate further decreases nutrient uptake.
- **New proteins.** The genetic engineering process itself creates new proteins. The majority are harmless. Many are damaging over time. And a few are as toxic as the deadliest biological weapons known to man (they're both made from extremely toxic exotic proteins).
- **Goes hand-in-hand with glyphosate.** GMO crops are used in combination with glyphosate, radically enhancing a GMO's toxicity.

- **Massive organ damage, quickly.** Rat studies show the first organs to be damaged by GMOs are the liver and kidneys, because a mammal's body treats the foreign proteins as toxins, not a food, thus placing enormous stress on detoxification systems.
- **Shuts down detoxification.** GMOs shut down C1 metabolism (a detoxification pathway), which depletes glutathione and prevents plants and animals from breaking down formaldehyde.
- **Premature aging.** Ranchers say their two-to-three-year-old cattle that should be prime beef are being downgraded, as if they were 8–10 year-olds, as a result of eating GMO feed laced with glyphosate.
- **Cancer.** Professor Seralini's studies show that GMOs cause enormous tumors to grow in rats shortly after small exposures.
- **Transgenes spread like a slow-moving plague.** GMO genes contaminate non-GMO crops, soil microorganisms, animals, our microbiota and our own DNA. In the case of "Bt toxin," this causes infected organisms to produce the toxin inside its own cells.
- **Rise of new pathogen.** A new pathogenic entity found in GMO soybean and corn feed is causing widespread infertility, spontaneous abortions, and stillbirths in cows and other livestock. It threatens more than just dairy and beef production. About the size of a small virus, and unlike any other microorganism, scientists have yet to determine exactly what the new entity is. It contains no genetic information and replicates similar to a prion (which are thought to cause "mad cow disease"). But technically, it's non-living, so it's very hard to eradicate. *How do you kill something that replicates and infects other organisms, yet is not living?* As a result, many dairy farms are experiencing 40–50% spontaneous abortions in cows, on top of 15–20% infertility. This has US cattle ranchers, their veterinarians, and health agencies around the world desperate for answers.

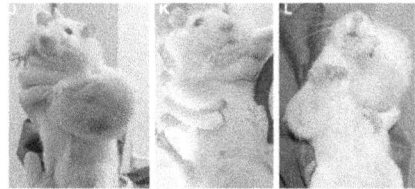

What is genetic engineering?

Genetic engineering in commercial agriculture is the process of artificially forcing the genes from one organism into the DNA of another. The two organisms are often completely unrelated life forms and could never mate and reproduce in nature. For example:

Gene: Snippets of DNA coding that tell the nucleus of cells how to make proteins, organs, systems, and the organism. Genes are instructions to produce physical traits and (indirectly) behaviors.

- Spider genes have been injected into goats in the hopes they could be milked to get spider web protein to make bullet-proof vests.
- Scientists have spliced cow genes into pigs, so they grow cowhides.
- They've put human genes into corn to make spermicide.
- (For their own morbid entertainment?) genes from a luminescent jellyfish have been put into pigs to make them glow in the dark.

Unnatural combinations like these are the reason that industry can no longer call some end products of genetic modification simply a *plant* or an *animal*. Instead, they contain the genetic material of both plant *and* animal, or plant *and* bacteria. So the end product of a genetic experiment must be called a genetically modified *organism*. Add to that a complete disrespect for Nature, plus hideous intentions, and you've got cringe-worthy abominations that would be right at home in a sci-fi horror movie.

The two most common genetic modifications in agriculture

For food crops, there are two main categories of genetic modification: those crops modified to tolerate (resist) glyphosate exposure (about 85% of all GMOs made today), and those modified to produce a bacteria-derived poison called "Bt toxin" (Bacillus thuringiensis). These operate by rupturing an insect's stomach when they eat the GMO "plant."

The problem with each of these scenarios: (1) glyphosate is extremely toxic over time because it ties up beneficial minerals and inhibits enzyme activity essential to plants and animals; (2) the other kind of GMO unavoidably poisons its consumer with Bt toxin. There's no getting away from either situation, because neither glyphosate nor the Bt toxin can be neutralized or washed off. If you eat the GMO, you're surely being poisoned by GMO proteins and their companion chemicals.

Only 9 GMO crops are widely commercialized. But their derivatives are found in about 30,000 products (80% and rising)

- soy (about 95% of all soybean production)
- corn (and most corn products, except popcorn)
- cottonseed (for oil and animal feed protein)
- canola (for oil and animal feed protein)
- sugar beet (as sugar and beet pulp for animal feed)
- papaya (Hawaiian and Chinese)
- zucchini
- yellow crookneck squash
- alfalfa (for feeding livestock and human consumption)

To give you an idea of how broad GMO use is in our food supply, soy is used in thousands of foods as a cheap filler (e.g., milk substitutes, dietary supplement powders, protein bars) and as lecithin emulsifiers in bakery products. While corn is used in dozens of food types, animal feed, ethanol production, and high fructose corn syrup production. Canola and cotton-seed are used in cooking, or as an ingredient. Sugar beet is used to make 60% of US sugar. And alfalfa is quickly taking over the animal feed industry as a main source of protein and nutrients for herbivores such as cows.

Man's understanding and control of genetic engineering is primitive

GMO companies want us to believe genetic engineering is an exact science that they control from conception to execution to long-term effects. But nothing could be further from the truth as we'll soon see. Genetic engineering, as it's practiced today, is still a highly unpredictable, poorly controlled "throw-it-against-the-wall-and-see-what-sticks" experiment. Most of the time, they have no idea what's going to happen when they do an experiment, let alone predict its long-term effects. They are virtually blind to the relationships that genes have with one another.

In Big Ag's arrogance and greed, they concern themselves only with the gains to be had, and let others deal with the consequences. The big 6 GMO companies – Monsanto, BASF, Bayer, Dupont, Dow and Syngenta – reap the rewards of pushing GMOs and force the entire planet to pay the price.

Nature engineered grace and mercy into DNA, in that some genes regulate or suppress, rather than create

Some genes are meant to control others – especially under adverse circumstances. Some turn on physical traits or bodily functions. Others regulate, or modify, the expression of those genes. While other genes are inhibitory, preventing gene functions from expressing themselves at all.

So when those regulatory genes are left out of the "splicing and dicing" experiments of modern genetic engineering, you circumvent the organism's innate ability to adapt to environmental changes, overcome adversity, and keep potentially harmful traits from expressing themselves.

Safeguards like these are built into the genetic code of all lifeforms. But when you treat DNA as if you were a supreme being who can do no wrong, you tend to forget you're working with a fraction of a fraction of a fraction of the intelligence, experience and foresight as that of its original design. When scientists force the DNA of one species into that of another life form, they omit the gene sequences Nature incorporated into that genome to keep the gene(s) of interest from producing undesirable outcomes under certain circumstances.

Sadly, biotech companies are infected with a narrow-minded *"survival of the fittest, and let others worry about the consequences"* mentality. This makes them think they can combine individual genes with the organism of their choice and end up with all good attributes and no bad. However, genes rarely act alone. Instead, they work as teams. Families of genes work in concert with one another to produce families of functions and traits that change, based on what's happening in their environment. The problem is, GMO companies don't have a clue how individual genes regulate the expression of others, let alone the dynamics of gene families.

Genetic engineering and complex computer systems respond to changes in unpredictable ways

As a computer system becomes more complex and interdependent, you lose the ability to predict what one change will do to other elements of the system. Even developers of a complex computer system who were intimately involved in the designing, programming, building and debugging cannot predict exactly what will happen when a single change is made somewhere in the system.

One change in input causes chain reactions that surprise even the most far-sighted of developers. This is widely known and generally accepted in the design of complex computer systems. It's for this reason that critical systems in medical imaging, nuclear power plants, and aviation are operated extensively in test environments before new versions are entered into service with real-life ramifications.

Now consider human DNA (or any higher life form). Human DNA is inconceivably more complex and interdependent than any computer program. There's no way any human can predict exactly what will happen when you insert gene sequences into the DNA of another organism. For example, legend has it that creators of life on this planet experimented for some time to arrive at higher life forms that were compatible with the environment and other life forms present. Even entities possessing supreme intelligence had to experiment to get more of what they wanted, and less of what they didn't, when engineering new life forms. It is said that chimeric human-beast hybrids depicted in ancient mythology were genetic experiments that just weren't right for the earth for one reason or another.

Bottom line: No one can predict the long-term consequences of mixing DNA from entirely different life forms. That's why studies done by GMO companies to show safety have been as short as possible. They most certainly have found out through their unpublished research that the longer a study goes on, the greater the likelihood of serious long-term consequences that can't be misrepresented, covered up, or otherwise eliminated by "massaging the data."

And you know what, these kinds of outcomes are exactly what we're experiencing in our rates of chronic disease that correlate perfectly with the introduction of GMOs and glyphosate in our food supply.

How are GMOs made?

GMOs are engineered in a lab by first isolating a portion of an organism's genetic code that produces a trait with commercial value to the agrochemical company. This packet, or sequence, of genetic material (which is not always clearly defined) is called a "gene." The most widely used gene comes from a bacterium that makes genetically modified soy, corn, cotton or canola resistant to glyphosate through the production of

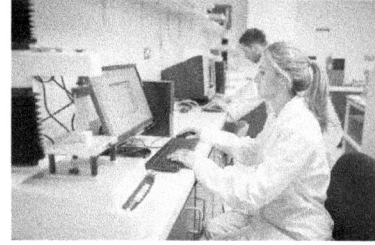

an enzyme called "CP4 EPSPS." We'll use this kind of end goal to illustrate how the genetic engineering process works:

- After isolating a gene of interest from its brethren, engineers usually add a fragment of another gene, called a "promoter," to activate the gene and mark their beginning on a strand of DNA. Otherwise, the gene would have little to no effect. In this case, the promoter gene comes from a plant virus (as most do).

- Engineers then add a third gene fragment from a petunia to make sure the enzyme offering glyphosate resistance goes to the right place in the GMOs cells, and does what engineers want it to do.

- Determined to make it all work, scientists then add a fourth gene fragment from another bacterial species to tell protein-production processes, and replication processes, where that snippet of code ends and the next begins.

- Together, these four snippets of genetic information, taken from four separate organisms, form a gene "cassette," which is everything needed to create the desired effect when that unit of code is inserted, or "transplanted," into the DNA of a foreign organism.

- Engineers then coat tiny pellets of gold or tungsten with millions of copies of those gene cassettes (which we'll call a *gene* for simplicity), load those pellets into a tiny gun of sorts, and bombard millions of recipient cells in culture with those nano-sized pellets.

- This GE process forcibly injects the desired "transgene" (as the newly relocated gene is now called) into a random spot in the host cell's DNA. Perhaps one in a million host cells successfully integrates the new transgene into one of its chromosomes as intended.

- Technicians continue this process until they find a host cell/transgene hybrid that can survive, replicate, and express the gene as desired, as well as not produce too many mutations or adverse effects.

- One of the major problems with this process is that experimenters only reject plants that are visibly deformed, or don't grow properly – not those that have intangible, but invisible, issues such as new toxins or compromised immunity that only show up under stress.

- Provided the previous steps go according to plan, they then need to separate new GMO cells from the millions of original cells. So, concurrent with the first gene insertion, engineers add a fifth snippet of code that offers antibiotic-resistance into the gene cassette. That way they can kill the original cells with an antibiotic, leaving only genetically engineered cells.

- When all that is achieved, they clone those GM cells repeatedly to make a plant in much the same way that stem cells replicate, differentiate, and grow into a complete organism.

Genetic engineering is based on a false belief, disproven 60 years ago

The entire GMO industry still operates on the misconception from the 1950s that each individual gene controls one physiologic feature or function – one gene, one function. We now know that's not true. It's a flawed assumption proven incorrect when science sequenced the human genome starting in the late 1980s.

Geneticists around the world fully expected human DNA to contain around 100,000 genes when the Human Genome Project began. But, when the sequencing was completed, they were shocked to learn there are far more features and functions in the human body than there are genes that supposedly control them – about 100,000 of them, yet only about 20,000 genes. This tells us genes have to control more than one feature or function. They must act in families. Specifically, their spatial relationship – where they sit on the double-helix in relationship to one another – and how they interact with influences in the environment, determines how each gene will be expressed.

Most important, some genes directly control a feature or function (through proteins that serve as a building material or control enzyme activity), while others activate, inhibit, or regulate the expression of genes in the first group (also through protein production). These four aspects of genetic engineering are the primary reasons why the genetic engineering process produces side effects that scientists cannot predict or control:

1. Random insertion of a gene messes up a DNA's sequence.
2. Regulatory genes are no longer present to inhibit or control that gene.
3. Geneticists don't know how the environment effects gene expression.
4. The cloning process poses problems that have yet to be solved.

Genetic engineering operates like a virus

A virus operates by injecting its genes into a host cell to make it do its bidding, contrary to what the host cell would do on its own. Viruses don't have their own equipment, such as a nucleus and cytoplasm, so they need to piggy back on host cells to survive and replicate. In a word, that's an infection. Genetic engineering, as it's practiced today, operates in much the same way as a virus: It injects genetic information into a host cell and makes it do things it wasn't *designed* to do, and would probably refuse to do, if asked.

Transgenes operate much like a virus, bacteria, or cancer in that they override genetically-endowed control mechanisms. This creates a lot of unwelcome side effects, such as the production of 10, 60 or 100 inappropriate proteins for each transgene inserted. Many of these never-before-seen proteins appear to do nothing. We don't know, because they haven't been observed for long. A few produce meager adverse effects. And some rare ones are as toxic as the deadliest poisons known to man.

Jeffrey Smith

"The process of insertion plus cloning creates massive collateral damage. There can be hundreds or thousands of mutations up and down the DNA. And hundreds or thousands of genes can change their levels of expression from that of the naturally-functioning plant. This creates unpredicted side effects. The [human] immune system looks at the highly unusual protein that's never occurred in nature before. It doesn't recognize it as anything that's nutritious or beneficial. So it perceives it to be a toxin, and attacks it as if it were harmful to your health."

Traditional plant breeding *vs.* modern genetic engineering

- **Selective breeding** accentuates desirable characteristics in a plant by repeatedly keeping those with the features we like through many generations, while discarding the ones that we don't – but always in compliance with Nature's rules. The genetics of most fruits and vegetables we eat are refined in this way.
- **Hybridization** mixes disparate species of plants through cross-pollination to gradually encourage the qualities we want, while discouraging the ones that we don't. Certain flowers are selectively evolved through hybridization.
- **Grafting** involves affixing a branch from one type of plant on to the trunk of another to make a mix of the two. For instance, the Japanese produce a pear-apple hybrid that's common in stores.

Over many generations, plants in traditional breeding programs such as these evolved to be bigger, better tasting, better in texture, easier to grow, more stout, consistent in size, or just different. They can become more nutritious. But whatever the form of traditional breeding, over time, plants evolved these desirable qualities *in partnership with Nature*.

Point being, traditional breeding merely selects genes from those that are available. Plants never get genes forcibly added to their DNA, in a random location, from a thoroughly divergent life form. This changes the spatial relationship of genes in the genome (an organism's complete genetic code). Just as important, regulatory genes never get separated from their partners, which preserves the wisdom in Nature's design.

On the other hand, genetic engineering combines gene sequences that never could, and never should, be combined. Just as bad, important inhibitory/regulatory genes that divert disaster before it occurs – they're omitted as standard practice in genetic engineering, leaving abominable combinations in their place. These unholy unions, as many would call them, combine to form revolutionary, and often dangerous, leaps in gene sequencing that product results akin to shooting in the dark.

Bottom line: Artificially injecting genes into the DNA of a completely unrelated life form is nowhere near the same as selective breeding programs that adapted plants to our liking over time. Not even close… despite what GMO proponents want us to believe. Modern genetic engineering is way too messy and unpredictable to shoot for certain objectives and get only that, with no more and no less. Remember, genetic engineers have no control over where transgenes settle in a host, so no one can tell you what the end result will be.

The natural sequence of DNA is no random accident

Geneticists have been in awe of the code contained in our DNA ever since Watson and Crick discovered its structure around 1953. That's because astute observers have realized that only supernatural intelligence could assemble DNA in the perfect order so that all the physical features and functional dynamics are expressed exactly as intended, and at the right time (i.e., conditional expression), while at the same time producing no coding errors or unintended consequences.

To foresee and engineer the outcomes and interactions of one creature's genetics is beyond genius. But for millions of creatures? That would take intelligence beyond comprehension. Indeed, Dr. Watson himself said the way DNA operates is so complex that there's no possible way it could have been arranged by chance and natural selection. Its combination of simultaneous complexity and refinement is just too perfect. Conversely, random mutation and natural selection would leave clues in the form of "bugs" in the code.

To this day, the biotech industry will still deny that GMOs had anything to do with its first mass-poisoning event

Genetic engineering's first fiasco: Starting in the late 1980s, thousands of people came down with bizarre symptoms that public health agencies could not explain. Fortunately, the symptoms were so unusual that they were not easily confused with other conditions. Otherwise, the supplement would probably still be on the market, and hundreds would be dead, perhaps 50,000 permanently disabled.

After ten years of fact-finding, medical investigators traced the condition back to a rogue protein found in a single brand of L-tryptophan (a natural supplement) that killed eighty, and severely injured perhaps 10,000 in extremely small doses. The fourteen natural brands of L-tryptophan made from non-GMO bacteria didn't have these problems.

The disease, called "eosinophilia myalgai syndrome," was almost certainly caused by genetically modifying a bacterium to produce twice as much L-tryptophan as usual. The company did this by giving the bacterium another copy of a gene it already had.

So how did the industry handle the situation? Commanded from high up to promote the biotech industry, the FDA failed to mention in their public statements that the supplement was made using genetic engineering. They proceeded to lay the blame on *all natural supplements* for the deaths and disabilities, and pulled all tryptophan off the market for a while. You see, at the time, Big Pharma had just started waging war against natural supplements in an effort to sell more pharmaceuticals. So they used the opportunity to make supplements look bad. They demanded stricter regulations to stifle the supplement industry.

Wild animals such as mice, squirrels, deer and elk refuse to eat GM corn, unless they're starving to death

When a wild rodent refuses to eat grain they have easy access to – that tells you something. We don't know exactly why. But it's safe to say they can smell the formaldehyde and/or Bt insecticide coming off the GMO corn. They probably don't like the tummy ache it gives them either. In any case, we know many wild animals are able to tell the difference between conventional plants and GMO plants engineered to produce the Bt toxin. Their survival instincts tell them something that escapes our senses.

Healthy animals died after grazing on Bt cotton

Prior to Bt cotton, farmers in India allowed their sheep, goats and buffalo to graze on cotton plants after harvest. But after the farmers made the switch to Bt-producing cotton, thousands of animals died within days of eating it. In one case, thirteen buffalo grazed on Bt cotton for a single day and were found dead three days later.

Genetic pollution

Industry observers shudder when they consider this set of facts:

- **Infectious.** They infect other organisms like a virus.
- **Inevitable.** Crop contamination is inevitable.
- **Persistent.** Transgenes resist degradation.
- **Allergenic.** They're extremely allergenic.

Horizontal gene transfer. Horizontal gene transfer (HGT, or "lateral" gene transfer) is the relocation of genes from one organism to another through some means other than reproduction. In this case, individual genes from a GE organism find their way into the environment and invade the DNA of another organism, infecting it like a virus.

It's thought to be a rare occurrence in multi-celled organisms incidental to: (1) cross-pollination, (2) movement through animals, (3) residual plant material left in the ground, or (4) the sharing of storage or transportation containers between GMO and non-GMO stocks. Industry reps claim that translocation of genes doesn't happen easily through these routes. However, any amount of HGT is unacceptable, because it means GE genes will eventually/inevitably be found in all sorts of places where they don't belong (like a slow-moving plague). HGT does happen easily and often in bacteria, though.

In the case of Bt-producing plants, their transgenes exit through the roots and get passed to microbial decomposers in the soil. Good and bad bacteria consume the plant material containing the transgenes, incorporating them into their DNA. They then produce those foreign proteins, which can be exchanged with other organisms.

So through varied means and efficiencies, transgenes can pass from one organism to another. They can go from soil bacteria to future crops on that land, from plants to animals, from animal products to our own gut bacteria, or from plant products to our microbiota.

What's worse, HGT is more likely to happen when leaky gut causes genetic material to enter the bloodstream in a partially-digested state – which glyphosate is notorious for doing. This leaves strands of genetically engineered DNA intact, which bacteria ingest to then produce Bt toxin.

But even more disturbing, it's well-documented that your gut bacteria then infect your own DNA with those transgenes, so **your own cells make Bt toxin inside you.** In fact, Bt insecticide/toxin was found in 93% of pregnant women tested at Canada's Sherbrooke Medical Center in Montreal. 70% of their unborn babies had the Bt toxin in their cord blood. And it's estimated the gut flora of 95% of the population now produces the Bt insecticide.

Vertical gene transfer. Vertical gene transfer is the endowing of genes from one organism into subsequent generations through reproduction. In the real world, it's cross-contamination through accidental cross-pollination. GMO crops interbreed with non-GMO crops and contaminate them for miles around… and there's nothing anyone can do to stop the spread short of growing indoors.

That's because GMO pollen is transported far and wide by bees, wind and animals. Under certain weather conditions corn pollen can travel up to 500 miles in a day and infect non-GMO crops, no matter how careful growers are to prevent cross-contamination. GMO genes are also eaten by animals and deposited miles away in their droppings.

So it's inevitable: Over a number of years, traditional crops will all become contaminated with genetically-modified DNA, as we're already seeing now. US national organic standards acknowledge this: A farmer won't lose their organic certification when a crop is contaminated up to a certain percentage (provided you make efforts to avoid this contamination).

Upsetting to say the least, that's why seed banks around the world were setup – to have a fallback cache of last resort should this nightmare scenario continue to play out the way it is now.

The burden to prevent cross-contamination is on independent growers. Courts have sided with Monsanto. They say it's the responsibility of an organic/conventional grower to setup portions of their own property to serve as buffer zones to decrease the opportunity for stray GMO pollen to contaminate their fields.

Monsanto uses this "burden of prevention" to intimidate and punish non-Monsanto growers for opposing them (i.e., not buying into their monopoly). To illustrate how aggressive they are, a couple of years ago, Monsanto was in the process of suing about 150 separate growers for "infringement" of their GE patents. Another 700 cases were settled out of court prior to that. Today, the total probably exceeds 1,000 separate cases.

All of which goes to show: Monsanto is extremely aggressive in crushing all opposition to their plans to take over worldwide food production. In practice, that means they don't just use patent protection defensively to protect what's rightfully theirs. Instead, they use patents and the courts as offensive weapons to terrorize and bully independent farmers into "playing ball" with them. In fact, they've openly stated their plan is to own and control the entire world's food supply with their GMO technologies – wiping heirloom crops off the face of the earth as soon as possible.

Dr. Michael Antoniou sums up GMO "safety"

"Based on the evidence as we have it now, no GMO crop of food can be categorically stated as safe to consume – especially on a long-term, life-long basis … and that any claims that there is a consensus on the safety of GMO foods … that the debate is over and that we should simply embrace them and welcome them – is totally unfounded. There is no scientific consensus."

The next wave of GMO absurdity: Gene editing and gene silencing

Knowing their current GMO products are losing effectiveness, regulatory acceptance and public approval, GMO companies are already working on the next generation of genetic engineering – when they haven't even begun to master the first. They're working on gene editing, which alters expression, and gene silencing, which turns them off. They go hand-in-hand to circumvent Nature's control mechanisms.

They figure these processes appear less foreign and manipulative because no genes are trans-located between completely unrelated organisms. In this second generation of genetic engineering, the focus is on transferring genes between subspecies. Therefore, it's somehow safer and less objectionable. To illustrate, the author/researchers of a recent paper said they only had to insert four genes into an organism to achieve their goal (whatever that was). However, they had to remove 4,000 genes to express the four that they wanted.

To top it off, agrochemical companies are petitioning government agencies so they won't be required to call an organism edited in this way *genetically modified*, because they're not taking genes from one organism and putting them into another (the present legal definition of "genetically modified"). Rather, gene editing and silencing merely turns genes on or off epigenetically (like through microRNA), instead of trans-locating.

In other words, do we as a society want to use the classical, intuitive *meaning of the words* "genetically modified," or should we permit Big Ag to use the inadequate *legal definition* (i.e., letter of the law), as defined decades ago by the USDA and EPA? For the foreseeable future, let's hope what happens in the lab, stays in the lab.

Genetic engineering wouldn't be complete without glyphosate

Some 85% of genetically modified crops are engineered so that you can practically soak the plant in glyphosate and it won't die. A much smaller minority is engineered to produce the Bt toxin insecticide within every cell of its anatomy.

Glyphosate has been an incredibly successful weed killer for the industry because, combined with Roundup-ready GMOs, it initially made weed control very easy. It's been instrumental in the creation of industrial-scale farms that grow monocrops such as corn and soybean, because it simplified the way they're grown, tended and harvested. And for the first few years, growers love it… that is, until unintended consequences such as sterile soils, resistant weeds, increased disease, and decreased stress tolerance catch up to them. Then they love it a lot less.

History of glyphosate

- **1964: Descaling agent.** In 1964, glyphosate was patented as a broad-spectrum chelator. It was first used to clean mineral deposits from industrial boilers and steam pipes because of its ability to chelate an extremely wide variety of minerals.
- **1969: Broad spectrum herbicide.** Seeing the potential in its ability to bind metals and kill plants, Monsanto applied for a patent to use glyphosate as an herbicide, receiving it in 1974.
- **2000: Original patent expired.** In 2000, the patent to use glyphosate as an herbicide expired. Foreign chemical companies started making glyphosate-based herbicides, which reduced its cost and increased its availability.
- **2005: Ripening/drying agent (desiccant).** Around 2000, glyphosate started being used as a ripening/drying agent, called a "desiccant," to prematurely end a crop's growing cycle and drying it out a few weeks before harvest. This makes it easier to pick up with harvesting machines, and keeps it from rotting prior to use.
- **2005: Burn down aid.** At around the same time, growers started spraying glyphosate on the post-harvest remains of non-GMO crops

Glyphosate
$C_3H_8NO_5P$

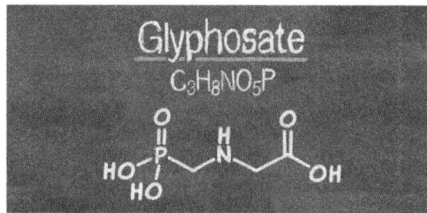

prior to burning the fields, which make it easier to ready the land for re-planting. Using glyphosate in this way has aggressively expanded its use on conventional crops, so its residues are now found on virtually all crops, everywhere.

- **2010: Broad-spectrum antibiotic.** Monsanto received a patent for using glyphosate as an antibiotic in 2010, due to its extremely strong ability to kill a broad spectrum of microorganisms. They had high hopes for this use in livestock that fell flat – mostly because glyphosate kills far more good bacteria than bad.

In summary, glyphosate use increased steadily from 1974 until 1996. But in 1996, its use skyrocketed when Monsanto introduced glyphosate-resistant GMO crops. That's about the same time dozens of human diseases started their steep upward climbs.

Glyphosate is the ultimate fast-acting poison for plants

Glyphosate (the active ingredient in Roundup) is a freakishly effective chelator that does most of its damage by tying up beneficial minerals that organisms need to drive their enzyme reactions, and thus their biology. This devastates biologic function so extensively, for so many life forms, that it's hard to believe it could be doing so much harm without the public being aware of its toxicity. Like other herbicides that chelate, glyphosate kills weeds through three mechanisms of action:

1. **Chelates minerals.** It chelates the minerals that plants depend on to run enzyme processes by which they grow, feed and protect themselves from pathogens, toxins and stress.
2. **Kills probiotic microorganisms.** It preferentially kills beneficial microorganisms that feed and protect plants.
3. **Stimulates pathogens.** It stimulates pathogen activity.

Mineral chelator. As a potent chelator, glyphosate ties up an extremely broad spectrum of minerals so they're not bio-available to the plant, including manganese, potassium, zinc, iron, calcium, magnesium and copper. It also disrupts the balance of nitrogen, boron and sulfur in plants. In doing so, glyphosate blocks the bioavailability of many positively-charged minerals. Like taking the key out of a car, minerals are then unavailable as activators for 291 enzymes that need a trace mineral to function properly.

As a result, glyphosate downregulates over 250 enzyme functions that life forms rely on for their biochemical processes. It upregulates about 30. And glyphosate produces these effects in incredibly small doses. These breakdowns interfere with biologic functions too numerous to mention, which then shut down the plant's resistance to all kinds of threats, including soil-borne pathogens, insects, toxins, malnutrition, and environmental stresses like drought.

Basically, glyphosate kills non-genetically engineered plants primarily by giving them a bad case of "plant AIDS" (immuno-deficiency). Pathogenic fungi then quickly overwhelm the plant and eat it alive. Unfortunately for consumers, genetic engineering does nothing to alter the chelating ability of glyphosate or the mineral absorption of crops. It merely helps GMO crops resist the pathogens that would ordinarily do it in. The net result is, the plant still ends up nutrient-deficient.

Broad-spectrum antibiotic. Glyphosate is an extremely broad-spectrum antibiotic that kills beneficial organisms in soil – including probiotic bacteria, mycorrhizal fungi and earthworms. These critters convert minerals into a bioavailable form, transport them to the plant, multiply the plant's absorption capacity, and limit pathogen populations, thereby protecting the plant from their attacks.

Stimulates pathogens. When the good guys in soil are wiped out by glyphosate, soil-borne pathogens have a feeding frenzy. Pathogens have alternative metabolic and immune pathways that allow them to survive glyphosate exposure better. **So it's not glyphosate itself that kills the plant. Rather, glyphosate weakens the plant's defenses in several ways, while at the same time amplifying the attack from the plant's enemies.**

This is why glyphosate can't kill plants in sterile "soil," or when a fungicide is applied to protect it: fungi is the real killer. In other words, glyphosate ties a plant's defenses behind its back so that pathogenic fungi and environmental stresses can beat up on it until it succumbs – taking as little as 2–8 hours.

As a result of this systemic spraying and weakening of crops by glyphosate, more than forty plant diseases are expanding in both geography and lethality, just within the last 5–10 years. At the same time, true weeds are becoming hardier – basically creating superweeds – because repeated glyphosate application selects for weeds that both survive glyphosate, and resist pathogens, better.

Plants suffer nutrient deficiencies, which they pass on to consumers

Glyphosate greatly reduces a plant's ability to take up nutrients, transport them around, and store them within their structure. Applications as low as ½ ounce per acre reduce uptake of iron by 50%, and manganese by 80%. At this tiny dosage, glyphosate inhibits internal movement of minerals by some 80–90%. According to one report, after one application of glyphosate, alfalfa lost 46% of its potassium, 26% magnesium, 52% sulfur, 49% iron, and 31% manganese. From the same report, soy beans lost 40% of their nitrogen content, 26% calcium, 30% magnesium, 27% copper, 48% manganese, and 30% zinc.

Glyphosate destroys the medicinal properties of plants

Glyphosate eradicates the healing ability of plants by blocking an enzyme pathway used by bacteria, fungi, algae, some protozoa, and plants to make important compounds in food. Bacteria and plants use this "shikimate pathway," as it's called, to manufacture an extremely active family of chemical compounds called "alkaloids" that give plants medicinal qualities, in addition to making many enzymes, hormones, signaling molecules, and other proteins. By blocking production of 4–6 of the 26 most important amino acids used in making proteins, **glyphosate robs plants of their innate ability to make medicinal compounds** that pharmaceutical companies observe in plants and try to replicate in their drugs, including

- antiparasitic (e.g., quinine)
- antiasthma (e.g., ephedrinc)
- anticancer (e.g., homoharringtonine)
- vasodilatory (e.g., vincamine)
- antiarrhythmic (e.g., quinidine)
- analgesic (e.g., morphine)
- antidiabetic activities (e.g., piperine)
- antibacterial (e.g., chelerythrine)
- mood stabilizing/neurotransmitter balancing (e.g., galantamine)
- antimalarial (e.g., quinine).

This epic instance of tunnel vision (or cold-blooded profiteering) contributes mightily to glyphosate's role in modern disease. By spraying 4.4 billion pounds of glyphosate into the environment every year, **we've wiped out the medicinal qualities that plants used to give us, before drugs highjacked our healthcare system.**

Glyphosate is not acutely toxic to mammals. But it is THE worst, given its ubiquity and sufficient time to cripple biologic functions

Acute toxicity is when a poison harms or kills you immediately, like cyanide or arsenic can. Chronic toxicity is when a poison wrecks your health gradually, like taking crack cocaine, chain smoking or alcoholism. That's why glyphosate has never been recognized as a toxin by regulatory agencies and its use restricted: governing bodies have only looked at its acute toxicity, not its chronic toxicity. In short, if you want to kill an organism with a functioning liver quickly, glyphosate is not your poison.

On the other hand, if you want to ruin a person's health slowly and surely over time – so as to avoid blame and liability – then glyphosate's your poison. In fact, Roundup's delivery system has been described as a perfect bioweapon. The World Health Organization (WHO) and the California Environmental Protection Agency (EPA) appear to agree: the

WHO decided to list glyphosate as a "known carcinogen" in animals, and a "probable carcinogen" in humans. Meanwhile, the California EPA issued a notice of intent to declare glyphosate a "known carcinogen," which Monsanto is fighting in court. Just think: If glyphosate/Roundup were used covertly by a terrorist group to wipe out the health of a nation, it would be classified as a weapon of mass destruction by our government, and treated as a threat to national security.

11 factors make glyphosate the perfect slow-killing poison for mammals

1. **Absorption.** Herbicides like Roundup add other (unlisted) ingredients besides glyphosate to make it penetrate the skin of plants.
2. **Multiplied toxicity.** "Adjuvants," as those other mystery ingredients are called, make Roundup 1,000 times more toxic.
3. **Concentrates in plants.** 80% of glyphosate accumulates in the growth points (roots, shoots, legumes, seeds) that animals and humans eat.
4. **Excretes into soil.** 15–20% of absorbed glyphosate is exuded through a plant's roots, into the soil.
5. **Perpetual use.** Growers used to rotate herbicides along with crops – depending on how long the herbicide took to degrade. But you can't do that with glyphosate. It's the only option. So farmers are stuck hammering glyphosate into plants and soil as it loses its effectiveness… and accumulates.
6. **Persistent.** Glyphosate is neutralized very slowly in soil, and degrades completely at an even slower pace.
7. **Reactivation.** After it's neutralized, glyphosate is reactivated by conventional phosphate fertilizer.
8. **Bio accumulates.** Glyphosate accumulates in humans and animals when they eat anything with glyphosate in it.
9. **Non-linear dose response.** Glyphosate toxicity declines the less of it you ingest. Then, at a certain point, it begins to climb again. This makes it disruptive to our hormonal system in miniscule doses.
10. **Water soluble.** Glyphosate dissolves in water and goes everywhere in the body that water does. Most toxins, in contrast, are fat soluble.
11. **Dissolves tight junctions.** Glyphosate dissolves the tight junctions keeping the barriers of the body intact (gut, brain, kidneys and blood vessels). This causes leaky membranes all over the body, which leads to gut, brain, inflammatory, and immune system problems.

Glyphosate is 4,000 times more lethal to good bacteria than bad

Glyphosate is well-documented to kill microorganisms as easily in livestock such as cattle, horses, pigs, sheep and poultry as it does in soil – and at doses as low as 0.1 part-per-million. Consequently, it was patented as one of the broadest, most potent antibiotics ever in 2010 – albeit slower-acting than conventional antibiotics. The list of microbes that glyphosate is known to kill from the patent is voluminous. So there's no reason to think it doesn't do the same to our good bacteria.

However, unlike conventional antibiotics, glyphosate is far stronger at killing good bacteria than it is pathogens. In fact, it takes 4,000 times the dose to kill pathogens as it does beneficial bacteria because pathogens have alternative metabolic pathways to survive the exposure. This preference for killing probiotic bacteria contributes chronically to corruption of the microbiome, neurotransmitter imbalances, and neurological disorders.

In livestock, glyphosate is killing the beneficial bacteria that normally keep the botulism bug (Clostridium botulinum) under control in cows' stomachs. That's why botulism deaths are spreading like the plague in herds across America.

As a result, glyphosate is corrupting our microbiomes over time. Glyphosate weakens and kills small populations of beneficial bacteria every time we ingest food, water, air, or any substance containing any glyphosate. Of course, the bacteria grow back between exposures. But this cycle continues day in, day out, for years, resulting in a gradual loss of good bacteria, and a takeover of pathogens that sabotage your health from within. That's why glyphosate is so devastating to our microbiome, neurotransmitter and hormone balance, and mental stability. It's also one of the leading causes of disease that we're now brewing in, yet fail to recognize and escape.

Glyphosate dissolves tight junctions, causing leaky barriers

Glyphosate makes cells of the gut lining produce more zonulin than they should (by up-regulating CXCR3 receptors, which enable gluten/gliadin to do their damage). Runaway zonulin production breaks down the tight junctions of the gut whose purpose is to open and close in a controlled manner to selectively let nutrients pass from the gut into the bloodstream. The gut then becomes porous and leaky – otherwise known as "leaky gut." To make matters worse, zonulin leaks into the bloodstream and travels everywhere.

Zonulin: Protein that modulates permeability of tight junctions of cells lining the intestinal tract.

As zonulin circulates, it dissolves membranes throughout the body – just one cell thick – that are supposed to act as protective barriers against intrusion of toxic chemicals, heavy metals, pathogens, and undigested food. With leaks occurring through the blood-brain barrier, blood vessels and kidneys, your whole body becomes a sieve to harmful substances. This is what makes glyphosate public enemy #1 in the rise of food sensitivities, digestive disturbances, autoimmune conditions, malnutrition and neurological problems.

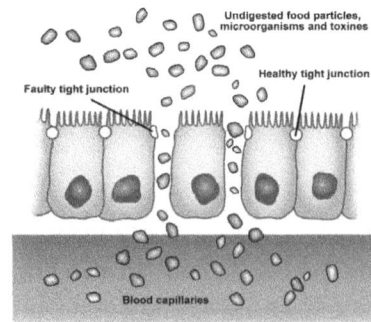

Undigested food particles, microorganisms and toxines

Healthy tight junction

Faulty tight junction

Blood capillaries

INFLAMMATORY, IMMUNOLOGICAL, AUTOIMMUNE AND NEOPLASTIC REACTIONS

Image used under Creative Commons 4.0 license. Author: BallenaBlanca.

Glyphosate causes a hormonal "non-linear dose response"

Government health agencies create regulations based on the traditional assumption that toxicity declines as you ingest less of a toxin, until it becomes non-toxic (and thus "safe"). Biologists call this a "linear dose response." In basic terms, it means *the dose makes the poison.*

Unfortunately, this is not an accurate description of how glyphosate affects the body in real life. Instead, glyphosate toxicity decreases with exposure level, until you get to a certain point. Then, counter-intuitively, it levels off, or goes back up. This means a larger dose can trigger a healing response such as apoptosis (cell-suicide) so that injury is repaired. Whereas as a smaller dose does not damage cells or the endocrine system enough to ever activate a healing response. Thus, cell damage persists. For this reason, reducing your intake could make your problems worse.

To name a few, an incredibly small dose of glyphosate can cause issues with sex hormones and fertility, insulin reception, metabolism and weight, as well as hormones that regulate brain function. In particular, glyphosate is known to disrupt estrogen function in women, dramatically increasing the incidence of breast cancer. And it collapses testosterone levels in men, severely decreasing sperm quantity and quality.

Glyphosate kills the bacteria that help make neurotransmitters

Essential to neurologic function, beneficial bacteria in the gut make aromatic amino acids we can't make on our own – including tyrosine, tryptophan, phenylalanine, L-dopa and 5-HTP. These amino acids are the building blocks of the essential neurotransmitters dopamine, serotonin, epinephrine, and norepinephrine that run brain function. Therefore, glyphosate promotes mental health disorders through this pathway:

1. Glyphosate preferentially kills good bacteria that make aromatic amino acids.
2. Shortages of aromatic amino acids = less neurotransmitters for the brain.
3. When brain circuits don't have the electro-chemical juice to fire properly, our neurology malfunctions, which we call ADD, anxiety, depression, autism, obsessive/compulsive behaviors, bipolar, learning disabilities, social delay, eating disorders, sleep problems, anger management issues and cognitive decline.

Glyphosate impairs detoxification in all living organisms

It does this by disturbing the cytochrome P450 enzyme pathway (CYP), which is a family of 20,000 enzymes (aka "metalloproteins") that act as oxidants and catalysts – thus reducing detoxification in bacterium, plant and animal cells. Humans have about 57 of these CYP enzymes directly controlling our detoxification system's ability to neutralize and remove toxins. They're essential for normal physiological function. On the other hand, chronic, degenerative diseases occur when glyphosate blocks their ability to oxidize toxins and deport them. For instance, a dysfunctional CYP enzyme system constricts bile flow. Low bile flow chokes off a major pathway by which toxins leave the body.

Glyphosate moves through the environment with ease

Most toxins are fat-soluble (lipophilic), which means they tend to dissolve, travel and accumulate in *fat* much more easily than water. In living systems, toxins tend to collect in fatty tissues and bio-accumulate up the food chain. But, terrifying to people who understand the implications, glyphosate is the opposite. It's one of the few toxins that's water soluble (hydrophilic). It has an affinity for *water* instead of fat.

That means glyphosate travels easily through the air, water, soil, plants, animals, and our bloodstream. In other words, there's nothing stopping glyphosate from moving through the environment and contaminating every nook and cranny of the planet and its inhabitants, because it has an all-access pass to go places inaccessible to most poisons.

Glyphosate's toxicity can linger for decades

Despite Monsanto's claims, glyphosate degrades with great difficulty in the environment. It can remain toxic for a generation or more. So even though its toxicity to plants, animals and people may be disabled temporarily by soil microbes or chelation – losing half its original toxicity over 1½–22 years – its bioactivity can be revived to do more damage. Like dormant zombies, glyphosate hides out underground, waiting to be raised from the dead. Conventional phosphate fertilizer brings inactivated glyphosate back to life, restoring its former toxicity – even years later – which is why you may see glyphosate toxicity returning years after a grower switches to bio-friendly farming.

So whether land has been producing or dormant, glyphosate toxicity sticks around for decades, and is harder to eradicate than zombies that won't take no for an answer. In fact, Monsanto was found guilty of deceptive advertising in two lawsuits over false claims that Roundup is biodegradeable, which is simply not predictable. In summary, evidence clearly shows that glyphosate accumulates in the environment for years. You can disable most of its virulence temporarily through years of exposure to environment forces. But conventional fertilizer wakes it up. So, under most real-world conditions, glyphosate remains highly toxic for a very long time, wherever it is. It needs to be banned completely.

Commercial farming releases megatons of carbon into the ecosystem

Globalists want us to think that fossil fuel use causes climate change. They say the greenhouse effect is the result of CO_2 from cars and industry accumulating in the atmosphere. While the burning of petroleum (which does not come from dead dinosaurs or plants) is certainly not doing the planet any favors, it does trick people into looking at one thing the globalists want us to blame and abandon: *using petroleum for energy* to another that few know anything about: *commercial agriculture's side effects*.

The latter would probably be the bigger influence of the two, *if* the planet were warming, *if* burning petroleum products was causing it, and *if* atmospheric carbon caused a greenhouse effect. However, they aren't. These are half-truths used to deceive and manipulate the masses. First off, plants thrive when they get more CO_2 because it's their oxygen. Second, secret programs have been controlling the weather for decades because weather is the most powerful weapon of them all.

Consequently, most weather catastrophes – including floods, droughts, hurricanes, tsunamis, and sub-zero temperatures in Texas – are man-made to serve some purpose. These people even came right out and said it in the 1960s: they wanted to use environmental destruction (aka "weather warfare") as a fear and control tactic. Why would anyone believe the global elite are too kind and compassionate to do what they set out to do? That's willful ignorance, if you ask me. But I digress.

See "The Report for Iron Mountain" to read how the globalists, in the absence of an existential threat such as a war, were going to purposely create environmental catastrophes to control every facet of people's lives.

Commercial farming – particularly glyphosate – is adept at killing microorganisms that keep carbon in the soil, where it belongs. Killing soil microbes releases millions of tons of carbon into the atmosphere every year, because **each acre of biologically-active land contains ten to twenty tons of carbon-rich biomass**.

Industry is only required to test glyphosate itself for toxicity, not Roundup's full formula

As toxic as glyphosate may sound, it's not good at penetrating a plant's skin when sprayed on plants by itself. For this reason, herbicides require helper chemicals that act as antagonists, or "adjuvants," that break down the skin of the plant, get inside cells, circulate throughout, and cause lethal reactions. These surfactant/adjuvants massively increase glyphosate's toxicity. In the case of Roundup's newest formulation (of three or four), the full formula is 1,000 times more toxic than glyphosate alone.

However, because Monsanto doesn't declare the other toxins to be active ingredients, they're not required to list them on the label, or test them for toxicity – either individually, in combination, or as a complete formulation. Monsanto alleges by omission that the other ingredients are inert, thereby escaping regulation and liability (nice trick, if you can pull it off).

That's how Monsanto has sidestepped testing Roundup's complete formula for years, even though the full formula is what actually gets sprayed onto crops, and what we end up ingesting. To this day, industry-sponsored research studies only glyphosate, while independent, honest research makes a point to study *real products*, the way they're used in practice.

EPA has raised the "safe" limit of glyphosate repeatedly

The EPA has repeatedly increased the allowable "safe" limits of glyphosate because its potency is wearing off, weeds are becoming stronger, and growers are being forced to use more and more to reach a lethal dose. So, what's been happening is, Monsanto, every so often, goes to the EPA and asks them to raise the permissible limit in order for the levels reached in harvested crops to pass inspection.

Crazy as it may sound, this is not being done as a result of any safety studies, or even lies that sound real. Rather, it's because (1) chemical companies have to keep using more to get the same effect, (2) they beg the EPA to raise the limits, and (3) they simply let them. For example, in 2013, the limits were raised on some food crops by 30-fold! Just as senseless, the EPA and FDA routinely disavow any responsibility for the increases. Their disclaimers say something to the effect of: "We do no independent testing. We rely solely on the manufacturer's promise that these levels are safe."

Glyphosate and neonicotinoids are causing bee die-off

Bees are dying in record numbers. Bee populations are down an average of 50% nationwide – called "colony collapse disorder." And, as Einstein said, we have about four years to live after the bees go because they pollenate so many of our mainstay crops. Glyphosate and neonicotinoids (a class of insecticides sprayed on GMOs and conventional crops) contribute to colony collapse disorder by

1. depleting plants and their pollen of minerals through chelation;
2. killing bees' own gut bacteria (lactobacillus and bifidobacteria), which prevents them from digesting their honey;
3. they can't find their way back home after foraging because glyphosate upsets their endocrine-based navigation system.

These herbicides and pesticides then combine with nnEMF pollution to injure enough bees to wipe out the hive.

Glyphosate is killing us all... slowly, but surely

When you deprive a living organism of minerals, you ravage its biochemistry (through enzyme inhibition), metabolism, detoxification, hormone function, immunity, fertility, and pretty much everything it takes to sustain a living organism. Examples: Poor enzyme function prevents you from breaking down food and metabolizing it properly, which makes you store that food as weight gain, instead of burning it efficiently. Decreased serotonin production damages the switch that tells the body to stop eating, further contributing to weight gain.

People have rightfully been worrying about 29 million pounds of conventional antibiotics such as streptomycin, tetracycline and penicillin being used in animal feed to prevent disease and fatten up livestock. But who even knows that we've been spraying 4.4 billion pounds of antibiotic each year on crops, roadways, driveways, gardens and waterways in the form of glyphosate? And its use is doubling every six years. This is why glyphosate deserves much of the blame for causing inflammatory and degenerative diseases spreading like wildfire since about 2000. In fact…

The growth curves of 30+ degenerative diseases match the introduction of glyphosate and GMOs

When you plot the occurrence of dozens of diseases on a graph, and compare them against the introduction of glyphosate and GMOs into our food supply, they match almost perfectly. Statistically, they reach a correlation coefficient greater than 0.925 (or "R" value, where 1.00 is 100% perfect correlation). And this isn't just for one disease, but over 30 diseases suspected to be caused by glyphosate and GMOs, including…

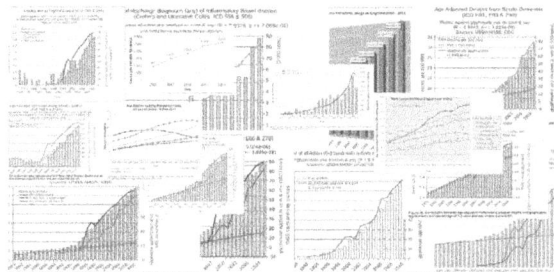

From the paper: "Genetically engineered crops, glyphosate and the deterioration of health in the United States of America," by Nancy L. Swanson, et al., published in "Journal of Organic Systems," 9(2), 2014.

- autism (R=0.9972 for glyphosate)
- ADHD (R=0.9466 for glyphosate)
- dementia (R=0.9942 for glyphosate)
- Celiac disease (R=0.9759 for glyphosate)
- obesity (R=0.96).
- anxiety (R=0.95 for glyphosate)
- Alzheimer's (R=0.9373 for GE, 0.917 for glyphosate)
- Parkinson's (R=0.9516 for GE corn and soy, 0.8754 for glyphosate)
- renal failure (R=0.9775 for glyphosate, 0.9674 for GE corn, soy)
- diabetes (R=0.9547 for GE corn and soy, 0.935 for glyphosate)
- stroke (R=0.9827 for GE corn and soy, 0.9246 for glyphosate)
- hypertension (R=0.9607 for GE corn and soy, 0.923 for glyphosate).

Many more diseases line up almost as well: Allergies, asthma, arthritis, dermatitis, autoimmune diseases, bipolar, birth defects, many cancers, chronic fatigue syndrome, Crohn's disease, gluten intolerance, infertility, inflammatory bowel disease, leaky gut, miscarriages, multiple sclerosis, and sudden infant death.

Now, you may say one or two diseases lining up could just be a coincidence. But all these chronic diseases rising at the same time, and the same amount, as glyphosate? The only explanation is an extremely pervasive, recently introduced, toxin that we're all exposed to. It pretty much has to come from something in the food supply and/or the environment. What other influence could possibly match introduction dates, growth curves, and expected effects of glyphosate to observed causes of disease?

Glyphosate causes gruesome birth defects, kidney failure and cancer

Three Rivers region (near Yakima), Washington State, 2008: Invasive weeds were clogging the three rivers supplying water for residents and irrigation. Wanting to get on top of the situation, county officials made the fateful decision to dump glyphosate into the rivers to kill the weeds.

Two years later, horrendous birth defects skyrocketed due to glyphosate's strong ability to disrupt the endocrine hormone system of pregnant mothers and their unborn babies. Investigators discovered that glyphosate in the drinking water caused serious endocrine-related deformities like anencephaly where the baby is born with most of its brain and cranium missing (images omitted to spare you the disgust). Seasoned midwives who noticed the shocking rise have been told to keep their mouths shut so they don't upset anyone.

- Similarly, frogs in glyphosate-rich waterways are showing up with grotesque mutations like extra legs and conjoined bodies.
- In El Salvador, Sri Lanka, Panama and Nicaragua, 1 out of 4 sugarcane workers is expected to die from kidney failure due to glyphosate use as a ripening agent – 20,000 affected.
- Research shows the 90-mile stretch of the Mississippi River, from Baton Rouge, LA to New Orleans, deposits 90% of the glyphosate and crop chemicals collected from farmlands feeding into the Mississippi River. This is causing the highest cancer rates of any population group in the civilized world – prompting some to call it "Cancer Alley."

Glyphosate toxicity summary

- Glyphosate weakens a plant's ability to feed itself.
- It compromises its defenses directly.
- It kills microorganisms that support the plant, which supports pathogens that attack the plant.
- As a chemical cocktail, Roundup is great at breeching a plant's skin.
- The full formula is massively more toxic than glyphosate alone.
- Glyphosate concentrates in parts of the plant that we eat.
- It contaminates the soil and makes minerals unavailable to biology.
- It lingers for decades.
- It dissolves tight junctions, causing leaky membranes all over the body.
- It tampers with hormones, neurotransmitters, detoxification, metabolism, and most physiologic functions in the body.
- It does all this in extremely minute quantities.
- It's also killing bees.
- And it's wrecking the environment on a planetary scale.

Fortunately, when you stop eating GMOs, symptoms go away

What was once *circumstantial evidence* or *interesting observation* is rapidly becoming *scientific fact* through "challenge-rechallenge" testing because 'on-off-on' testing is considered valid scientific proof of causality. In this case, when practitioners recommend that their patients – particularly children – stop eating GMO foods, a wide variety of symptoms suddenly disappear, including GI disorders, food sensitivities, allergies, hyperactivity, brain fog, autism symptoms, rashes, aggression, depression, headaches, fatigue, infertility, kidney damage, liver damage, diabetes, high blood pressure, skin problems, weight problems, and immune system problems.

Germane to GAPS in particular, experts in the field now believe Celiac disease has very little to do with gluten itself and a lot to do with GMOs and glyphosate. To illustrate the real-world results, one health professional that Jeffrey Smith talks about in "GMOs Revealed" saw symptoms in 5,000 of her clients vanish when they eliminated GMOs. Fortunately, more and more peer-reviewed papers are coming out connecting GMO foods to symptoms and diseases. Most are conducted and published outside the US, but the truth has a way of spreading.

Reducing glyphosate exposure

Many non-GMO crops contain as much glyphosate as the GMO crops, if not more. Most major non-GMO crops now have toxic levels of glyphosate, because it's used as a ripening and burn-down agent. Affected crops are sprayed just days before harvest to increase yield, so you can't simply choose to go non-GMO and avoid exposure. To a lesser degree, many organic crops are also contaminated with trace amounts of glyphosate due to environmental residues such as rain, soil, water table, and air pollution – not from intentional spraying.

Certified "Glyphosate-Residue-Free" by The Detox Project. Established in 2015, this certification assures consumers that produce, packaged foods, and supplements are low in glyphosate. Let's hope it takes off. Conclusion: We need to apply pressure to food companies, grocery stores, public health agencies, agrochemical companies, and lawmakers to get rid of GMOs and glyphosate. Only by choking off their funding AND outlawing their usage will we get them out of our food supply. We need to quit glyphosate and GMOs completely to survive as a species. I don't think half-measures will do much.

Where's the glyphosate story headed?

As of the year 2000, the patents covering glyphosate have expired. China now produces most of the world's glyphosate. This makes glyphosate-based herbicides cheap and readily available. So the methods developed and promoted by Monsanto are now being used throughout the world.

This is causing widespread injury to the health of large populations around the world. Leaky gut, brain, kidneys and body, as well as an avalanche of common, complex diseases stemming from these conditions are now world-wide health crises needing immediate attention.

In 2013, a small section was snuck into a large appropriations bill at the last minute that protects Monsanto from being sued, and its products banned. The "Farmer Assurance Provision" of the Agriculture Appropriations Bill (Section 735 of H.R. 933, dubbed by watchdog groups the "Monsanto Protection Act") effectively prohibits federal courts from banning the sale and planting of genetically-modified organisms, as long as the GMO was/is legal to make and sell at the time.

Article about the rider that protects GMOs: (foodfirst.org/the -monsanto- protection-act-of- betrayal/).

The legislation was not permanent, but it does several detestable things: It proves that bioengineering companies know the damage their products are doing, and are taking steps to shield themselves from liability. It encourages more of the same. It also sets a dangerous precedence that bioengineering firms can get away with willful destruction of people and planet, as long they can pay for laws to be enacted, and we as consumers allow it to happen.

More recently, Roundup sales are down 12% in one quarter to $1.1 billion as more knock-offs enter the market, and more people wake up to the biological effects of glyphosate. But sales are still huge. Look at the herbicide/pesticide wall of any home improvement store, and you'll see most of it is devoted to glyphosate-based products.

Many countries are rejecting huge shipments of glyphosate-tainted product – even when that crop absorbed it accidentally. Germany recently rejected one million pounds of almonds because it was tainted with excessive glyphosate absorbed from soil used in a prior season. Even more encouraging, countries around the world have studied the science and the injuries being done to their people, and have either banned the use of glyphosate within their borders, or are seriously considering it – including Sri Lanka, El Salvador, Russia, Mexico, France, Netherlands, Bermuda, and Richmond, CA.

Scientists are working on soil remediation products that break down glyphosate

It's a race against time. Can chemists develop degradation/remediation agents before our runaway use of glyphosate wipes out what remains of the planet's life support systems? Will corrective remedies in development even make a dent in glyphosate contamination of our soil, hydrological cycle, and air? In the meantime, people's health will be under attack for decades to come – even if glyphosate use were to stop today. If we don't change course soon, half our population will experience diseases that threaten the survival of the human race.

The flawed science and dirty politics of genetic engineering (GE)

How Big Ag increases their profits from GMO technology and practices

Crucial to any discussion on the virtues and vices of GMOs is how Big Ag companies set themselves up for bigger profits. This is a story of infiltration, deception, intimidation, and buying favorable regulation.

- **Selling GMO seeds.**
- **Selling chemicals** that work with the seed, such as glyphosate, 2,4-D, and dicamba. The bulk of agrochemical company profits used to come from selling chemicals. Now it's royalties on GE patents.
- **Far more repeat sales.** Farmers have to buy new seed every year.
- **Monopoly market control.** Monsanto uses every dirty trick in the book to exert unfair control over growers, competitors, markets, government agencies and nations.
- **Government subsidies** (for GMO sellers) as insurance payments.
- **Market expansion.** Big Ag companies can undercut all others due to large-scale farming practices, GMO seeds, and glyphosate being used as a competitive advantage. That's forcing growers around the world to get on-board with their technologies and practices or be crushed by competition wielding a huge price advantage.

These expanded revenue streams can easily multiply their profit potential ten or twenty-fold. Nothing wrong with being ambitious. Rather, it's the unethical strategies, the harm to human health, and their ruthlessness we should be worried about. A perfect example: Monsanto has been caught saying behind the scenes that they want to control all of the world's food supply by influencing the White House, English Parliament, and French Parliament, etc. They plan on eliminating all natural seed in the process – effectively controlling the food supply of the entire world with their proprietary products. What's more, they've demonstrated not only a complete disrespect for Nature and all life in carrying out their agenda, but also a "biggest bully" mentality as a business model.

Monsanto has a long history of rigging research, hijacking regulatory agencies, and engaging in unconscionable behavior

- In 1983, the EPA started seeing a lot of fraudulent data coming in from the lab hired by Monsanto to test GMO safety.
- It got bad enough in 1988 and 1991 that the EPA took the lab to court for submitting fraudulent data to the government, including (1) falsifying laboratory notebook entries, (2) manipulating testing equipment so they didn't detect adverse results, (3) falsifying test results, and (4) substituting control groups from a prior study.

- In 1991, the laboratory director and 14 employees were hit with 20 felony convictions. The lab president was sentenced to 5 years in prison and fined $50,000. The lab itself was fined $19.2 million.
- 1993, Health Canada (Canada's equivalent of the USFDA) was evaluating bovine growth hormone (a genetically engineered product). Their senior scientist testified before their senate that Monsanto offered them a bribe of $1–2 million dollars to approve it without further study. The agency was being pressured to approve the drug, which they thought was of questionable safety. Her documents and notes were stolen from a locked file cabinet in her office.
- In 1995, the company prematurely ended a study when animals died from eating GMO corn.
- In 1996, the NY Attorney General charged Monsanto with false and misleading advertising.
- 2003, Kawata, Japan. Monsanto got caught reporting fraudulent safety-testing data.
- 2007 and 2009, the French High Court convicted Monsanto of false advertising claims of biodegradability, increased yield, and environmental benefit.
- And, for good measure, in 2016, Monsanto settled multiple lawsuits out of court, to the collective tune of $700 million, for poisoning residents of a town near their plant with PCBs.

However, these penalties and public humiliations were mere slaps on the wrist compared to what the GMO companies have unlawfully gained through their misdeeds. Specifically, the "science" and manipulation that the EPA relied on as a basis for determining "substantial equivalence" and GRAS (generally regarded as safe) of GMOs have allowed agrochemical makers to sidestep any need for safety testing, ever since the designations were misappropriated around 1996.

That means the entire GMO industry doesn't have to test any new GMOs they want to introduce, because Monsanto lied, cheated, bribed, coerced or defrauded their way into getting the GRAS designation in the first place. And it's been that way ever since. What's more, foreign regulatory agencies have relied on EPA and FDA determinations as precedence (excuse) to form their own policies.

Seven ways that Monsanto misleads, deceives and defrauds

1. For many years, the only studies supposedly proving the safety of GMOs were conducted by the companies themselves. GMO companies paid for and conducted the studies themselves. Just as suspect, no one outside the EPA and FDA was allowed to evaluate the way the studies were designed, conducted and analyzed for years because it was all kept secret. The EPA and FDA just took Monsanto's word for it when they said GMOs were safe. Consequently, Monsanto's scientists could blatantly cheat in their study. For instance, feeding their control animals food that had just as much glyphosate as the food given to test animals.

2. GMO makers prohibit almost everyone from studying their seeds – except their own scientists. GMO companies use every means at their disposal to stop others from studying their GMO seeds – going so far as to force their growers to sign a contract stating they won't study the very crop that they're growing in their own field, for any reason (without the company's written consent) – even to see which crop is better. For this reason, researchers have had great difficulty obtaining GMO seed to study. In fact, one research group spent an entire year looking for a legal way to obtain GMO soy seed from Monsanto.

3. Virtually no studies have been done on humans. Instead, we get to find out how destructive glyphosate is to human health after the damage is done by: (1) seeing our own family members be hurt or debilitated; (2) hearing stories of others being injured in exposés; and (3) collecting statistics from independent sources. We have to extrapolate from animal studies how harmful GMOs and glyphosate are to human systems.

Sobering fact: Studies that were *funded and conducted* by Monsanto consistently find that GMOs are safe and non-toxic – using their study criteria, data collection and conclusions. On the other hand, dozens of *independent* studies show GMOs cause grave organ damage (particularly kidney and liver damage), massive pre-cancerous tumors, immune system failure, holes in the GI tract, allergic reactions, infertility, and much more.

4. Monsanto kept their studies as short as possible to avoid the health effects they didn't want published. The longest safety study that Monsanto conducted on glyphosate and GMO crops was three months (rats live about 2½ years). Some were 30 or 60 days. One was as short as seven days. However, Professor Seralini's studies found breast cancer, prostate cancer, testicular cancer, and kidney cancer started showing up at the four-month mark in rats exposed to glyphosate or GMOs.

What a coincidence: Serious diseases started showing up weeks after Monsanto's longest studies concluded. Maybe they knew something they didn't want others to know? They could plead innocent and say the World Health Organization calls for toxicity tests to last 90 days.

Or, maybe this happened: A multi-billion-dollar corporation with the sophistication of Monsanto found out *what* adverse effects happen, and *when*, so they can simply design their study around the adverse effects. That's what savvy companies do. They don't leave things like this up to chance. What are the odds that a century-old, multinational corporation with a virtually unlimited budget just got lucky and happened to end all their studies weeks before adverse effects started showing up?

5. GMO companies fight labeling tooth and nail because they don't want anyone studying the long-term health effects via retrospective studies. If you don't know who is eating what, you can't tell looking backward whose health is being harmed by GMOs and whose is not. That applies to health consumers, study participants, patient populations, or any way you choose to group people. You also can't do anecdotal research (personal stories) to form hypotheses to test in future research.

In other words, when you don't have a well-defined, *unaffected* "control" group to compare/contrast against an *affected* test group, it's impossible to conclude much of anything from such a study. Your observations and conclusions are scientifically meaningless. In this case, it's impossible to gather statistical evidence and connect *cause* (GMOs) with *effect* (dysfunction and disease). And that's exactly the way GMO companies like it. They want to keep you ignorant and compliant at best, chronically ill and addicted at worst. (Tobacco companies used a similar strategy of deceit and confusion for decades until they were stopped.)

Plus, *not knowing* detaches GMO companies from all liability. If you can't trace your symptoms, disease or death back to those that caused the harm, then you can't assign any blame or assess any damages, now can you? Contrast that with smoking and cancer, where you have a well-defined control group (non-smokers) that you can compare against a well-defined user group (smokers) in order determine causality looking backward.

Bottom line: Besides a moral right to know so that people can choose, the practical reason GMOs should require labeling is so that people with severe allergic reactions can prevent GMOs from ruining their health. In fact, GMOs and glyphosate are a greater health concern than the two biggest food allergies people suffer from today – gluten and casein – because GMOs and glyphosate are largely responsible for causing gluten and casein sensitivity in the first place.

Unfortunately, agrochemical companies do everything in their power to prevent you from having knowledge and choice because it's bad for business. They want to price as many families out of the non-GMO market as they can through extra costs that companies must pay to maintain their organic status (which gets passed on to consumers). Recent regulatory efforts are even trying to make food companies incur extra cost to label their foods GMO-free, while GMOs would require none.

6. Monsanto tells two different stories, depending on who they're talking to. When talking to the FDA, media and consumers, Monsanto says their genetically modified organisms are "substantially equivalent" to conventional/traditional plants. They claim their GMOs are generally regarded as safe (GRAS), and should be treated as such for the purposes of market approval and subsequent regulation (or lack thereof). If true, their GMO products don't need to be tested at all before being put on the market. And they escape any sort of enforcement actions, and legal liability, because they were legal to sell when first introduced.

On the other hand, when Monsanto addresses the US Patent and Trademark Office, they say their genetically modified seeds are new (meaning substantially different) and contain useful innovations – both legal qualifications to secure patent protection. Therefore, they should be entitled to ownership, exclusive use, and twenty years of protection under international intellectual property laws.

They want to have it both ways: They're asserting both substantial similarity and substantial difference, which means they're lying to one of those groups. They might argue the genetic code of their GMOs are different for the purposes of novelty and beneficial effects, but no different in terms of harmful effects. But how could their crude gene splicing produce exclusively benefits without producing any negative effects? And how on earth could they possibly know the full extent of both, considering the complexity of mammalian biology?

You would have to know everything there is to know about genetic engineering, have absolute control over the process, and possess the clairvoyance to know what will happen combining genes that have never been combined before. I'm going to call "B.S." on that one. In effect, they're claiming ownership of all the differences that benefit the company, while denying/dismissing any differences that hurt the company's case for receiving GRAS designation. Very convenient, to put it mildly.

7. Monsanto likes to claim they've reduced pesticide use. GMO advocates like to pat themselves on the back by saying they've reduced pesticide use by 15% in certain US crops since 1995 (before GMOs). However, that's a slimy way to spin the facts. Specifically, growers in France reduced their pesticide use to 12%, and herbicide use to 82%. Sounds fantastic. Unfortunately, what they did is simply rearranged where and when it's applied, and neglected to tell anyone in their PR campaigns.

Instead of measuring how much insecticide is sprayed on a crop, certain GE crops now produce Bt toxin in every cell of their anatomy. Farmers may spray a crop less while it's growing, but total exposure to the end consumers is often much more, because the plant makes it in every cell of its structure. And there's no way to wash it off. Another tactic: A highly toxic group of insecticides, called "neonicotinoids," are sprayed on GMO (and conventional) seed to protect it in storage and transport. That enables them to leave that application out of the numbers.

FDA's own scientists doubted the safety of GMOs from the start

In 1998, The Alliance for Bio-Integrity sued the FDA and forced them to divulge 44,000 pages of internal documents. These documents – from the same time period that Monsanto was first trying to get GMOs approved for sale – revealed that the overwhelming consensus among scientists at the FDA is that GMOs carry abnormal risks.

They felt GMOs might create allergens, novel toxins, and nutritional problems. They urged their superiors to require testing with whole GMO foods. And when they saw drafts of proposed policies that would allow GMOs to be released into the market with little to no safety testing, or future regulation, they objected. They urged their superiors to change course. Basically, Mike Taylor – then in-charge of policy-making at the FDA – ignored the science, ignored the scientists, denied the existence of the scientists' concerns, and set forth a policy that allowed GMOs to be put on the market in a way that creates unprecedented risk for human beings and the environment.

Conclusion: FDA memos prove there was NO consensus among industry experts that GMOs were safe, as Monsanto and the FDA had claimed. Instead, their own memos (which are now in the public record) prove there was serious doubt within the FDA's own ranks. Officials at both Monsanto and the FDA flat out lied about there being a consensus in the industry. They used this fabrication as the basis for GMOs receiving GRAS status around 1996, which stands to this day.

See Jeffrey Smith's documentary "GMOs Revealed" to learn more about GMOs.

Results of early testing to establish European safety standards

In the mid-90s, the world's leading expert in plant biochemistry, Arpad Pusztai, PhD, at the top nutritional research laboratory in the UK, received €1.5 million to develop a method to test the safety of GMOs. This testing methodology was intended to be incorporated into European Union law as the test that GMOs had to pass in order to be sold throughout Europe. He had about twenty-five researchers working with him at three institutes.

- **Rats in Group 1** were fed potatoes genetically modified to produce the Bt toxin insecticide *from within.*
- **Rats in Group 2** were fed organic, naturally-grown potatoes.
- **Rats in Group 3** were fed organically-grown potatoes *externally sprayed* with the insecticide that GMO potatoes make internally.

The results: In ten days of eating GMO potatoes early in their lives, the rats in Group 1 had slower growth, problems with internal organ development, pre-cancerous cell growths, smaller brains, partially-atrophied smaller livers, smaller testes, and damaged immune systems. But, to their surprise, the group eating the potatoes manually sprayed with the insecticide did not have these same problems.

This led Dr. Pusztai's team to conclude that it was the process of genetic engineering itself, and its unpredicted side-effects, that were responsible for the rapid and permanent damage to the rats' internal organs and development – not the insecticide itself. The insecticide alone did not cause dramatic injury. Instead, **something intrinsic to the process of genetic engineering caused the damage that the rats had suffered.**

The study continued for another twenty months. Though his research was not designed to study cancer, when the rats started developing massive pre-cancerous tumors beginning in the fourth month, he was obligated to extend the study to the rats' full lifespan by European science rules. Near the end, many rats did indeed come down with cancer. But the toxicological aspect of the study didn't use enough rats to be considered statistically significant. So the cancer findings were dismissed as irrelevant. Their conclusions: Dr. Pusztai's team demonstrated that GMO potatoes did not kill rats right away. Instead, the process of GMO engineering causes serious health problems, including cancer, over time.

Dr. Pusztai spoke out against GMOs, but Monsanto didn't like what he had to say

He shared his concerns about GMOs and was a hero at his prestigious institute for about two days. The press was going wild. Here was a well-respected mainstream scientist saying that we should not treat people as guinea pigs… and that he personally would not eat GMOs from then on, based on what he had discovered.

Shortly thereafter, the director of Dr. Pusztai's institute allegedly received two phone calls from the UK Prime Minister's office. The next day, Dr. Arpad Pusztai was fired from his job after 35 years. He was silenced with threats of a lawsuit. His laboratory was locked. His materials were destroyed. His team was disbanded. And they never implemented the protocols his research was intended to codify into law. Instead, a campaign was launched to destroy his reputation in order to protect and promote the reputation of biotechnology.

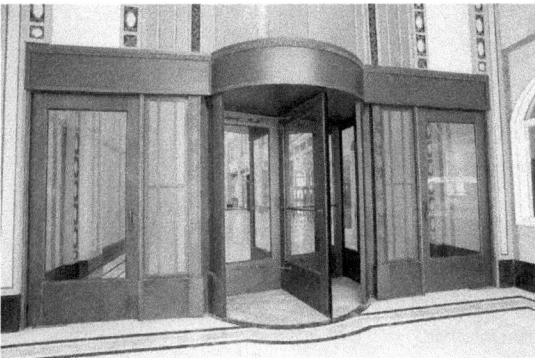

The infamous "revolving door" between government agencies and the companies they're supposed to regulate

Big Ag and Big Food are notorious for infiltrating government agencies through political appointment so they can get crucial rules/regulations/approvals passed that are instrumental to their long-term plans. These insiders go back and forth between high posts in government agencies, and the corporations they're supposed to regulate.

Let's use Monsanto as an example of how this works.

- A trusted, high-level insider is chosen to infiltrate a government agency and do Monsanto's bidding.
- Monsanto uses their political influence (usually at the presidential level and above) to get them appointed to a powerful position in-charge of making precedence-setting decisions. Sometimes, a position is created inside a government agency specifically for them.
- After achieving their objective at the agency (e.g., FDA), the insider returns to the company to be rewarded with a cushy, high-paying job.
- When the giant multi-national needs another "insider job" done, they repeat the process.

That's how the most inane, controversial decisions affecting mass populations have come into being the last few decades. Perfect example: Mike Taylor could serve as the poster-child for the revolving door.

- 1976. Attorney for FDA.
- 1981. Attorney for Monsanto.
- 1991. Deputy Commissioner for Policy, FDA.
- 1998. Vice President Public Policy, Monsanto.
- 2009. Senior Advisor to FDA Commissioner.
- 2010. Deputy Commissioner for Foods, FDA.

How Monsanto and Big Ag companies hijack government agencies and the regulatory process. They…

- install agents in public health agencies to get their approvals passed
- use intimidation and litigation to bully small, independent farmers
- silence critics by controlling medical journals
- stop real research by controlling funding to colleges and institutions
- take unethical advantage of intellectual property laws prohibiting anyone from studying their seeds because they're patented.

Dr. Don Huber knows of no peer-reviewed studies proving the safety of GMO crops, companion chemicals, or the products they produce

Dr. Don Huber: Professor Emeritus plant pathologist, Purdue University

"When a group of us [scientists/researchers] met with top USDA administrators, they assured us that they based all their decisions on peer-reviewed science. When we asked them if they would share any of that, they have been unable to produce any. There are many papers – both clinical papers, as well as peer-reviewed scientific papers … that show just the opposite. We have some recent papers that document what many of those health effects are. I know of no studies that will establish the safety of either the genetically engineered proteins, or the chemicals we're consuming in ever-larger quantities as a result of those genetic engineering processes."

Debunking the promises of GMOs

Fiction: Genetic engineering improves crop yield. Truth: Bio-friendly farming is better than genetic engineering at improving yield, nutrient density, and many other attributes. Dr. Don Huber estimates most conventional crops are expressing only about 25–30% of their genetic potential in yield. In other words, they could be producing three or four times their present yield – as well as growing faster, more nutrient-dense, and with more resistance to threats and stresses – given perfect growing conditions.

In real-world conditions, growers that switch to bio-friendly farming see an average of 79% increase in yield, dramatically improved nutrient profiles, increased resistance to disease, up to 65% less water used, reduced chemical runoff and contamination downstream, as well as many other benefits. Of course, this requires a change in ideology and methodology to make the switch – composting, for example.

Point being, we don't need genetic engineering to feed the world, strengthen crops' defenses, or get adequate nutrition for ourselves. Nature has science and industry beat, for the foreseeable future. And Dr. Elaine Ingham's real-world experience in bio-friendly farming techniques prove these concepts valid and very attainable.

Dr. Elaine Ingham: World's leading soil biology researcher, characterized "The Soil Food Web," author of the USDA's Soil Biology Primer.

Big Ag spokesmen tell you all you need to know about the improvements that GMOs claim to offer: 'GMO traits are absolutely useless unless they can be put into the very best conventional seed varieties.' Which is another way of saying traditional breeding is what creates most improvements. Biotech companies then tweak Nature's product to gain proprietary control over the commercial version. Nature does almost all the work, and GMOs are taking credit where credit is not due. What's more, GMO technology is not needed for attributes that consumers consider most valuable.

Feeding the hungry in Third World countries has nothing to do with yield. It's about economics, food quality and politics. Feeding the world's hungry has never been about growing *enough* food to feed everyone. That's never been <u>the</u> problem, or even <u>a</u> problem. Over the past 50-plus years, traditional breeding techniques have been spectacularly successful at increasing volume and consistency of yields. So, believe it or not, traditional farming techniques could potentially support 15 billion people, or more. We could probably feed 11 billion people right now with natural growing methods. On the other hand, genetic engineering fails miserably to beat Nature's best.

The real issue is that the hungry in Third World countries can't even afford to buy the crappy food that wealthier nations refuse to eat – let alone buy food that's high in nutrition, low in contaminants. Feeding the world's hungry has very little to do with quantity, as far as production and transportation are concerned. Rather, cost, food quality and political complications are the bigger challenges derailing the noblest intentions.

More accurately, World Economic Forum types use hunger and scarcity as tools to gain power and control over others. Restricting the supply of essentials, such as food and energy, is a tried-and-true method of increasing their control over populations. The hungrier, poorer, and more desperate that a person is, the more receptive they are to the rule of tyrants and dictators that control the scarce resources. As a result, you tend to do what you're told when you can't feed your family.

Bottom line: There is no shortage of food, and there never has been since agriculture met machinery. Instead, food quality, its costs, and getting it into the hands of those in need – those are the real problems that need to be solved, not yield.

GMOs three biggest benefits for *agrochemical companies*: They increase chemical company profits, they perpetuate a demand for their products, and shift power from individual growers to big corporations.

GMOs two (supposed) benefits for *growers*: They simplify weed and pest control. And they make the growing process more consistent and predictable, thereby allowing more mechanization and larger farm size.

Conclusion. GMOs exist solely to sell more chemicals and make more money from their patents. In the process, Big Ag and Big Food aim to make everyone dependent on them. Whereas, anything they do that happens to support health and life is just a talking point they weave into their PR. Or, to put it even more bluntly, they're in the death and disease business, masquerading as health and life. So don't be surprised by how cold-blooded their tactics are. They *do* kill things for a living, after all, with their herbi<u>cides</u>, pesti<u>cides</u>, and insecti<u>cides</u>. Food for thought.

Big Ag sees the whole GMO game as a race against time

Big Ag companies and their captured agencies know with 100% certainty that GMOs and glyphosate destroy the health of all life on earth, chronically. They're just hoping that GMO science can survive its technological adolescence before: (1) the public catches on to the harm being done, (2) we stop buying genetically modified products, and (3) the funding dries up from sales, investments, subsidies and grants.

They're well aware of the damage they are doing. But they have a serious case of The God Complex, which emboldens them to keep the charade going as long as possible in the hopes that one day they will under-stand gene regulation better, control the insertion and cloning processes, and thus produce the outcomes they want with fewer side effects. They think if they can keep the deception going just a few more decades, by that time, they will have mastered the complexity of genetics, and have God-like power to create life at-will, with all 'pros' and few 'cons.'

You see, at the top of the power structure, globalists are big believers in "apotheosis," which means *man becomes God*. And whether you believe in the idea or not, the important thing is *they believe it*. And they act aggressively on those beliefs. In either case, genetic engineering in its current form, is the riskiest gamble Nature has seen since nuclear weapons. And every living thing on earth is a test subject. It's my belief that glyphosate and GMOs are so chronically toxic that they will inevitably be banned world-wide. I suspect the industry sees their day of reckoning is coming. But until that day comes, their strategy is to use every dirty trick in the book to keep the con going as long as possible, while we pay the price.

We've beaten GMOs before, and we will beat them again
In the last 15+ years, the following GMOs have failed
- Genetically engineered tomatoes.
- GE wheat. Growers refused to adopt GE wheat because they know the US exports 50% of its production, and foreign countries will reject it.
- GE rice ("golden rice" variety recently released).
- GE biopharmaceuticals (vaccines in food).
- GE bentgrass (however, GE bentgrass escaped confinement so the USDA choose to deregulate it!).
- Use of GE bovine growth hormone to enhance milk production of cows has been dramatically reduced.

Dozens of countries have banned or restricted the sale of GMOs
After doing their homework, scientists in at least twenty-six countries have found GMOs to be too harmful to be cleared for use – including Switzerland, Australia, Austria, China, India, France, Germany, Hungary, Luxembourg, Greece, Bulgaria, Poland, Italy, Mexico and Russia.

Significant restrictions on GMOs exist in about sixty other countries, including fifty that require labeling. Two superpowers have already pushed back against GMOs – not out of fear or for political reasons, but because it's a smart move: China refuses to feed GMO products to its military personnel, while Russia has banned all production and sales of GMO products in the country, period.

The anti-GMO movement is gaining traction
Non-GMO Project Verified: Independent organization that certifies GMO-free status.

When a product earns the "Non-GMO Project Verified" certification its sales are shown to increase by 15–30%. Collectively, sales of Non-GMO Project Verified products rose from $348 million to $1.2 billion – in one year. Jeffrey Smith says all it will take for Big Food companies to turn their backs on GMOs is for them to see a decline of 5–10% in sales that they can directly attribute to consumer refusal of GMOs. It's happened all over Europe already. Several years ago, when negative publicity and public outcry showed up in company earnings reports, many multi-nationals dropped GMOs completely (many sell in Europe and the US).

Stop buying GMOs and they'll stop making them

- Stop buying GMO foods.
- Buy "Non-GMO Project Verified" products. Many consumer advocates consider the Non-GMO Project Verified label to be the most trustworthy certification currently available.
- Or choose certified organic.
- Visit Jeffrey Smith's Non-GMO Shopping Guide: www.nongmoshoppingguide.com.
- Or avoid the at-risk ingredients listed on Jeffrey Smith's webpage titled "Invisible GM Ingredients": www.nongmoshoppingguide.com/invisible-gm-ingredients/.
- Tell grocery stores and food companies that you've stopped buying these questionable foods because they're horrible for your health.
- For extra credit, apply pressure to lawmakers to ban GMOs and glyphosate to get them removed from the food supply completely.

You can cut your exposure to herbicides and pesticides as economically as possible by buying only those organically-grown vegetables and fruits whose conventionally-grown counterparts are most likely to have been sprayed due to how vulnerable they are to threats. On the other hand, buy conventionally-grown (non-GMO) produce when the crop is not sprayed as much because it doesn't need to be. You can find lots of these "Clean Fifteen" and "Dirty Dozen" lists on the Internet, such as that put out by the Environmental Working Group.

6

REDOX SIGNALING AND INFLAMMATION
How Oxidation, Reduction and Inflammation Keep the Body Tuned-up, or Cause it to Break Down

Ever wonder how 35 trillion host cells, and 100 trillion microbiota, live together as one organism?
The answer is *communication* lets trillions of microscopic cells – such as your cells and your gut microbiota – live together as one macroscopic organism – as they do in you, an animal or a plant. It's really quite remarkable when you think about it, because without exquisite communication and control systems keeping all the members of the choir on the same page, singing the same tune, it would be utter chaos on so many levels.

Imagine what would happen if each cell selfishly did whatever it wanted, whenever it wanted. Imagine cells calling for help and their calls going unanswered. That's the difference communication makes in ensuring the body's needs are being met at all levels.

In the same way that many channels of communication are needed to run households, businesses, armies and countries – many channels of communication are needed to orchestrate the body's essential functions. Clear lines of communication are needed to protect and care for its citizens, repair damaged facilities, allocate resources appropriately, and manage activities benefitting the group. Without coordination and cooperation at many levels, complex organizational structures would not be possible.

More than anything, that means having a variety of ways one member of a group can get a message to another – be they peers, or managers higher up the chain of command. It's *communication* – or *signaling*, in the case of biology – that turns many individuals into one well-functioning organism.

To name three forms of communication you've heard about, but probably haven't thought about quite like this…

1. **Neurotransmitters** conduct signals along nerve pathways using electro-chemical signaling molecules, such as dopamine and serotonin.
2. **Hormones** regulate the activity of organs at a distance via messenger molecules sent through the bloodstream.
3. **DNA** transmits the organism's genetic blueprint into the construction of proteins, cells and organism.

Redox signaling

Just as important to our physiology, there's one communication system most people know nothing about. It's so new to science most people in the general population have never even heard of it, despite the fact it's essential to all life on earth. And that system is the network by which communication happens at a cellular level, called "redox signaling."

Conveyed through compounds called redox molecules, mitochondria make one type of redox molecule, called *oxygen* redox molecules, while bacteria make another, called *carbon* redox molecules. Each makes its own type of redox molecules for its own purposes, thus forming two distinct communication networks. Mitochondria make and use *oxygen* redox molecules (aka free radicals, reactive oxygen species, or oxygen radicals) for signaling among human cells and mitochondria, while bacteria make and use *carbon* redox molecules for signaling between each other and cells of the gut.

The body uses redox signaling to

- **protect** against damage from foreign invaders and toxins
- **detect** damage after it happens, and tell the immune system how much
- **repair** cells when the damage is reversible
- **replace** cells when the damage is beyond repair
- **adjust** efficiency of energy production and metabolism
- **adapt** to seasonal changes.

It's through this communication network that biologic systems read conditions inside and outside of cells, and do what they need to do. Conversely, when communication breaks down, bodily systems can't respond to threats when, where, and how they should. Threats include foreign frequency stress, food mismatches, oxygen deprivation, toxin damage, infection, malnutrition, DNA mutations, and water contaminated with deuterium or fluoride.

This new science of redox signaling is a major advancement in our understanding of how dysfunction and disease materializes. And the discoveries of just the last 10–15 years represent a giant leap forward in reversing them. Before we proceed, let's define mitochondria.

Mitochondria

Mitochondria are essential to every member of the animal kingdom because they make a biochemical used to meet its energy demands: ATP. Through ATP production, mitochondria also produce redox signaling molecules that allow cells, mitochondria and the immune system to talk to each other.

About 200 to 5,000 of these mitochondria live inside each of our cells – most cell types anyway – equaling 30% of a person's dry weight. They take care of the cell in so many ways (or not). However, they are their own life form (organelles, actually) and possess their own DNA. So they ride along inside each cell. Yet they live, reproduce and die separately from their host's cells. Basically, the more mitochondria you have, and the healthier they are, the more energy you can produce, and the better your cells operate in many ways.

Conversely, depressed mitochondria equate to chronic low energy, poor cell-cell communication, reduced cell repair, and accelerated aging. Unfortunately, mitochondria populations weaken (1) as you age; (2) when toxins and disease mutate their DNA; (3) when you lack sleep and exercise; (4) when their communication network breaks down; and (5) when the both of you are malnourished, among other reasons.

Oxidation and reduction overview

Over the last 20–30 years, you may have heard wellness coaches and marketers talk about how free radicals and antioxidants greatly influence health and longevity. They are the yin and yang of the "oxidation-reduction" cycle in the rapidly emerging field of oxidative medicine. Unfortunately, what started out as a misleading half-truth has blossomed into a fully-flawed belief system that few think to question today.

Redox reaction with electron transfer

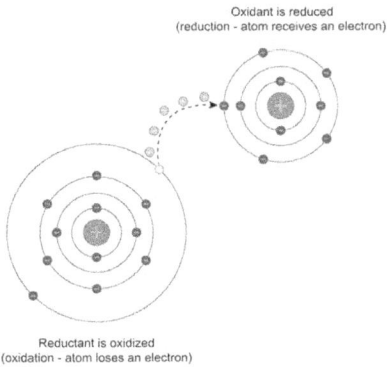

Oxidant is reduced
(reduction - atom receives an electron)

Reductant is oxidized
(oxidation - atom loses an electron)

Oxidation-reduction: Simply put, oxidation and reduction describe the exchange of electrons.

Electrical charge: Electrons are negatively charged. So *removing* electrons through oxidation increases positive charge and acidity, while *adding* electrons through reduction does the opposite: it increases negative charge and alkalinity. This is important because most pathogens, toxins, and free radicals are in their comfort zone when positively charged and acidic, while antioxidant activity fights those threats by donating electrons, thereby increasing a tissue's negative charge and alkalinity.

Oxidation is the "stealing" of electrons from a molecule – or an *increase* in the state of oxidation. So molecules with a propensity to oxidize substances are called "oxidants." To illustrate, when oxygen takes electrons slowly from iron, that's a form of oxidation we call rust. When a flammable material burns or explodes – again, with oxygen – that's oxidation happening rapidly right before our eyes.

Oxidants: In biological systems, oxidation destabilizes the matter inside cells by stealing their electrons, which makes them blow apart in a hurry unless they find an electron to pair up with to zero out their charge. Employed for their ability to obliterate, oxidants are used by our immune systems as the ultimate antimicrobial, detoxifying agent.

Cell Attacked by
Free Radicals

Normal Cell

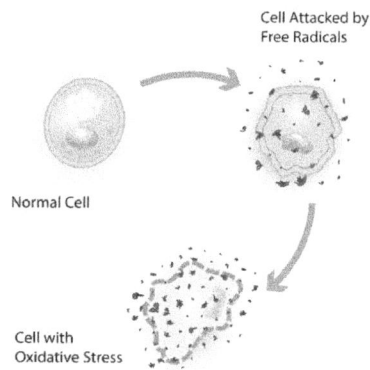

Most oxidants, as the name suggests, are predominantly
oxygen-based molecules, so they're called reactive oxygen
species or oxygen radicals. Some of the best-known oxidants
in the functional medicine field are oxygen, chlorine dioxide,
ozone, and hydrogen peroxide. Nitrogen and sulfur also form
their own less-diverse reactive species, such as nitric oxide.

Cell with
Oxidative Stress

Free radicals: When a molecule with a balanced pair of electrons gains
or loses an electron due to oxidation or reduction, the resulting molecule
can become a free radical because of its extra, unpaired electron, which is
highly reactive and potentially damaging to cells. Its destructive effect on
cells is why the public was taught to fear free radicals in the 1980s–2010s,
and why we were instructed to get plenty of antioxidants to combat free
radical damage. Most, but not all, reactive oxygen species are free radicals.

Reduction is the opposite of oxidation. It's the giving of electrons, or
a *decrease* in the state of oxidation (hence the term "reduction").

Reductants: Molecules that give up their extra electron in chemical
reactions are called "reductants," or reduced species (RS).

Antioxidants (stricter definition) are tiny molecular catalysts that make
oxidants give their extra electron(s) to reductants, thereby neutralizing them
both of electrical charge and biological reactivity. The body's naturally-
produced antioxidants such as glutathione can perform tens of millions of
these reactions per minute. Reactive oxygen species and reductants then
turn back into salt water (from which they came). More loosely defined,
antioxidants are any substance that reduces free radical damage.

Redox: Not too long ago, redox scientists realized that saying the words
oxidation, reduction, and *reactive oxygen species* out loud made them sound
like nerdy chemists who use big words to confuse or impress people. So
they came up with a cooler sounding umbrella term to describe the
players and processes. The field swapped and shortened oxidation-
reduction to "redox," which is short for REDuction-OXidation. And it
seems to have a ring that's right for the mainstream.

Redox signaling molecules: Reactive oxygen species/free radicals
(ROS), and reductants/reduced species (RS), are collectively called
"redox signaling molecules" or just redox molecules. In particular,
mitochondria's *oxygen redox molecules* are by-products of metabolism that
form a major communication network between mitochondria and human
cells. Their signature trait is they have one or more unpaired electrons.

Similarly, bacteria make "carbon redox molecules" as by-products of
their metabolism, which they use to communicate between themselves
and cells of the gut lining. Carbon redox molecules are the
communication medium of the microbiome.

Oxidative stress: Oxidative stress is the amount and duration in which
oxidants outnumber reductants. Oxidative stress can be damaging when

you don't have enough antioxidants and reductants available to neutralize oxidation – particularly, in chronic, uncontrolled circumstances. On the other hand, oxidative stress can be beneficial when used therapeutically.

Why oxidation and reduction matter

Oxidation and reduction are fundamental to life as we know it, because biochemical reactions revolve around the exchange of electrons. Redox reactions are integrally involved in energy production, healing, immunity, detoxification, hormonal response, youth, and support of the microbiome… when they work properly. And they cause a lack of cell repair, a long list of chronic, degenerative problems and accelerated aging when they're not.

So redox reactions are more than important to all life on the planet; they're essential. Life would cease to exist very quickly without oxidation and reduction. Oxidation and reduction, or redox signaling (they're the same system), is one of the biggest, most important stories for medical science to study today, and you to learn about, in our ongoing effort to get healthy and stay healthy.

We used to think free radicals were harmful by-products of exercise

Until just a few years ago, wellness experts believed that *free radical oxidation* harmed cells and accelerated the aging process… and that was all there was to it. Researchers and educators basically thought aerobic exercise and inefficient energy production make reactive oxygen species by accident. Because free radicals are good at destroying things, they believed the resulting oxidation is responsible for randomly injuring cells and making us age before our time. Therefore, we needed to protect ourselves against this sort of cell damage by eating foods high in antioxidants, or take them as a supplement.

But science has since come to its senses as research has revealed that we shouldn't think of reactive oxygen species as harmful by-products of metabolism that you need to eliminate, else they harm cells and cause premature aging. Instead, they're made for a very good reason – many beneficial reasons, actually. Researchers have come to realize that the body uses oxidants in a controlled manner to selectively repair or replace injured cells, depending on the extent of damage. Even more pertinent to the discussion, redox molecules are created to communicate what's happening inside the cell.

So redox molecules are both the communication network of the mitochondria, and the disinfectant that wipes out unwanted material to make way for healthy, new cells. But, up until just 15–20 years ago, scientists didn't realize that a healthy system purposely makes an equal amount of destructive oxidants and restorative reductants to maintain balance. In other words, good health is a balanced redox system.

In fact, large amounts of both reactive oxygen species and reduced species are made when you exercise. So, oddly enough, taking a redox molecule supplement does many of the same things that exercise does, whereas ingesting antioxidants right before you exercise blocks some of their benefits by neutralizing some cleansing and restoration.

We used to think antioxidants only came from food

We now know our own cells make large quantities of antioxidants that are far superior in reach and capacity to those supplied by foods. In fact, most antioxidants that come from foods can't get inside cells, so they don't do what scientists thought they did. Vitamin C is an exception. That said, antioxidants like vitamin A and E do offer some benefit quenching free radicals in the blood and extracellular matrix – colorful vegetables being their richest source. However, that's only half the story.

Extracellular matrix: Supportive structures and biochemicals outside of cells (e.g., collagen, enzymes, glycoproteins, and minerals).

As a compensation mechanism in the body, raw vegetables increase alkalinity through their calcium, magnesium, potassium, sodium and iron. The compounds formed from these minerals become a reserve of alkalinity, or buffer, that the body uses to raise pH level when the blood becomes too acidic (low pH). It's a standby method to adjust pH level that complements a vegetable's antioxidant effect.

That is, **redox reactions and pH regulation both deal with electron balance.** Together, they are big reasons why raw, naturally-grown vegetables can be good for you. Unfortunately, food companies tend to exaggerate the benefits of antioxidants taken in isolation – similar to the way drugs try to replicate a natural substance's active compounds, and the way some vitamin supplements are promoted. Whichever way it's presented, redemption in a pill or a potion *sells* with a good story behind it.

In any case, antioxidants from food can be good for you when used intelligently. They're just not as all-powerful as those the body makes internally. To give you some perspective, dietary sources contribute about 4% of the body's total supply of antioxidants, while internally-produced glutathione, by itself, represents about 85%, and is much stronger.

Our new understanding of oxidation and reduction

We now know oxidation and reduction is a carefully orchestrated, essential process the body uses to rectify injury and degradation, so repair processes have a pristine environment in which to rebuild. Without oxidation and reduction healing you, you'd have mere hours to live – mere minutes without redox happening in the electron transport chain.

Oxidation and reduction are fundamental to human life because the body uses oxidation to destroy everything it deems undesirable – including microbial pathogens, toxins, heavy metals, dead cells, and unrepairable cells. However, oxidants are like wild beasts in that they're useful when kept under control, a destructive nuisance when they get out of control.

Cells communicate and heal with redox molecules

Like a vast military operation with lots of moving parts, mitochondria need excellent communication to perform efficiently and effectively under all conditions. Through redox signaling, the body is able to:

- detect when cells are under stress
- tell DNA to activate coping mechanisms
- call in the immune system to fight off threats
- repair mildly damaged cells
- hit the self-destruct button on badly damaged cells
- regulate hormonal response
- fine-tune mitochondrial metabolism
- and turn off coping mechanisms after a threat subsides.

When cells become damaged for any reason, they enter a state of oxidative stress. High amounts of reactive oxygen species are the "S.O.S. distress signal" that tell cells and systems there's a problem that needs to be fixed, where it's coming from, and how dire the situation is. Like smoke coming from a burning building, the more oxidant molecules the immune system finds leaking out of cells (because they were never neutralized by antioxidants and reductants), the more emphatic the distress signal is deemed to be.

After the situation has been resolved, the lack of free-floating redox molecules inside and outside cells prompts the nucleus and the immune system to turn off coping mechanisms and go back to business as usual (i.e., homeostatic balance). So it's through mitochondrial redox signaling that the nucleus "reads" the condition of oxidative stress occurring in the cell and can activate a variety of genetically-controlled coping mechanisms to deal with the threat and restore balance to the system.

Of course, most of the time a cell reads its status report and realizes it's fine and doesn't need repair. Still other times, cells take a look around and realize they're different from that of the host organism. They realize they're a cancer cell and need to be sacrificed to protect the health of the whole.

But the thing is, without the proper vocabulary with which to communicate, cells don't even realize what a healthy cell is supposed to look like, compared to a cancer cell. They don't talk to each other fluently about their status and needs. And they don't relay that information to the organ systems that need to know, such as the immune system. All of that is the job of redox signaling molecules – known to most of the world as free radicals.

Summary: In the same way that analyzing a car's exhaust tells a mechanic how well an engine is running, the ratio and volume of ROS to RS indicates whether the cell is happy or distressed. Mitochondria, cell nuclei, and organ systems can then use this information to activate healing or turn it off.

Here are 12 "buttons" the nucleus can push to call for help

List is from Dr. Gary Samuelson's paper "The Science of Healing Revealed," pp. 45–46.

1. **The DNA Repair** "button" mobilizes the DNA damage detection-and-repair crew.
2. **The Antioxidant Boost** makes more antioxidants to neutralize the potentially harmful surplus of oxidants.
3. **The Intercellular Communication** strengthens lines of communication between cells.
4. **The Increase Blood Supply** dilates blood vessels to cells that need more resources.
5. **The Stronger Cell Adhesion** makes cells hold more tightly together.
6. **The Inflame Tissue** stops damage from spreading.
7. **The Secrete Antibiotics** deploys antibacterial substances.
8. **The Stop Cell Division** prevents damaged cells from replicating.
9. **The Send Distress Call** sends a distress signal to the immune system.
10. **The More Energy to Repair Crew** brings in more energy for repair processes to work with.
11. **The Prepare Cell for Shutdown** places the decision to euthanize a cell with its neighbors.
12. **The Master Shutdown** kills and demolishes the cell.

That's basically healing at a cellular level

These genetically-controlled processes, activated by the nucleus in response to redox distress signals, are the mechanisms whereby cells are instructed to activate repair processes when repairable, or make way for their replacements when gravely injured. These are the mechanisms that heal cells and stave off the aging process. A perfect example is button #12. The body is supposed to shut down attempts to repair cells after two hours if they were unsuccessful, then turn on cell suicide (apoptosis). But poor redox signaling disables this programming, allowing damaged cells to persist and replicate. In a word, that's aging.

Oxidative therapies use oxidation and reduction to heal and renew

- hyperbaric oxygen chambers
- chlorine dioxide
- ozone therapy
- hydrogen peroxide
- exercise.

Exercise benefits the body by enhancing oxidation, reduction and redox signaling

Exercise is oxidative stress. Oxidative stress is like exercise. At the same time, the ability to sustain exercise is determined by mitochondrial production capacity, antioxidant capacity, and a balance between oxidation and reduction. Most important of all its functions, exercise is controlled oxidation. Meaning, exercise produces a cleansing and renewal effect at a cell level. That's *why* it's good for you, and *how* it benefits the body. It leads to very important mechanisms of cell regeneration, aerobic capacity, and speed of recovery.

You see, exercise makes mitochondria burn fatty acids or sugar along with oxygen to power cells. Through this process, energy production in the mitochondria makes large amounts of reactive oxygen species (aka free radicals) that act as both universal cleansing agents (that need to be neutralized) and immune-system messengers.

Exercise, oxygenation, and the resulting capacity for oxidation and reduction also help improve electrical charge and pH balance. Electrical potential improves cell wall permeability, hydration, nutrient exchange, and detoxification. In conjuction, breathing from exercise balances pH because O_2 alkalizes, while CO_2 acidifies. These factors promote either a high state of health and healing when they're present, or disease conditions that favor pathogens and breakdown of cells when absent.

The point is, exercise, oxygenation, and oxidative activity are precious to your wellness. But the other half of the story is that it takes time to build up a capacity for exercise, which is largely dependent on antioxidant capacity and completion of the redox cycle. Otherwise, you experience extended recovery time and overuse injuries pushing yourself too hard when you're out of shape.

Through redox molecules (reactive oxygen species and reducing species), exercise dramatically increases protection of cells, healing of cells, balance, and a laundry list of good things. When well-controlled, oxidative reactions represent most of the body's mechanisms of healing and anti-aging. Conversely, when those systems are overwhelmed or fail altogether, like ROS not being neutralized properly, then oxidative damage becomes the mechanism of imbalances, exposure to genetic weaknesses, breakdowns, and rapid aging.

To sum it up, exercise is oxidation. Exercise is cleansing and rejuvenation on a cellular level. But exercise needs to be matched up with an equal amount of aerobic fitness, which is determined by your mitochondrial strength, your body's capacity to neutralize free radicals, and balance between oxidation and reduction. You need all that to sustain aerobic exercise. Otherwise, you get too much breakdown and not enough repair. So, basically, aerobic capacity is brought about by a redox signaling system that performs well under load.

Both cell-cell communication networks come from mom

As Doug Wallace, PhD taught us, you inherit all your mitochondria from your mother. Each human egg has some 100,000 mitochondria, which is more than any other cell in the human body. On the other hand, the 200 or fewer mitochondria in sperm are seen as foreign and selectively destroyed after the egg is fertilized. Mitochondria then reproduce as welcome guests inside most new human cells made. Which means all the mitochondria you will ever have descend from that original batch in the egg.

A curious consequence of this process is that you acquire half your redox communication ability from your mother *at conception* in the form of mitochondria and the oxygen redox molecules they make in cells. And you inherit the other half of your cell-cell communication from your mother *at birth* in the form of bacterial microbiota and the carbon redox molecules they make in the microbiome. That is, when a baby is born conventionally, friendly bacteria from the mother's birth canal seeds baby's digestive tract with starter cultures. Over a baby's first few weeks, those initial bacterial colonies populate their GI tract and make the carbon redox molecules that form the communication network of the microbiome.

So, as it turns out, fathers are almost useless in the world of redox communications. Their role happens on the sidelines of all the action.

What happens when your redox system fails?

Poor cell-to-cell communication causes breakdowns and failures to occur in protection, detection, repair and replacement, which leads directly to

- slow cell repair
- low energy
- premature aging
- immune system dysregulation
- autoimmune problems
- neurotransmitter and hormone imbalances
- psychological disturbances
- chronic inflammation.

This failure to communicate collaborates with other anomalies to make chronic, degenerative disease possible. First conspirator is a lack of energy. That starts the degeneration process. The second is impaired redox functioning so cells and mitochondria can't tell there's a problem brewing. Meaning, cells can't protect themselves from injury in a state of poor redox signaling. They don't know they've been injured. They don't call for repair mechanisms. And cells don't replace themselves when they ought to.

These imbalances and repercussions express themselves symptomatically wherever the body is lowest in energy, or hardest hit by the ensuing hormonal, neurological and immunological stresses – taking their toll as

- poor brain function in autism, Parkinson's and ADD
- digestive disorders like irritable bowel syndrome and Crohn's Disease
- insulin dysfunction in diabetes

- nerve damage in neuropathies
- cardiac weakness in heart disease.

The damage of all these conditions is sustained by a failure of cells to communicate and repair appropriately, which, for most intents and purposes, is the same as *chronic inflammation*. Chronic inflammation more or less equals loss of cell–cell communication. They're nearly one and the same.

The human body has incredible repair mechanisms, but they're useless without effective redox signaling

Our DNA (which mostly codes for proteins) is almost identical to the way it was decades ago. Our machinery for cell repair is the same. Our enzymes for detoxing haven't changed. Everything is the same as it always has been. But lately, our body's repair kit is doing a miserable job at keeping us running smoothly.

The systems are sitting there, ready to kick into action. But if the signaling network goes down, cells can't protect themselves like they're supposed to. They can't marshal the resources they need for routine maintenance. And, equally bad, cells don't even realize when they've been injured, let alone call for help.

With our rate of injury so high, and our rate of repair so low, cells are not repairing and replacing themselves like they used to. So they're accumulating toxins and DNA damage, rather than continually rejuvenating themselves like they should. Those imperfect cells then go on to replicate in an unrepaired state. Yep, you guessed it; that's aging and disease.

Rate of injury *vs.* rate of repair

Cells in your body are constantly being injured and killed every minute of every day. At the same time, the body's healing mechanisms continuously repair damaged cells, and replace dead cells with healthy new ones. So there's always some rate of injury happening versus some rate of repair.

That ratio determines your ability to stay well. It greatly influences your energy level – physically and mentally. It controls your recovery time from exertion, injury and illness. It has a lot to do with your rate of detoxification. And it's a primary factor in the rate at which you age biologically.

The point being, both of those states – damage and repair – can change quickly through interventions, or gradually through natural processes. But you seldom notice any of these changes because the human body has a built-in buffer zone of coping mechanisms – a reservoir of healing capacity – that's designed to favor life and healing, until your compensation mechanisms are stretched past their limits of competency.

So you only notice three conditions:

1. When your rate of **new injury increases rapidly** due to some event or circumstance (e.g., a major infection or massive toxin exposure).
2. When **repair has fallen far behind** and injury is clearly winning (i.e., the basis of disease).
3. When your rate of **healing improves quickly** through a lifestyle change such as a healthy new diet, an exercise program, or getting out of a bad relationship.

You see, complex organisms are designed to start their lives with a full bucket of life force, if you will. They (should) spend the majority of their lives with healing capacity to spare in the form of compensation mechanisms, emergency procedures, and various workarounds the body employs to cope with sub-optimal conditions. It's only when injury exceeds the body's ability to repair by a wide margin that you see acute disease take place, or you die.

In daily life, however, you typically don't notice a gradual expansion or contraction of your healing or repair, because your buffer zone absorbs slow changes with any excess healing capacity you may have. Your body just does its normal healing thing and you're none the wiser.

But our multitude of sins against Nature have stretched our coping mechanisms to the limit

Our excesses and irresponsibilities have exhausted our healing capacity at all levels – cell, organ system, individual, society and planet. So now the majority of people are living their lives on a razor-fine edge between health and sickness, with dangerously little safety margin to spare.

That's an important concept to internalize, because the slightest new insult in nnEMF exposure, diet, lifestyle choices, or internal milieu can push a person into disorder. In case you hadn't noticed, that very situation is occurring all around us in our personal lives, social circles, healthcare systems, and every health statistic you'd care to measure.

To venture a guess, I'd say probably 40% of the population is slightly over the edge into the disease/dysfunction side (minor disease), 20% is well into disease (intractable disease), 25% is slightly on the desirable side of health (occasional health problems/annoyances), and 15% of the population has a decent amount of extra healing capacity to overcome new insults.

In other words, almost everyone is on the verge of manifesting a chronic, degenerative disease. Those in jeopardy just can't see it. So as soon as the body uses up the last trick it has in its arsenal to keep you running problem-free, serious disease suddenly appears out of nowhere, and we blame it on bad genes, diet and misfortune.

High blood-sugar raises insulin, which triggers inflammation

Basic biology says the hormone/endocrine system regulates blood-sugar level by releasing insulin to let sugar into cells. Insulin also causes the liver to store sugar for future use. But did you know that eating sugar makes mitochondria crank out free radicals as a by-product of ATP production?

The problem is, the more broken-down your energy production system gets to be, the more ROS tends to be made relative to reductants. Those extra reactive oxygen species increase chronic oxidative stress, which can threaten cells all over the body with oxidative damage, including insulin-producing beta cells in the pancreas.

To protect itself from this rapid burst of oxidative damage, the pancreas is designed to pump out insulin as fast as it can in order to store that sugar in the liver, instead of burning it immediately and overwhelming the system with free radicals. Unfortunately, it has the opposite effect. What ends up happening is, insulin drives the sugar into cells faster and more furiously, which only increases oxidative stress and inflammation as by-products of metabolism.

So, basically, eating lots of refined carbs and sugar is like pouring gasoline on a fire. **It's a sugar-induced explosion of oxidation** that can only be controlled (hopefully) by flooding the system with insulin to stash sugar in the liver. This isn't a problem when antioxidant supplies can handle the increased oxidative load. But, more and more often, that's not the case as our population loses its healing capacity, and sugar consumption rises.

Thus, you've got yet another factor, among many difficult to avoid, that increases inflammation… another coping mechanism stretched to the limit. This is one of several vicious cycles involving redox reactions that elevate and perpetuate inflammation. In this case, with antioxidant and redox reserves exhausted throughout the body, insulin conspires to keep the destruction phase of inflammation going longer than it's supposed to.

Frequent high levels of insulin then cause the battle between inflammatory *destruction* and *repair* to rage on continuously. Elevated blood sugar from blue light and nnEMFs also help keep the wheels on this cycle spinning. Of course, constant demand for insulin also contributes to diabetes (another pathway whereby poor redox signaling turns into disease).

Chronic inflammation drives degenerative diseases

Chronic inflammation is integrally involved in creating most disorders involving the immune system, hormonal system, heart, brain, digestive tract, and cell repair – basically, everything that happens in the body. This is because **the majority of damage that a disease causes is not done by the pathogen or problem itself, but by inflammation the body employs to fight the threat.**

In other words, most infections, toxins, and disease processes are not the thing that does the most harm. Instead, the body's own threat annihilation system – inflammation – is far stronger at wiping out friendly cells than the menace itself. When it persists, unchecked inflammation causes the symptoms we collect into categories and call disease.

In fact, practitioners that know their stuff realize that most modern diseases, barring trauma, are nothing more than a variety of different ways and places that chronic inflammation exhibits itself in the body, as repair fails to keep up with injury. Therefore, a failure of cells to repair themselves completely is what causes modern disease (as well as aging). And that's caused by inadequate energy production, combined with poor redox signaling, which results in chronic inflammation and unfinished repair. They're partners in degeneration, with chronic inflammation being the culprit that actually "pulls the trigger."

Cancer cells are a quintessential example of what happens when inflammation persists and cell's distress signals go unanswered. Cancer is believed to take place after a cell has borne the brunt of some 20,000–25,000 unrepaired injuries to its DNA (i.e., failure to repair/replace).

How inflammation heals

The body uses inflammation to repair pretty much any sort of damage that can happen anywhere in the body, including:

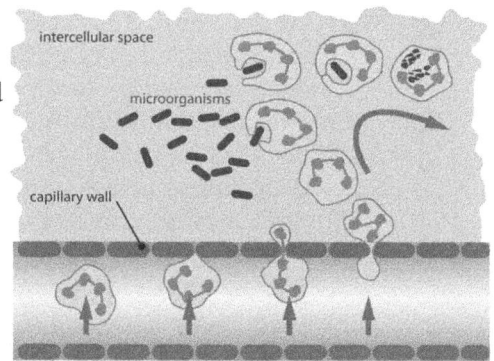

- cuts, bruises and overuse injuries
- damage to bones, muscles, tendons, blood vessels and internal organs
- microbial infection
- radiation damage
- chemical and heavy metal poisoning
- as well as ordinary wear and tear.

It does this by first increasing permeability of blood vessels so immune cells, such as white blood cells, can pass through the vessel wall to fight invading pathogens. This also lets more blood into an area, which we call swelling. Swelling makes movement painful, thus limiting mobility and further damage.

Barring outside intervention, inflammation then launches an oxidative attack on everything in the area that the immune system doesn't identify as your own healthy cell. Through oxidation, the first stage of inflammation kills infectious microorganisms, neutralizes toxins and heavy metals, and it destroys your own damaged, diseased and dead cells.

When inflammatory processes are working correctly (i.e., acute inflammation), the first phase of inflammation eventually shuts down and the second phase takes over. In the second phase of inflammation – the repair phase – unhealthy cells and debris are replaced with new cells and collagen fibers (made from protein and cholesterol).

On the other hand, when inflammation doesn't let up, both phases stay active at the same time – destruction and creation. And that's the leading cause of chronic, degenerative disease today: inflammation that doesn't stop destroying tissue, which is itself caused by poor redox signaling and a lack of energy from the mitochondria.

But the mind-blow you need to know is that **pain and swelling are integral parts of the healing process. If you prevent pain and swelling from running their course – like with anti-inflammatory painkillers, icing, elevating, compresses, or fever reducers – then full healing may never take place because you shortcut the healing process.** Believe it or not, **pain itself actually stimulates healing by kicking the immune system into action.**

This is why so many people today suffer from chronic pain issues that linger too long, or never end: they've interrupted the healing process so many times throughout their life – with drugs that block inflammation and pain – that injuries and inflammation become more or less permanent.

Acute inflammation *vs.* chronic inflammation

There are two kinds of inflammation: acute inflammation, which is temporary and beneficial, and chronic inflammation, which is persistent and harmful. Acute inflammation heals and protects you on a daily basis from threats that can damage tissue, such as cuts, bruises, infectious organisms, ordinary wear and tear, oxygen deprivation, and toxin exposure. Everyday occurrences like exercise and sun exposure also turn on inflammation without you even knowing it.

Through acute, fast-acting inflammation, the immune system gets called into action. It wipes out the threat in a matter of days to months using a four-step process whereby: (1) oxidants *destroy*; (2) antioxidants team up with reductants to *neutralize* the oxidant; (3) redox signaling partners with the immune system to *repair or replace* damaged cells; and (4) when that process is finished, if everything's working properly (i.e., complete healing and the redox signaling to match), inflammation shuts down, and the body resumes normal operation.

On the other hand, chronic inflammation is where the same processes get activated, but they're unable to turn themselves off. Step 4 *shut down* kind of starts, but is never completed. Instead, the first three stages get stuck in a vicious circle of destroying and repairing cells repeatedly, which can smolder along unbeknownst to you for years, or even decades.

The reason the immune system is not able to turn itself off after the initial burst of activity is due to one or more of the following circumstances:

1. Your antioxidant system is overwhelmed

First, some significant insult takes place requiring the immune system to use its oxidative stress tool – often between the ages of ten and thirty. This could be a sports injury, a nasty infection, or an acute poisoning event such as a major round of vaccines.

In this situation, cells don't have antioxidant and reductant reservoirs large enough to neutralize the oxidation being done. So the repairing and replacing of damaged cells is done slower, and less completely, than it should. Cells then eke by and reproduce themselves in a partially-damaged state, which is frustrated by lingering attempts by the immune system to simultaneously *destroy* with low-grade oxidative stress and *heal* using redox signaling and repair processes.

This smolders along underneath your conscious awareness until later in life your cells are being injured by oxidative stress faster than they're able to heal. At that point, you get symptoms that bother you. But, all the while, you've had chronic inflammation you only noticed occasionally (like an old knee injury that only hurts when it starts to get cold out).

2. Pro-inflammatory exposures sustain the situation

- You eat pro-inflammatory foods, such as refined vegetable oils.
- Leaky membranes cause poor digestion, food sensitivities, immune system hyper-activation, and autoimmune conditions.
- You continue to stress that old knee injury with the help of anti-inflammatory painkillers or other medications.
- You come down with a long-term illness such as Lyme's disease.
- You continue to take in toxins faster than you release them.

3. Fewer reductants, diminished redox signaling capacity, and a shortage of energy all prolong inflammation

As we age, we lose mitochondria. Scarcity of mitochondria means fewer reductants get made, diminished redox signaling capacity, and not enough ATP for all bodily processes. Plus, the mitochondria that do stick around age with us. Their DNA accumulates damage just like ours does.

As our mitochondria age, our once-balanced blend of oxidants-to-reductants tends to tip toward a surplus of oxidants, and a deficiency of reductants. That pushes us increasingly in the direction of oxidative stress as we grow older. However, too much of either one – oxidation or reduction – results in unregulated oxidation and cell damage. To complicate matters further, inefficient redox signaling sends unclear messages to the nucleus, which then makes fewer antioxidants.

In this situation, any sort of severe or prolonged damage can cause the immune system to dump oxidant into an area that it's not able to clean up properly due to reductant and/or antioxidant deficiency. So as oxidative stress, positive charge, and acidity build up in the cell, the clarity of the message conveyed by redox molecules declines.

From that point on, the immune system's oxidative response becomes its own worst enemy. Oxidant is dumped in the area to start the clean-up process, but cells don't have antioxidant reserves large enough to clean up the oxidation. Full healing never takes place. The immune system senses something's wrong, but it gets confused by the mixed signals, and failure of its tools to do their jobs properly. So it continues to promote the destructive component of inflammation, as it tries in vain to rebuild as best it can.

Neither side – destruction or healing – is able to prevail while the immune system is caught in a vicious cycle of antioxidant/reductant deficiency and imbalanced/unclear redox messaging. That's what's happening when acute inflammation turns into chronic inflammation. And that's how chronic inflammation causes disease. It's the failure of cells to repair or replace themselves effectively. Cells then continue to live and reproduce in an unrepaired state. That's most of what drives modern, degenerative diseases today – including heart disease, arthritis, Alzheimer's, cancer, diabetes, and GAPS conditions.

GAPS: Coined by gut-brain health pioneer Dr. Natasha Campbell-McBride, Gut and Psychology Syndrome conditions are gut imbalances, such as leaky gut and gut dysbiosis, that cause impaired brain function, such as ADD, autism, anxiety and depression.

Negative charge and alkalinity are synonymous with health and healing. Positive charge and acidity create inflammation and disease

If you had to pick only one metric to assess your relative state of health or sickness, electrical charge and pH belong near the top of that list. You can think of the two as pretty much the same thing in the body, because they're like dance partners. When oxidation steals electrons, cells and atoms gain positive charge. That means more corrosion, greater instability, and inflammation that doesn't know when to quit. It means your cells and atoms are literally falling apart and not repairing themselves efficiently, which is imbalance, sickness and aging, in a nutshell.

On the other hand, when your immune system is good at making antioxidants, and it has all the electrons it needs for reduction, the atoms in your cells stay happy and whole, instead of falling apart. We call this *neutralizing, quenching,* or *extinguishing* oxidative stress. This translates into better cell-cell communication, inflammation that starts and stops appropriately, and healing capacity to spare.

On the other side of the scale, acids have more protons than electrons, which gives them a positive charge. The more

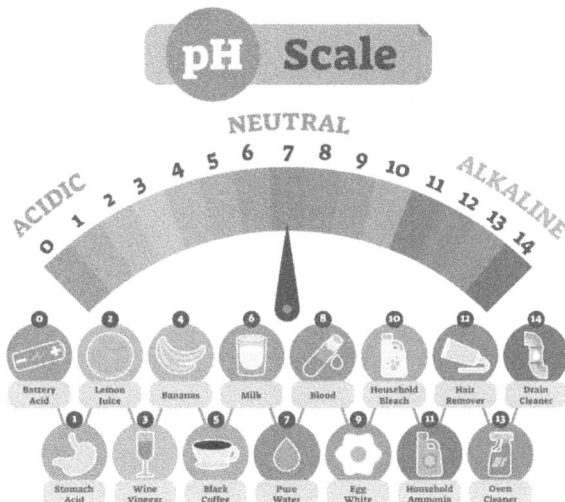

pH Scale

NEUTRAL

ACIDIC   0 1 2 3 4 5 6 7 8 9 10 11 12 13 14   ALKALINE

0 Battery Acid 2 Lemon Juice 4 Bananas 6 Milk 8 Blood 10 Household Bleach 12 Hair Remover 14 Drain Cleaner

1 Stomach Acid 3 Wine Vinegar 5 Black Coffee 7 Pure Water 9 Egg White 11 Household Ammonia 13 Oven Cleaner

protons a substance has, the more acidic it is. And the opposite is true: the more electrons something has in relation to protons, the greater its alkalinity. Hence, many alkaline foods and substances are famous for their healing/antioxidant effects.

In short, extra electrons are *negative charge* and *healing capacity* through oxidation quenching, and helping the immune system know when to shut down inflammation (alkalinity supports cell-cell communication). While at the other end of the spectrum, electron deficiency is *positive charge* and *poor healing ability* through corrosion, lack of light energy (electrons hold light energy), and failure to realize that inflammation is not working the way it should. Acidity aids and abets breakdown.

Disease is made possible by a shortage of energy

A shortage of systemic energy is involved in nearly every disease process. When cells don't have enough energy to do what they should be doing, they behave and replicate improperly. This makes organs malfunction, which we experience as dysfunction and disease. A form of energy widely used by the body is ATP. ATP is made in mitochondria, and is used to run dozens, if not hundreds, of systems and processes in the body. This is why mitochondria are often described as being power plants of the cell.

To illustrate why ATP availability matters, a large percentage of GAPS individuals, having been born with weak mitochondria, are genetically predisposed to energy deficiencies. In a state of energy deficiency, environmental exposures then pull the trigger to cause full-blown disease. Whether that exposure is from heavy metals, industrial chemicals, infection or antibiotics, these individuals can't make enough energy to overcome the environmental insult and pay for energetic needs, as well as luxuries.

When there is not enough of a broadly used energy currency to go around, something's got to give. In autism, that often means higher brain function and detoxification will be sacrificed to supply basic life support and repetitive muscle movement.

The body's energy needs are many, but supplies are limited

- **Basic life-support.** Heart, blood vessels, lungs.
- **Physical activity.** Muscles and nerves.
- **Brain function** (5% of body weight, consumes 20% of the glucose).
- **Digestion**.
- **Replenishing biochemicals** such as neurotransmitters and hormones.
- **Fighting infection.** Innate and adaptive immune response.
- **Cell replication.**
- **Muscle repair after exercise.**
- **Fighting aging**.
- **Detoxification.** Heavy metals, chemicals, metabolic waste products.

Of course, this is a fluid hierarchy of priorities that changes in response to shifting demands – the result being occasional conflicts, postponements, or cancellations of bodily processes. For instance, the GI tract puts digestion on hold when you exercise on a full stomach. Mental acuity drops in the latter stages of an endurance race when muscles need energy more than the brain. And the body throws every task that it can on the back burner while it's fighting a life-threatening illness like cancer or HIV-AIDS.

Point being, systems and processes are always vying to get their share of a limited supply of energy coming from food, sunlight, water and grounding/earthing. But when there isn't enough energy to satisfy every expenditure, the body must make choices and accept sacrifices. Compromises of this nature determine the way in which chronic disease affects you and your healing efforts.

Coming back to autism, the factors converging to put a person on the spectrum *lower* the production of energy in its various forms, while increasing demand, if anything. You can tell how bad the shortage is by counting the number of areas affected, and how high up the ladder they go. Nearly every physical and mental process is impacted.

Quick tip: ribose

Ribose is a 5-molecule sugar (table sugar is six) that the body uses as a building block to make ATP. It helps mitochondria make more energy on a cell level, which the body uses for dozens of processes. Ribose is an excellent supplement because it's reasonably strong (as natural supplements go) and very easy on the body. It's available over-the-counter and is lower on the glycemic index then regular sugar. I highly recommend it to improve your energy level – either therapeutically for conditions of chronic low energy, or as part of a daily routine.

Oxygen redox molecules
How food becomes ATP and oxygen redox molecules

Animals like us can't access any energy directly from the food we eat. Instead, we need our bacteria, mitochondria, and multiple processes to transform diverse energy caches, such as sugars and fats, into fewer forms that are more universally-accepted throughout the body, such as ATP, electrons and light.

In the mouth, chewing and saliva begin breaking down solid food. Next, the stomach uses hydrochloric acid and enzymes to turn pulverized food into a nutrient soup. Bacteria and enterocyte cells of the gut lining complete the digestive process. Food constituents go through the gut wall and enter the bloodstream. The liver then collects those nutrients from the bloodstream, converts them into simple fat or sugar, and returns them to circulation.

Once inside the cell, metabolic processes such as glycolysis deconstruct glucose or fat molecules to make precursors for the electron transport chain in mitochondria. Mitochondria finish the job of energy extraction and conversion by burning these base materials in the presence of oxygen to make ATP and a small percentage of oxygen radicals.

Note how many steps there are between the food you eat and fuel that your cells can use. Unfortunately, as we age, we lose about 1% of our mitochondria population per year. In that decline, so goes our energy production and redox signaling capacity. So by the time we're 70–85, we're down to 10% of the energy and healing capacity that we had as teenagers. And since mitochondrial redox molecules are the communication medium of cell repair, perhaps half of the aging process is a result of diminished redox signaling and repair.

The smartest scientists thought stable redox molecules were impossible
Around the late 2000s, researchers had been studying redox reactions intensively for 10+ years. At that time, some 100 scientific papers were published every month on the subject of redox reactions, representing about 300 months' worth of research produced every thirty days.

The consensus was that it could not be done: *redox molecules, stabilized outside the body.* The reason is, when mitochondria make reactive oxygen species, they only live a fraction of a second. They're so reactive they bond immediately and they're gone. So the idea of stable redox molecules – both inside or outside the body – was preposterous to researchers studying them. But that didn't keep one adventuresome startup from trying. Unfortunately, after $15 million dollars and twelve years of trying, the best they could do was keep oxygen redox molecules stable for ten minutes. But that wasn't long enough to make a viable product that consumers could benefit from. They went bankrupt.

But then Gary Samuelson, PhD (medical atomic physicist) did the impossible: having access to the first team's research materials, he took 18 months to develop a method to keep oxygen redox molecules stable for well over a year. Ultimately achieving a half-life of two years, Samuelson created a product that did things in the body that had never been done before. The product, called Asea, was launched in 2010 as a network marketing company. It was the first redox signaling supplement of its kind.

Asea™ (for mitochondrial communication)
Redox signaling molecules, in supplement form, offer wellness seekers huge improvements in cell-cell communication, healing, and anti-aging because redox signaling initiates so many things that cells do (and would like to do). To a large degree, the redox signaling system can either giveth life when it works well, or it can taketh away when it fails to perform as well as it did when we were young.

Asea™ helps

Disclaimer: This description of how Asea works is not approved or endorsed by the company that makes Asea. It is based on information available around 2015–2018. I have no association with The Company.

- **Protect.** Increase antioxidant effectiveness by 5X, thus raising your defenses against toxins, infections and aging.
- **Detect.** Makes cells aware when they're damaged.
- **Repair.** Activates genetic switches to make new proteins to repair damaged cells.
- **Replace.** Prompts un-repairable cells to kill themselves, and tells neighboring cells to fill in the void.
- **Hormone reception.** Normalizes hormonal response.
- **Detoxification.** Upregulates detoxification through NRF2 activation.
- **Energy.** Regulates mitochondrial productivity, thereby increasing energy production in the cell.

Independent research shows that Asea increases athletic performance – as measure by VO_2 max, ventricular threshold. One of its main mechanisms of action is that it mobilizes fatty acid stores (presumably from the abdomen) for cells to burn during exercise. Fat burning produces about twenty times more ATP than glucose.

By increasing fluency of redox signaling, middle-aged to senior adults (who have reduced redox signaling) can increase their mitochondrial population by 10–30%. That means individuals of this age can reverse many years of cellular degradation in terms of endurance, speed of recovery, sense of well-being, and healing capacity. This is why academics and users are so impressed with what Asea can do – though children and teenagers who have abundant redox signaling probably won't notice a huge difference.

Carbon redox molecules

Produced by the metabolism of bacteria, carbon redox molecules send and receive information related to the wellness or sickness of cells in the microbiome. In doing so, the awesome intelligence of the microbiome is transmitted through carbon redox signaling. Rich in minerals, carbon redox molecules also provide nutrients for bacteria to grow. This makes bacteria caretakers of the microbiome and their host. Carbon redox molecules are the microbiome's greatest strength when diverse and fully fluent. Conversely, they are the microbiome's Achilles heel when depleted and uncommunicative.

How bacteria make and use carbon redox molecules

Each of the tens of thousands of bacterial species makes 10–15 distinct carbon redox molecules as they metabolize food, resulting in hundreds of thousands to a million unique varieties. Dubbed "carbon snowflakes" due to their extremely varied molecular structures, carbon redox molecules are both a communication medium for cell-cell signaling, and they're a source of minerals for microbiota, like a compost-rich soil.

Each carbon snowflake has its own specialized role in cell-cell communication. Like words of a language, each variant communicates a slightly different message, for different purposes, and does things that others can't. This fluency of communication permits an unimaginable variety of messages to be broadcast to members of the entire community. For example, when redox signaling is present, depleted populations may realize they're endangered and ask neighboring species for more room to grow. Abundant populations relax so that rare species can go on a growth spurt.

But if redox smoke signals are absent, those bacteria can't tell how many of their kind are left. Without clear communications, they're not able to sense when more of them are needed. Hence, they stay endangered, or go extinct. This is one of the main mechanisms by which diversity in the gut has plummeted. Conversely, when probiotic bacteria are able to sense an overgrowth of pathogenic microbiota like candida, they sound the alarm for the whole probiotic team to start making more anti-fungals, anti-virals or anti-bacterials to knock back the decomposers.

The human gut used to host 20,000–30,000 species of bacteria

A booming intestinal ecosystem in a healthy person once contained the biodiversity you might see in a coral reef or thriving rain forest. The human gut used to host perhaps 20,000–30,000 kinds of bacteria – some say as much as 100,000. However, modern society's questionable ways have taken a toll on that variety and balance. Antagonists include

- herbicides like glyphosate
- chemical fertilizers
- antibiotics in meat and medicine
- industrial toxins such as bisphenol-A, PCBs and phthalates
- pharmaceuticals like NSAIDs, birth control pills and steroids
- heavy metals in personal care products.

So, today, you'd be fortunate to have 10,000 species – as evidenced by a 2010 NIH study, which mapped the genome of the human microbiome. It took 44 participants to reach 10,000 species of bacteria – down to ½ to ⅓ of what it used to be. This narrowing of species has put an enormous dent in the microbiome's ability to protect us from tight junction injury and toxin exposure, as well as take care of the gut, which then takes care of us.

Lack of diversity in the microbiome starts in the soil

For millennia, traditional farming techniques supported diversity in the soil through manure, polycultures, crop rotation and composting. But now, Big Ag grows (1) one crop on a plot of land year after year, (2) using inorganic chemical fertilizers and (3) crop amendments like glyphosate, (4) in an increasingly lifeless soil food web. These unnatural actions destroy microlife in the soil. A broken ecosystem in the soil then gives a plant fewer nutrients and more toxins to pass to its consumers.

Fewer nutrients in a plant mean less nutrition for our beneficial bacteria to feed on. That means rare species, which are skilled at digesting trace minerals, get malnourished and neglected. So, in a state of: (1) starvation, (2) blindness to their endangerment, and (3) slow repopulation, rare species of bacteria are under pressure to disappear from our microbiome. Meanwhile, human antibiotics devastate our microbiomes acutely, while toxins in our food, water, air, medicine and personal care products beat up survivors on a daily basis.

Diversity of species, and fluency of communication, gives the microbiome strength and resiliency – not just an absence of pathogens

This is one of the rare cases where the natural healing community, in the 1990s and 2000s, failed to understand the microbiome almost as much mainstream medicine, because both groups had flawed beliefs. Namely, the presence of pathogens is *a* problem in gut dysbiosis, but it's not *the whole* problem, leading to disappointing results. The truth of the matter is, diversity of species and fluency of communication give the microbiome its ability to nourish the body and protect you from injury. Let's see how a few of the popular approaches to improving gut health in the 1990s and 2000s have worked out.

Probiotic supplements. When probiotic supplements first became popular, health professionals thought they would do a lot more good for people than they actually have. Eager to use this promising new healing tool, practitioners of all types recommended that their clients take probiotics to rebalance their gut flora and hopefully reverse their chronic gut issues. But the results have been mixed.

Many would say their pathogen overgrowth, like candida, seemed to recede at the time they took the probiotic. Symptoms subsided and they felt better for a while, but not necessarily well. So probiotics helped a good number of people, a fair amount, temporarily. A modest percentage of people in thousands of studies showed marginal results. But most healers now admit that probiotic supplements don't get your gut anywhere near fully healthy, whether taken alone, or in combination with other things.

Probiotic supplements did not meet people's admittedly high expectations when they first hit the scene because their ingredients are contrived due to labeling standards. You see, most "controlled" formulas give you three to seven strains of bacteria, and thus limited benefits. On the other hand, probiotics made from wild sources will naturally have a wider variety of robust species – although their populations can't be named and quantified on a label the way man-made ones can. As a result, mass-produced probiotics are generally weaker and less complementary to the digestive tract, and therefore not as efficacious.

Digestive enzymes, hydrochloric acid (HCL) supplements, and acid-blocking drugs have shown similar results. Many folks have found them useful in treating symptoms, but not one of them has solved digestive disorders indefinitely. The reason is, probiotic supplements, acid blockers, acid enhancers, and digestive enzymes are trying to solve the wrong problem. They're close. And you may relieve some symptoms being in the right ballpark. But restoring cell-cell communication looks like it's more valuable to the microbiome than simply driving pathogens out, or covering up symptoms for a while. Diversity appears to benefit the GI tract most – even more than strength of individual species.

In contrast, almost all commercial probiotic supplements are made from a small number of bacteria species sourced from cow intestines and cultured in isolation. The problem is, those bacteria are not prevalent colonizers of the human intestinal tract due to vast differences in pH, digestive enzymes, and overall design (i.e., four stomachs instead of one).

But, as crazy as it sounds, ingesting cow bacteria can provide some benefit for a really screwed up microbiome that's filled with the microbial equivalent of weeds such as candida, klebsiella, pseudomonas and E. coli. Microbiota from cows can do some of the things that our native bacteria do. But nowhere near the whole shebang of systemic benefit needed to support immaculate health. Bottom line: It's better to get biodiversity back in the microbiome than the artificial environment of (most) probiotic supplements, digestive enzymes, acid enhancers or acid blockers.

Fermented foods follow the same rules

Most store-bought fermented foods such as yogurt, sauerkraut and kimchee are made from a very limited number of bacterial species added as starter cultures (usually one or two species). This applies pressure to the microbiome to narrow its diversity of species. Yogurt is the naughtiest of the bunch due to having only two bacterial species, high sugar content, casein, and a bare minimum of fermentation time. Plus, yogurt's digestive benefits tend to be greatly oversold by food companies, giving you a false sense of security.

In contrast, you don't add any starter culture when you ferment vegetables the wild way. You simply let the microbes that found their way onto the surface of the vegetable go the work. Doing it naturally like this, you may get hundreds of potent, soil-based microbes joining the party. So, in summary: Wild fermented veggies are great for you. Standard fermented veggie products are good for you. And conventional yogurts and fermented dairy products give you some benefits to go with some drawbacks.

Tight junctions and leaky membranes
Protective membranes in the gut, brain, blood vessels, kidneys and liver are held together by tight junctions

Membranes. Membranes are a specialized layer of tissue just one cell thick that acts as a firewall between an organ's exterior (pre-absorption) and its interior (post-absorption). At just 50 microns – about half the width of a human hair – they function as a barrier against unauthorized entry, as well as serving roles in nutrition, hydration, detoxification and immunity. At its simplest, membranes actively keep harmful things out, while letting beneficial things through. The entire GI tract is protected by these dynamic, intelligent membranes that run from your sinuses and mouth, to your throat and stomach, through the small and large intestine, all the way out your rectum. Every major organ in your body relies on a membrane to separate its "outards" from its innards.

Tight junctions. Just as important, every cell in every membrane is held to its neighbor by a set of interlocking protein fibers, called *tight junctions*. These cross-linking fibers act like Velcro: they open and close when the immune system wants to send cells through the membrane to fight threats on the other side.

Tight junction intelligence. That ability to open and close on purpose is what gives membranes the intelligence that they lose when tight junctions are damaged by excessive zonulin.

Zonulin. Zonulin production is hyperactivated when the gut wall is exposed to toxins and certain pathogens. Unfortunately for modern humans, overproduction of zonulin breaks down the tight junctions. That means excess zonulin is the most potent and prevalent mediator of leaky gut, leaky membranes, food sensitivities, autoimmunity and GAPS conditions, as well as a major contributor to chronic inflammation and disease.

Probiotic bacteria protect tight junctions from injury
- They: protect you from tight junction damage by gobbling up toxic peptides that raise zonulin level
- control pathogens that stimulate zonulin production
- increase production of DDP4 enzyme that breaks down zonulin, after it's been made
- nourish and protect enterocytes that line the gut wall
- reduce inflammation and immune activation of the GALT
- provide minerals (in redox molecules) that support microbiota
- support diversity of carbon redox molecules that are the communication network of awareness, defense, repair and replacement of microbiota

Sources of tight junction injury

The biggest threats to tight junctions are glyphosate, gluten, NSAID pain-killers like ibuprofen, steroids, and pathogens such as candida, clostridium difficile and cholera. Tragically, these are everywhere. Glyphosate, for example, is the active ingredient in most herbicides. That means it's in our soil, drinking water and organic food. It's in our blood, mothers' breastmilk and urine. You can't avoid it. In fact, recent reports say 75% of the world's rainwater contains harmful levels of glyphosate.

And we have the US EPA to thank for setting up the regulations that allow (practically dare) Big Ag, Big Pharma, and Big Food to assault us chronically with this existential-level poison. Just one example of the toxicity ceiling being raised for no good reason: In 2013, the US EPA passed a **30-fold increase** in the allowable limit of glyphosate on many US food crops... just because the chemicals companies asked for it.

How glyphosate and gluten cause leaky membranes, allergies, chronic inflammation and degenerative diseases

The diagram below illustrates how toxins in the diet, and pathogens in the gut, trigger a cascade of events that: breakdown tight junctions, turn membranes leaky, induce food intolerances and autoimmunity, increase chronic inflammation, and cause dysfunction throughout the body.

How that pathway to disease gets turned on: Gluten (gliadin), glyphosate and pathogens introduce toxic peptides into the intestinal tract that make gut mucosa produce way too much zonulin. Zonulin dissolves tight junctions in the gut wall whose purpose is to keep the gut virtually impenetrable to inappropriate material. This is what causes leaky gut. Hyper-permeability of the gut then leaks zonulin into the bloodstream, which goes everywhere. Zonulin proceeds to attack membranes all over the body, resulting in leaky blood-brain barrier, blood vessels, kidney tubules, liver cells, and more.

Meanwhile, just behind the gut wall sits the gut associated lymphoid tissue (GALT, for short), which makes 80% of the immune system's antibodies. Broken tight junctions expose the GALT to all the hazardous substances in the digestive tract. This irritates the lymphatic system, which exhausts its antioxidant reservoirs, dysregulates the immune system, and unleashes chronic inflammation. And, as just discussed, unrelenting inflammation drives all degenerative diseases, most noteworthy for this audience: ADD and GAPS conditions.

Diagram used courtesy of Dr. Zach Bush.

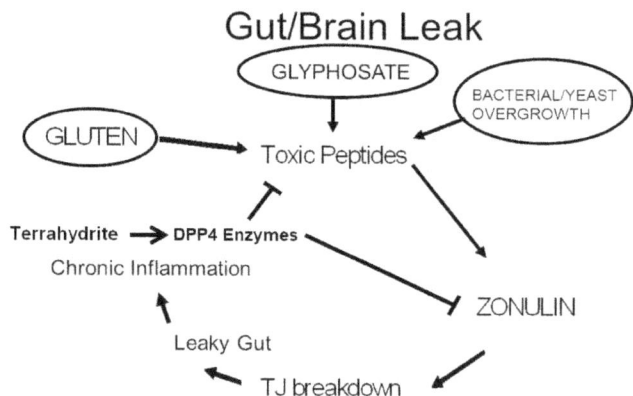

Gut/Brain Leak

Dr. Zach Bush on *how you can tell if you've got a leaky gut*
"If you've got a gut, and you live on planet earth, you've got a leaky gut. That's pretty much where we're at right now."

Other effects of broken tight junction and leaky membranes
Tight junction injury spreads imbalance, toxicity and dysfunction throughout the body, which shows up as a loss of membrane integrity/intelligence, dehydration, nutrient deficiency, and loss of cellular communication. Leaky membranes affect the body in many ways:

Mitochondrial insufficiency lowers electrical charge. When mitochondria slow down (concurrent with diminished redox signaling), the cell loses electrical charge. Electrical charge is what pulls water into the cell. So as mitochondrial activity goes down, dehydration goes up inside the cell (where it counts).

Collecting and directing fluids where they need to go. Leaky membranes impair cell function through dehydration. When membranes lose selectivity over what they let through *vs.* what they block, membranes lose their intelligence. They lose their ability to control where fluid goes in the body. You could be drinking eight glasses of water a day. But if the colon can't pull water out of your food properly, distribute it to cells via the bloodstream, and get it into cells the way it should – all tight junction dependent – you could suffer dehydration in the cells. At the same time, water is the vehicle that takes nutrients into cells, and waste out, thus nutrient deficiency goes up, while detoxification declines.

Nutrient surpluses and deficits. Each cell type has its own nutritional requirements. Muscles crave protein (as amino acids). Nervous system cells love fatty acids and cholesterol. Thyroid cells are big fans of iodine. And liver cells can use all the antioxidant vitamins they can get. Mismanagement of water causes some cells to get more nutrients than they can use (becoming toxic in excess), while others downstream are starved because they were supposed to get those nutrients delivered to them. So no one's happy when membranes fall apart.

Immune system irritation in the nose creates seasonal allergies. When you have intact membranes in the sinus passages, you can breathe pollen and pet dander all day long and not have a problem. But when permeable membranes let allergens into the sinus tissue (where they don't belong), the immune system in the sinuses overreacts. It responds by releasing antibodies to fight the intrusion of foreign material, which triggers the release of histamine. That's what seasonal allergies are: nasal sinus irritation, followed by histamine release. Of course, conventional medicine combats this effect by (chemically) blocking histamine, which fights the symptom, not the source.

Increased nnEMF sensitivity: A growing percentage of people are sensitive to nnEMF pollution because of the damage that glyphosate, gluten, and various pharmaceuticals do to tight junctions. What's happening at a cell level is, when tight junctions disintegrate, cell signaling goes down, cells can't sync their vibrational frequency to each other. The whole fabric of the membrane loses vibrational coherence. When that happens, stray electromagnetic frequencies become the predominate vibration they're exposed to. So instead of healthy frequencies supporting a cell's well-being, cells are violently shaken at rates that injure, confuse, and extinguish them.

Fortunately, Nature hid the antidote to man's self-destruction in the ground beneath our feet

In 2012, William Vitalis showed Dr. Zach Bush a white paper about soil science, hoping to learn why half of Dr. Bush's patients responded well to a plant-based diet, while the other half didn't get better, or even got worse.

As Dr. Bush flipped through the pages, a molecule jumped out at him that looked similar to the compounds he had been studying involving communication of the mitochondria – only this molecule was predominately made of carbon, instead of oxygen. The molecule looked like it had greater redox signaling potential. And it looked to be significantly more stable than redox molecules from mitochondria. Might this have been used for cell-cell signaling by whatever it was that made it? Might it be used therapeutically if they could find out how to make it in volume?

It took his group two weeks to find out that the molecule, from soil, was indeed made by a bacterium, and it definitely had signaling potential. This led Dr. Bush to realize that bacteria have a communication network, first of all. And it's the same whether they live in soil, or in a mammal's digestive tract. These were brand-new ideas to medical science. The field was already studying mitochondria and their redox signaling molecules. But bacterial redox molecules had yet to be discovered and studied properly. That begged the investigation into what carbon redox molecules are designed to do, and what they potentially could do, when put to good use.

Dr. Bush's team invented a way to make carbon redox molecules

Knowing it would be darn near impossible to find someone with a perfect microbiome today, Dr. Bush went about finding soil that had the diversity he was looking for, yet wasn't polluted with chemicals. That ruled out wet climates, and soil exposed to air. He ended up finding highly compressed, fossilized remains of soil, buried in the desert Southwest of the United States. Dating back fifty million years, this layer of "lignite extract" is eight feet thick and biologically inert when it's pulled from the ground.

He took the carbon-rich sediment back to his lab, and a colleague of his taught him how to reanimate its bioactivity by restoring its mineral ratios and amino acid balance back to that of living soil. When he did that, voilà, the oxygen and hydrogen binding sites woke up, restoring the molecule's functionality as a medium of communication. What's more, the compound was shelf stable. So, finally, here was the very same signaling system that bacteria use for their communication – in a bottle, and non-perishable. Think of what it could do.

Carbon redox molecules become a viable product

The first order of business with any new substance intended for human consumption is to test it for toxicity. So Dr. Bush applied the compound to kidney tubule cells. He was amazed but not surprised to find out that it's one of the least toxic substances ever discovered – even less toxic than water. You can drown in it, but exposure to ridiculously high concentrations just makes extremely sensitive cells live longer.

The next thing Dr. Bush did after getting carbon redox molecules into a stable and non-toxic form is he tested them on cancer cells. A burst of reactive oxygen species shot out from the mitochondria, indicating the need for oxidation was detected and deployed. Then he put the compound on healthy control cells and the exact opposite occurred: ROS production went down – meaning less oxidation was needed and produced. This meant that if cells were unwell, more potent healing mechanisms were mobilized to accelerate repair and replacement. But if cells were healthy, the immune system reduced the oxidative stress load.

This shocked and amazed him and his team even more than the toxicity results, because it was the first time any of them had seen a substance produce two completely different reactions, based on what cells needed. Further research has revealed that bacteria do indeed use carbon redox molecules for cell-cell signaling. And the diversity found in ancient ecosystems can be supplied as a supplement. Keep in mind, the idea of stable, renewable carbon redox molecules was brand-new to the literature in 2012.

But, eventually, the magnitude of the discovery hit him: When you repair tight junction injury, you can fix leaky gut. Integrity of the gut lining then enables the microbiome and GI tract to nourish the body as intended, and protect the immune system from dysregulation and overactivation. This could have a huge impact on the mental and physical well-being of those reliant on commercial farming, organized medicine, and ways of our modern world. It could reverse a lot of the damage being done to us, or protect us from it.

Dr. Bush points out that ION Gut Support™ (formerly Restore) does not treat cancer, or any disease for that matter. Instead, it reestablishes the redox signaling network by which bacteria communicate, proliferate, and support the health of the gut. That helps the body to look after itself.

Dr. Bush then asked a pivotal question

"What happens if we stop trying to micromanage and over-engineer our gut bacteria (e.g., with probiotics) and, instead, just give back the cell-cell signaling the gut is supposed to have?"

ION Gut Support™

ION Gut Support™ does at least six things to repair tight junctions and create a thriving ecosystem in the gut:

1. Breaks down toxic peptides that trigger zonulin production, and zonulin itself (after the gut makes it), protecting tight junctions.
2. Restores the communication network between bacterial species.
3. Rebalances minerals in the microbiome so enzymes work.
4. Increases glutathione production 1,200% in the gut.
5. Increases stem cell activity by 30% in the gut.
6. Neutralizes toxins in the gut 10 to 50 times better. endorsed

1. Carbon redox molecules in ION Gut Support™ keep the membranes in your body well protected against tight junction injury. This seals your gut lining and heals the microbiome. By repairing gut permeability, ION Gut Support™ reduces food intolerances, chronic inflammation, psychological disorders, and autoimmunity.

2. Helps bacteria talk to each other and the immune system. Fluent communication between bacteria makes the group aware when pathogens have overgrown, so the good guys can go into rapid replication and drive pathogen populations down with antimicrobial compounds.

3. Rebalances the mineral composition of the GI tract to that of a healthy gut – like natural fertilizer for the microbiome. This makes micronutrients available for the production of enzymes that drive cell function. When you have diversity in your microbiome, a lot of health problems go away for good. The microbiome can then revive its balance and numbers from the 5,000–10,000 species it has today, to something closer to the 20,000–30,000 species ideal, once present in humans.

These efforts create a cascade of protective and restorative effects in previously corrupted systems. For instance, **(4)** when terrahydrite touches the wall of the small bowel, there's a **1,200% increase in glutathione** production in a matter of hours (the body's most powerful antioxidant). **(5)** One tablespoon of terrahydrite increases **stem cell activity by 30%.** And **(6) detoxification,** hydration, and nutrient absorption are also improved.

Bottom line: When the gut has what it needs to thrive – that is, when man gets out his own way and lets Nature do the driving – the body's innate intelligence knows what needs to be done, and it has the equipment to do it. ION Gut Support™ helps accomplish that, so long as toxins are an unavoidable part of our lives.

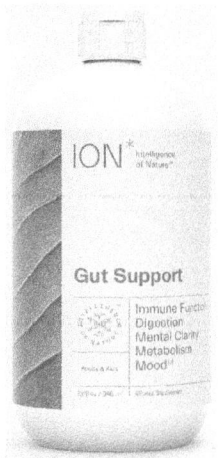

Disclaimer: This description of how ION Gut Support works is not approved or endorsed by the company that makes ION Gut Support. It is based on information available around 2015–2018. I have no association with The Company.

Redox molecules are here to stay

Of course, you still need to eat well. Dr. Bush reminds us that having perfect membrane function is not a license to eat whatever you want. You still need to eat well, and avoid the bad stuff.

Plants love ION Gut Support™. Not unexpected, but still fascinating to watch, ION Gut Support™ makes plants grow faster. This is exactly what we would expect, considering the raw material in ION Gut Support™ is the very same bacterial communication that promoted ancient plant growth, once-upon-a-time.

Scientists recently discovered sensors in the gut. They found out that neural dendrites, which are remote extensions of the brain, actually poke through the lining of the gut, and collect information about the microbiome, without a membrane between them. Presumably, the brain and nervous system are literally reaching into gut's ecosystem with nerve sensors to gather intel about what's happening in the GI tract.

It's possible that carbon redox molecules transmit messages to the brain through these neural dendrites about the gut's microbiota, contents, and enterocyte cells. This may be one of the reasons that brain function is enhanced when ION Gut Support™ seals the gut wall and rebalances the microbiome. It could be why concentration, sleep quality, memory and brain fog improve when people take ION Gut Support™.

The field of redox science has only just begun. The last 15–20 years have taught the wellness community new methods of repairing, defending, and resisting aging with redox signaling. Gary Samuelson, PhD, Dr. Zach Bush, and their teams have successfully learned how to stabilize redox molecules and present them as supplements to wellness seekers around the world. The field has learned a great deal over the past decade-and-a-half. Yet, many believe we've only uncovered the tip of the iceberg in understanding how redox molecules can be used in and outside the body.

———— ⟳ ————

PART 2

———— ❧ ————

Microbes and Our Corrupted Guts

7

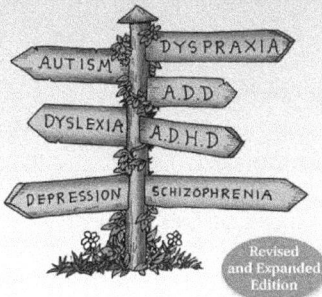

Gut and Psychology Syndrome

Natural treatment for

AUTISM · DYSPRAXIA · A.D.D · DYSLEXIA · A.D.H.D · DEPRESSION · SCHIZOPHRENIA

Revised and Expanded Edition

Dr. Natasha Campbell-McBride MD,
MMedSci(neurology), MMedSci(nutrition)

A MOTHER'S DETERMINATION TO HEAL HER SON STARTS A WORLDWIDE AWAKENING

When Dr. Natasha Campbell-McBride started talking about the gut-brain connection 20 years ago, pretty much everyone laughed at her

But not anymore. Her teachings that once seemed peculiar and speculative are quickly proving to be scientific fact. Today, there's millions pouring into scientific research and the development of commercial products supporting gut health. The gut-brain connection seems self-evident now that esteemed institutions, doctors and media are talking about it. Meanwhile, big money interests have hopped on the bandwagon in developing probiotic supplements and cultured foods, such as yogurt and kombucha.

You see, all truth goes through three stages: First, it's ridiculed. Then, it's violently opposed. Third, it's generally accepted as being the obvious truth – as if everyone knew it all along. As a result, Dr. Natasha suddenly (after twenty years) finds herself at the forefront of a worldwide revolution in understanding the connection between the gut, the brain, and the body.

What inspired Dr. Natasha to get into medicine, and then gut-brain health?

At 18 months of age, Natasha came down with a very serious bout of food poisoning and almost died. She lost a lot of weight and had terrible digestive problems. So her parents sent her to live with her grandparents, at their village in the Ural Mountains, where they had a small family farm with livestock, poultry and a garden.

Her grandmother, who was a village healer, herbalist and therapist, took her in and cured her. And she cured Natasha with diet... with food. As she grew up, Natasha would spend school holidays in the village with her grandmother, observing how she would cook, prepared food, and use food as medicine. Natasha would observe her grandmother helping villagers not only their health problems, but family and life problems as well. She always had good advice.

Natasha was very impressed seeing the world of good that a healer can do in the lives of others, so she decided to follow in her grandmother's footsteps. In 1984, Natasha Campbell-McBride graduated with honors as a medical doctor from Bashkir Medical University in Russia. She later earned a post-graduate degree in neurology, and practiced five years as a neurologist, three years as a neurosurgeon.

Just a few years into her career, she noticed an unlikely coincidence in her patients

She noticed that most of the patients she was seeing for neurological conditions also had severe digestive disorders. But, to her disappointment, medical specialists don't usually talk to each other to understand how bodily systems interconnect, and how they could fix the problems presented to them. Instead, specialists tend to treat bodily systems as separate and unrelated.

In her case, neurologists don't talk to gastroenterologists to make connections between the brain and the gut. As a result, Dr. Natasha's observation that most psychology patients have terrible digestive problems might have remained coincidence and speculation in her mind, had life not thrown her this curveball: At three years of age, things went horribly wrong for her son. His behavior and social skills grew increasingly abnormal. He was diagnosed severely autistic.

When she discovered her own profession had nothing to offer them besides coping strategies, she, as a mother, refused to accept that. She threw herself into intensive study about how autism originates in the body. She went back to university, studied everything she could find on the subject, and spoke to hundreds of people. Eventually, she came up with answers and solutions to reverse autism in her child. And, with her son's full participation, she cured him. Today, her son is a healthy, happy young man – fully recovered and leading a normal life. They've forgotten about autism long ago.

This trial by fire is what led Dr. Natasha on her personal and professional journey. She earned a second post-graduate degree in human nutrition from Sheffield University in the UK. As she worked with her son to correct his challenges, she returned to work and started treating other children with autism and learning disabilities to great success. News spread, and people with all sorts of psychiatric conditions began to seek her out.

Today, Dr. Natasha's many years of investigation and treatment became a program that explains and corrects the root causes of many psychological and physiological disorders. It's called G.A.P.S., which stands for both Gut and *Psychology* Syndrome, as well as Gut and *Physiology* Syndrome.

The concept of GAPS is revolutionizing our understanding of chronic, degenerative disease, because it explains the mechanisms of action by which disorder in the digestive tract becomes mental, physical and autoimmune challenges in the body. The GAPS healing protocol tells you how to use food, probiotics, and detox protocols to heal the root causes of modern disease, at the source.

Dr. Natasha is now recognized as a world-leading authority on treating children and adults with learning disabilities and other mental disorders. As a pioneer in describing the gut-brain connection, she is an in-demand speaker, author, and advocate for the natural treatment of autism, ADD/ADHD, dyslexia, dyspraxia, depression and schizophrenia. Her books include: *Gut and Psychology Syndrome*, *Put Your Heart in Your Mouth*, *Vegetarianism Explained,* and *Gut and Physiology Syndrome.*

GAPS was born out of Dr. Haas' Specific Carbohydrate Diet

Renowned American pediatrician, Dr. Sidney V. Haas, invented the Specific Carbohydrate Diet (SCD) in the first half of the 20th Century. He treated over 600 celiac patients with excellent results. After at least a year on the regiment, he saw no relapses, deaths, crises, pulmonary events, or stunting of growth in his patients.

In 1951, he and his son, Dr. Merrill P. Haas, published their results in the medical textbook *The Management of Celiac Disease.* Shortly thereafter, The Specific Carbohydrate Diet was generally accepted as a cure for celiac disease, which was described within. Unfortunately, in those days, celiac disease was not well understood or clearly defined, which resulted in many disorders of the gut being classified as celiac disease. Later, celiac disease came to be defined as gluten intolerance, which then excluded a large percentage of digestive disorders from the definition of celiac disease.

Problem was, because the medical community thought gluten intolerance and celiac disease were one and the same, the gluten-free diet was soon proclaimed to be the treatment of choice for celiac disease. So the SCD diet was dismissed as no longer being relevant. That effectively ended all research into finding treatments for inflammatory gut conditions that fell outside the box of celiac disease, because they thought they had the cure.

Following the mix up, the Specific Carbohydrate Diet would have been forgotten, were it not for a desperate mom that found success treating her daughter with the diet. Elaine Gottschall's little girl suffered from severe ulcerative colitis and neurological problems, and went to see Dr. Haas in 1958.

Two years on the diet turned out to be a smashing success. Elaine's daughter was completely symptom free, energetic and thriving. Eternally grateful to Dr. Haas and the diet for giving her daughter the gift of excellent health, Gottschall took up the mission of helping others using the diet. For years, she studied the biological effects of the diet on the human body, which culminated in her book *Breaking the Vicious Cycle: Intestinal Health Through Diet.* Since then, she and her book have helped thousands of people overcome Crohn's disease, ulcerative colitis, celiac disease, diverticulitis, and other digestive disorders.

Along the way, many children have also reversed their behavioral difficulties such as autism, hyperactivity and night terrors. All of which helped Dr. Natasha refine the SCD diet over years of clinical practice into her own version tailored to today's gut dysbiosis and mental health issues. But curiously, it was her patients that dubbed her food-based diet the "GAPS diet."

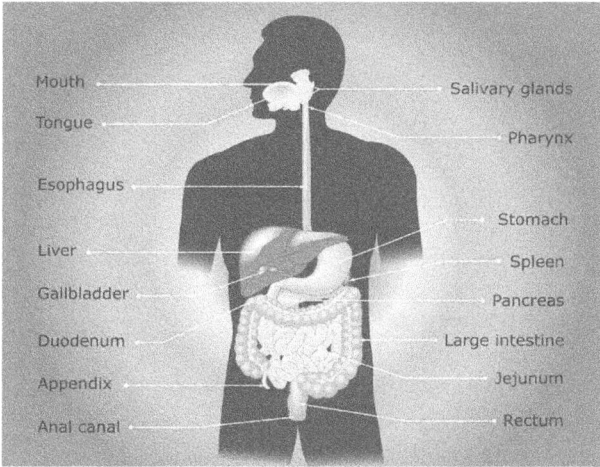

Mouth • Salivary glands
Tongue • Pharynx
Esophagus
• Stomach
Liver • Spleen
Gallbladder • Pancreas
Duodenum • Large intestine
Appendix • Jejunum
Anal canal • Rectum

8

THE HUMAN DIGESTIVE TRACT AND COMMON PROBLEMS

The digestive tract plays major roles in digestion, assimilation, detoxification, elimination and more

The gastrointestinal tract (GI tract) is the most underappreciated system in the human body, considering all that it does for us. The GI tract consists of several organs that run from the mouth to the anus that are responsible for breaking down foods into smaller bits, separating useful substances from un-useful, and compressing waste material for removal.

For simplicity, we'll use the phrases "GI tract, digestive tract, or digestive system" almost interchangeably to describe organs that handle digestion. That said, when we talk about to "the gut," I'm usually referring to the small intestine, large intestine, in some cases supporting organs, and occasionally the stomach. We're going to focus most of our attention on the small intestine and large intestine (aka the colon or bowel) because the gut is where the majority of where wellness or illness is created in a person.

Hippocrates said, "All disease begins in the gut"

Modern humans now realize just how insightful he was in saying this. It may have taken two thousand years for minds to finally meet, but medical science has learned over the past two decades why gut health supports overall wellness, or contributes to the disease process. As for the general public, people once-resistant to trusting Nature and natural healing techniques are hearing about the gut-brain connection, learning the do's and don'ts, and are making wiser decisions such as avoiding oral antibiotics and eating fermented foods.

We've all heard it said: The most important thing in life is your health. Without your health, nothing else matters. Therefore, the gut is largely responsible for laying the foundation for a good life: energy, brain function, disease resistance, detoxification and longevity.

Conversely, almost all mental, physical and immune disorders are born in a disordered digestive tract. A corrupted gut, as I call intestinal imbalances, causes almost every chronic, degenerative disease. Specifically, the microbial populations residing in your intestines either nourish and protect you, or they poison you chronically and degrade your mental, physical and immunological capacity – depending on whether good bugs or bad ones predominate.

Terminology for the gut's community of microorganisms

Around the mid-late 2000s, the health community started calling the ecosystem of microbes in your gut the "microbiome," and the microbes themselves "microbiota" – after having been called "gut flora" or "microflora" for decades. Technically, the term microbiome means all the microorganisms living inside of you and out, that are not your own cells. But, more commonly, *microbiome* refers to just the microbes inside your intestinal tract.

This mass of microbes either work diligently to create a state of health-fulness in you, or they actively take it away from you, depending on which team the microbes play for. Most often, we call the friendly, helpful variety "probiotic," "beneficial," or simply "good bugs." While, we call the detrimental microbes "pathogenic" (meaning disease-causing), "invasive" (a bit of a misnomer, since they're always present to some degree), "unfriendly," or simply "bad bugs." When pathogens overpopulate the gut compared to good guys, I call this situation a *corrupted gut*. The technical term for a corrupted gut is "gut dysbiosis." Let's go over the anatomy, function, and dysfunction of the GI tract, so you can understand how digestion and absorption are supposed to work in a person.

The human digestive tract

The human digestive tract is a 30-foot-long tube, with lots of folds and bends, of varying surfaces and purposes, that runs from the mouth to the anus. The GI tract: centers around the (1) small intestine; upwards to the (2) stomach, throat and mouth; downwards to the (3) large intestine, and sideways to the (4) supporting organs.

In the business district of the gut, a semi-permeable section of the small intestine serves as our primary border between us and the outside world. The cells lining this section of the gut wall heavily influence what happens in all other areas of the body, because it is the membrane through which nutrition, hydration, toxins, and pathogens either enter the bloodstream and body, or they get blocked.

Equally important, a border is nothing without personnel to tend it. So this area is filled with a wide variety of microorganisms that we now call the microbiome. This microbial community actively detains and deports harmful substances. It maintains the physical integrity of the intestinal wall by nourishing its cells. And it helps feed the entire body through digestion and absorption.

Things you eat don't become part of you until they pass through the gut wall and enter the bloodstream

As food travels through the digestive tract, it's still effectively part of the outside world and inaccessible to the body. Food products have to get through the intestinal wall and reach the bloodstream before they can become internalized and nutritionally beneficial. Until this happens, food products are prepared for use by our microbes in the body's staging area of the gut.

Regulating this multi-stage process, the intestinal wall has a complex surface with lots of finger-like protrusions to optimize surface area and absorption capacity. If you were to lay the folds of the intestine flat, it would cover a tennis court, if not two. Enormous surface area is required to efficiently process the volume and variety of food particles passing through the gut. But, with huge territory, comes substantial risk.

With your bloodstream, immune system, organs, and brain function on the other side of that barrier, a lot of real estate can become vulnerable to unauthorized access. When selective permeability of the gut wall is intact, an expansive border is not a problem. But when the gut lining is porous and leaky, lots of territory is left undefended.

For this reason, Nature covered every square millimeter of our gut wall with a thick layer of bacteria and other microbial life, collectively called *microbiota*. These microbes form a barrier comprised of thousands of different strains of bacteria, yeasts, fungi, viruses, parasites and even mold – totaling 3–5 pounds and several trillion individual cells. But, as we in the Western world are learning one way or another, a healthy gut is becoming the exception, not the rule. Let's examine the architecture of the gut wall to learn why our health depends on it.

Image used under Creative Commons 4.0 license. Author: BallenaBlanca.

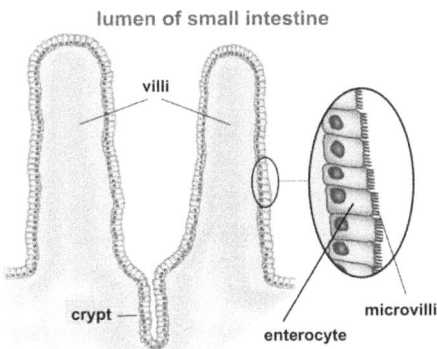

lumen of small intestine
villi
crypt
microvilli
enterocyte

Anatomy of the small intestine

The finger-like protrusions that line the gut are called "villi" (plural). And every "villus" (singular) is covered by a layer of "enterocytes" one-cell thick along its surface. Like wall-to-wall carpeting, enterocytes are the cells that complete the digestive process by breaking down food particles and letting them into the bloodstream. They also serve as a "castle wall" by blocking harmful substances from getting into the bloodstream and body.

Enterocytes work so hard at digesting and defending, they're only designed to live 3 to 5 days

Enterocytes are born at the bottom of "crypts," which are valleys between villi. Over the course of 3–5 days, enterocytes move up the villi like an escalator as they perform functions of digestion and absorption. When they reach the top of the villi, they mature, die and are shed.

Critical to digestion, each enterocyte has long hairs on its head called "microvilli" that perform the last steps of digestion. For this, microvilli produce enzymes that break down food particles into useful molecules. Maximizing digestion of the GI tract, these microvilli form a so-called "brush border" along the entire surface of the small intestine.

Now, one of the defining characteristics of Gut and Psychology Syndrome is ailing enterocytes. They weaken when malnourished and exposed to toxins and pathogens. Their journey time up the villi may then double, in which case old, decrepit enterocytes try in vain to do the work of healthy, young enterocytes. Plus, the hair on their heads gets fried, which prevents the microvilli's enzymes from completing digestion. As a result, food particles enter the bloodstream in an inappropriate form, rather than molecules ready to be metabolized by cells and mitochondria. Partially-digested proteins are notorious for causing problems because the immune system mistakes them for your own proteins.

Zooming back out, each enterocyte is firmly, but release-ably, joined to its neighbor by an adhesive-like protein called a *tight junction*, which acts like Velcro. Produced by enterocytes, zonulin regulates the permeability of tight junctions. It controls the timing and degree to which enterocytes open in its presence or close in its absence. Like a zipper, zonulin regulates the (1) passage of nutrients and materials through the gut *into* the bloodstream, (2) blockage of toxins such as heavy metals, and (3) transmission of immune cells *out of the bloodstream* into various tissues.

Unintelligent *vs.* intelligent filters

To appreciate what the gut lining does for you all day, every day, let's examine the way that conventional water and air filters operate. They are unintelligent filters that passively sort substances by size – basically arresting unwanted material larger than a certain diameter, while letting smaller material through that is desired downstream.

In contrast, the intelligent, living filters of the gut actively sort through *macro*scopic volumes of *micro*scopic-sized materials, in real time, to determine what's useful *vs.* harmful. Imagine for a moment every time you eat or drink – assessing each and every molecule you put in your mouth and knowing which have nutritional value and are permissible *vs.* which ones should be denied entry because they might harm cells and systems.

How do enterocytes manage the identification and sorting of millions of materials they may encounter… and do it so efficiently? That is innate intelligence on a level that most humans can't comprehend.

Leaky gut

When cells of the gut wall are unable to hold tight to each other, every toxin and immune system irritant entering your mouth is allowed to pass unchecked into the bloodstream and cause you mayhem – partially-digested proteins being the most destructive. The intestinal wall becomes a virtual sieve, leaking stuff into the bloodstream that doesn't belong there. This is the essence of the condition known as "leaky gut."

Think the body has no use for the appendix? Think again

Decades ago, medical experts presumed the appendix may have once served a purpose in man's ancient past, but we evolved out of it. Some doctors even removed the appendix when a patient had lower abdominal surgery, just to keep it from causing problems later. Imagine that: doctors did not notice the appendix doing anything special, so they figured it was useless and cut it out like a growth.

Well, wouldn't you know it? The experts were wrong... again. The appendix is not some evolutionary relic. It does have a useful purpose: it holds replacement bacteria to reconstitute the microbiome after injury. Like an emergency reserve of starter cultures, the body uses these stored bacteria to repopulate the gut after a major attack, like that from dysentery.

However, it can only distribute what it's got inside. So if your microbiome is corrupted, your appendix is likely to be as well. Maybe that's why appendixes appear to get infected and rupture? Makes too much sense. This could be why repairing a corrupted gut can be so difficult: the appendix helps maintain the status quo, no matter how corrupted the gut may be. And probiotic supplements can't repopulate the appendix directly. Their only access is via the gut.

How digestion works

Let's go over the four basic stages of digestion to give you an idea of what happens in a well-functioning digestive tract. And we'll discuss common problems occurring in GAPS individuals when certain steps malfunction.

Stage 1 of digestion: The mouth and chewing

Chewing starts the digestive process. The goal of the first stage of digestion is to break down food into particles small enough to fit through the esophagus. Chewing and salivation also pre-digest foods – particularly carbs – before reaching the stomach.

A common problem for GAPS individuals at the chewing stage is sensory processing difficulties. Many autistics have trouble chewing, tasting, and swallowing because their sensory perception is distorted. It's as if they're using the wrong code book to decipher signals, so their brain confuses what their nose, tongue, mouth, and throat is telling them about the food they're eating. As a result, they may not *smell* food properly to call salivary glands into action, *taste* it the way Nature intended it to taste, *feel* its texture, or *coordinate* swallowing appropriately.

The brain's sensory perception is so mixed up from blood-borne poisons such as acetaldehyde from candida, in addition to neurotransmitter imbalances, that foods feel and taste funny to them. The exceptions being gluten and casein, which have morphine-like effects on the brain. All of which leads to unusual, unhealthy, severely-restricted food preferences.

Stage 2: The stomach and nutrient soup

Stomach acid and digestive enzymes dissolve the connective structures of food to create a "nutrient soup." In the second stage of digestion, *stomach acid* made by the stomach lining, *bile* made by the liver, and *enzymes* made by the pancreas, dissolve connective tissue – thereby turning food particles into a nutrient soup called "chyme." Together, these digestive agents disintegrate the cell walls and extracellular matrix around meat proteins or plant fiber so that digestive processes can access their nutritious innards.

Five situations can derail digestion in the stomach:

1. **Low-salt diets decrease production of hydrochloric acid.** The GI tract needs the chloride in salt to make stomach acid. So salt deficiency turns down the acidity of stomach acid, thereby reducing the antimicrobial effect of stomach acid and letting pathogens into the gut. Low stomach acid also turns down bile flow, which inhibits fat digestion and absorption of fat-soluble vitamins A, D, E and K found in animal fat. One solution: season your food with sea salt.

2. **Dehydration inhibits stomach acid production.** You need water to make stomach acid. So drink more water no less than twenty minutes prior to meals.

3. **Too much water with meals dilutes stomach acid.** Limit water intake with meals. Resume drinking an hour to an hour-and-a-half after eating a good-size meal.

4. **Lack of digestive enzymes** impairs digestion in the stomach, contributing to problems associated with leaky gut. Enzyme deficiency can originate from a shortage of raw, fresh foods in your diet, pasteurization, irradiation, preservatives and processed foods. And it worsens with age, nutrient deficiency and toxin load.

5. Pathogens in your upper digestive tract can **paralyze the esophageal sphincter** with their poisonous waste products, causing acid reflux. Acid reflux prompts people to decrease stomach acid with drugs.

Esophageal sphincter: Valve that separates the stomach from the esophagus.

Stage 3: The small intestine and "ready-to-use" molecules

Microbiota, enterocytes and microvilli complete the digestive process by breaking down the nutrient soup into bioavailable molecules. After partially broken-down food leaves the stomach, digestion continues in the small intestine, and absorption begins. Stage 3 is working properly when gut flora, enterocytes, and microvilli deconstruct food particles into their smallest, most readily-absorbable forms of sugars, fats, proteins (as amino acids), vitamins, minerals, enzymes and other constituents. Molecules must be small enough to pass through the gut wall, be recognized by the immune system as friendly, get absorbed into cells and the interstitial space, and be of maximum nutritional value.

Let's examine how wheat and milk proteins (gluten and casein, respectively) are digested. Digestive juices in the stomach begin the process of breaking down gluten or casein into "peptides." Pancreatic juices in the small intestine continue deconstruction. "Peptidase" enzymes on the microvilli complete the digestion into useful molecules. Enterocytes pass the nutrient cocktail through the gut wall, into the bloodstream. It circulates through the bloodstream until it's absorbed into the intracellular space, and subsequently taken into individual cells.

Intracellular space: Collagen-connected space between cells.

Unfortunately, when the microbiome is corrupted, enterocytes and their microvilli can't produce peptidase enzymes that finish digestion, so gluten and casein peptides pass through the GI tract undigested. Partially deconstructed gluten and casein molecules – called "gluteomorphin" and "casomorphine," respectively – are absorbed into the bloodstream as-is. Chemically similar to morphine, these molecules intoxicate the entire body, and especially the brain.

In short, defective enterocytes, microvilli and zonulin cause: (1) poor digestion, (2) breeches in the "castle wall" that protect you from toxins and pathogens, and (3) inappropriate substances causing a cascade of injuries and imbalances throughout the body. Of course, pathogenic microorganisms are the primary source of gut wall dysfunction. These tiny troublemakers overgrow and suppress beneficial bacteria that would normally fortify the gut against these unfortunate circumstances. That's corrupted gut in a nutshell.

Another common occurrence in GAPS individuals at this stage is mal-absorption of fat. The gut wall is one big mucous membrane. And when it's attacked by pathogens, it produces extra mucous to protect itself. Food particles travelling through the GI tract then get coated with mucous, which shields them from bile and digestive enzymes, preventing them from being dissolved. As a result, fat goes undigested in severe cases of corrupted gut, which can cause pale, greasy stools, and deficiencies in fat-soluble vitamins A, D, E and K.

Stage 4: The large intestine and reintegration

The colon (aka bowel or large intestine) completes digestion and absorption. And it puts waste material together and eliminates it. How stools are made: (1) The colon takes food material that passed through the digestive tract undigested/unused (such as fruit and vegetable fiber), combines that with: (2) waste material from your own cells, (3) old and worn out bacteria leaving the microbiome, (4) remnants of spent biochemicals like hormones and neurotransmitters, (5) toxins expelled from the liver, and (6) toxins absorbed directly through the gut wall. (7) Excess water is pulled out of this mass of waste material to form stools (aka "bowels"). (8) Muscular contractions (peristalsis) move bowels through the colon and out in a bowel movement. That's the short version of how stools are formed and moved out.

The biggest problems seen at this stage in GAPS individuals are abnormal formation and elimination of stools. Fecal compaction, constipation, and diarrhea can lead to reabsorption and recirculation of toxins. Parasitic worms in the small and large intestine release their own toxins affecting the bowel region as well, particularly in autistics. The most common of their metabolites, morphine, paralyzes muscles of the intestine responsible for pushing stools through and out.

As if these problems weren't bad enough, rotting and reabsorption of compacted fecal matter sticking to the gut wall causes chronic poisoning and dysfunction in GAPS patients. On the bright side, when bowel motility improves – either by healing and sealing the gut, and/or by doing enemas or colonics – you remove a major stream of toxicity contaminating the body.

In summary, Stage 4 "bowel function" is the final stage of elimination for solid food waste and many toxins. If the bowels aren't moving, everything upstream stops too. And that's "nightmare scenario #2" of toxin retention, high body burden, and resulting toxicity (glutathione dysfunction is nightmare scenario #1).

9

MICROORGANISMS AND YOUR MICROBIOME

The human digestive tract is home to bacteria, yeasts, fungi, viruses, molds, protozoa and worms

We now call this mass of microbes in our digestive tract the *microbiome*. It weighs about 3–5 pounds and outnumbers our own cells between 1½ to 1, all the way up to 100 to 1, depending on who you ask. Most say it's 10 to 1. At that ratio, there's more than 40 trillion microbes inside us, making up 80% of the genetic material inside the human body. That's important because their DNA controls many aspects of our biology that we thought was run by our own genes.

By comparison, our own bodies have 1/10 the number of cells that they do, or 30 trillion. So we are just a shell… a habitat for this mass of microbes that are so fundamental to human health that if a person were to have their digestive system completely sterilized, they'd probably die, or at least be so disturbed mentally and physically that they wish they were dead.

Basic functions of gut flora

- break down food (aka digestion)
- produce vitamins
- neutralize or filter out heavy metals, chemicals and foreign pathogens
- help nutrients pass through the gut wall into the bloodstream
- modulate the immune system by protecting the gut wall and GALT.

To illustrate how important microbiota are to you, 90% of the digestive work happening inside of you is not done by human cells; it's done by bacteria. The salivary glands, stomach lining, pancreas, gall bladder and liver do make digestive substances that dissolve food into smaller particles. But most of the heavy lifting of digestion is actually done by bacterial enzymes. They eat the food that you eat and turn it into bioavailable minerals, vitamins, amino acids, redox molecules, and materials that support your cells and organs.

Your gut flora help make you the person that you are

We used to think physical and behavioral traits don't stray much from your genetic blueprint. Meaning, the person that you are is largely dependent on the genes that you inherit. But we now know that DNA makes you homo sapien, but within that framework, there is a lot of room for modification and interpretation. Gene expression is customized to your environment, courtesy of microbiota and epigenetics.

Scientists have identified about 500 species of pathogenic microbiota, and even more probiotic ones, that combine inside each person to form a community of microbes as unique as a person's fingerprints. Your microbial profile determines the nutrients you receive, detoxification capacity, health/sickness proclivities, energy level, weight, grace with which you age, and brain function.

But even more instrumental in making you who you are, microflora influence neurotransmitter and hormone levels such as serotonin, dopamine, testosterone and estrogen. Biochemicals like these influence your thoughts and emotions, not to mention behavior, social skills and learning. Your microflora initiate the psychology that we collectively call your personality. It's this pattern of thoughts, feelings and behaviors that make you the person that you are. Gut flora help to make us who we are through these mechanisms and more:

- **Neurotransmitters, hormones and other biochemicals.** Microbes contribute to production of neurotransmitters and hormones that control brain and nervous system function.
- **Toxin exposure.** Gut flora contribute to the health and integrity of the gut wall, blood-brain barrier, and other membranes.
- **Epigenetics.** They control how our genes are expressed.

Toxins and nutrition affect gene expression

Environmental factors such as toxins, nutrition, emotional state and stress level may influence gene expression even more than your own DNA. A striking example: Randy Jirtle's research at Duke University showed that exposure to bisphenol-A (BPA) caused pregnant mice to bear pups that were yellow, obese and diabetic. What's more, altered gene expressions like this were passed on to subsequent generations.

Bisphenol-A: Toxic chemical widely used in the manufacture of plastics.

This means that many of the physical, biochemical and psychological characteristics you thought of as "running in the family" are not genetic;

they're epigenetic. They get turned on at some point in a family's lineage by toxins and poor nutrition, combined with genetic susceptibility, and they stay switched on unless/until a concerted effort is made to reverse the damage by removing exposures and repleting with minerals and vitamins (many of which are made by probiotic bacteria).

Unfortunately for us, researchers believe that epigenetic alterations may take one to three generations to be triggered, and three generations to shut down in most cases. Fathers aren't excused from the process either. Their epigenetics can alter gene expression as easily as the maternal side.

Point being, the vitality of your microbiome and their DNA either helps protect you against toxin exposures when it's in a healthful balance, thus preserving your epigenetic code. Or, when corruption reigns in the gut, pathogens and their DNA amplify damage done to gene expression through gut leakiness, synergistic toxicity, poor redox signaling, and immune system reactions.

That's the multi-factorial cause-and-effect scenario that's confused scientists for so long. Medical science acts as if diseases and problems are caused by a single trigger. But that's seldom the way the body works. There's a lot of actions and reactions going on in the body at all times. And you have to understand that if you're to decipher what's causing good or bad situations.

The DNA of your gut flora is thought to be more influential than your own DNA at breeding health or sickness in you

The idea of your DNA being the sole factor in determining your genetic destiny is a leap of logic made decades ago, which lingers to this day. It's a presumption that's turning out to be less and less true the more that we learn about human gene expression.

The reality is, we're profoundly outnumbered genetically. The average person is made up of about 30 trillion human cells and 20,000 genes. By comparison, bacteria in a typical person's microbiome averages 1,000–4,000 species, 37 trillion cells, 2,000 genes each, possessing **2 million genes in total.** While our three mitochondria species average around 14 quadrillion cells, with 37 genes each.

Even more astronomical, scientists believe there to be 300,000 species of parasite living among us, with about 5,000 genes each, adding up to **1.5 billion genes.** Fungi have some 5 million species, with **125 trillion genes combined.** Yet we can hardly begin to pin down how many species of virus there are on earth. Guesstimates suggest there may be 10,000,000,000,000,000,000,000,000,000,000 species, possessing a lot more genes than that. So basically, our genes are infinitesimal compared to those of the microorganisms surrounding and inhabiting us.

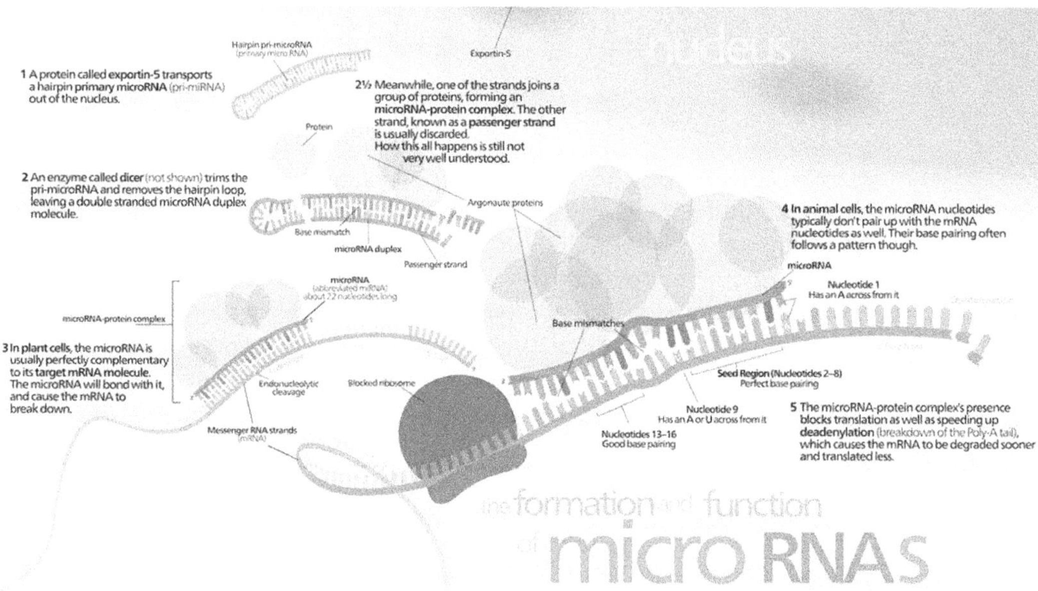
Hairpin pri-microRNA
(primary micro RNA)
Exportin-5
1 A protein called exportin-5 transports a hairpin primary microRNA (pri-miRNA) out of the nucleus.
2½ Meanwhile, one of the strands joins a group of proteins, forming an microRNA-protein complex. The other strand, known as a passenger strand is usually discarded. How this all happens is still not very well understood.
Protein
2 An enzyme called dicer (not shown) trims the pri-microRNA and removes the hairpin loop, leaving a double stranded microRNA duplex molecule.
Argonaute proteins
Base mismatch
microRNA duplex
Passenger strand
4 In animal cells, the microRNA nucleotides typically don't pair up with the mRNA nucleotides as well. Their base pairing often follows a pattern though.
microRNA
Nucleotide 1
Has an A across from it
microRNA
microRNA-protein complex
Base mismatches
3 In plant cells, the microRNA is usually perfectly complementary to its target mRNA molecule. The microRNA will bond with it, and cause the mRNA to break down.
Endonucleolytic cleavage
Blocked ribosome
Seed Region (Nucleotides 2–8)
Perfect base pairing
Nucleotide 9
Has an A or U across from it
Nucleotides 13–16
Good base pairing
5 The microRNA-protein complex's presence blocks translation as well as speeding up deadenylation (breakdown of the Poly-A tail), which causes the mRNA to be degraded sooner and translated less.
Messenger RNA strands
(mRNA)
formation function
micro RNAs

Image used under Creative Commons 3.0 license. Author: Kelvinsong.

DNA make snippets of microRNA that turn genes on or off

Geneticists say 99% of our genetic material doesn't appear to be doing anything. It's "junk DNA" that may have served a purpose in our ancient past, but is obsolete now. They didn't see it doing anything, so they assumed it's now expendable. When, in fact, many genes stay dormant until/unless until they're needed, in which case environmental triggers call them into action.

Snippets of genetic code made by DNA, called "microRNA," help regulate gene expression by activating or silencing the production of proteins. In doing so, microRNA control the expression of our own DNA into family traits. But here's the plot twist that surprised geneticists: About 15% of the microRNA found in our blood comes from bacteria, 15% comes from fungus, and the latest research says 5% comes from the food you eat – be it plant or animal-based. This means *your microbiome* influences your weight, energy level and insulin sensitivity. It controls your ability to detoxify, overcome environment threats, and much more.

It means the genetic content of your microbiome IS part of your genetic code – and that of your family. It just happens to be more fluid than your own DNA. This new science of epigenetics explains that your own DNA, and that of your microbiome, "load the gun" for traits to express themselves (potential). But it's exposures in the environment that "pull the trigger" and make traits manifest themselves. MicroRNA from external sources is one way by which *environment* influences our biology, and a core concept of epigenetics.

Microbiome diversity has plummeted, along with our trace mineral supply, defenses against toxins, and specialized job functions

Before the Industrial Age, people had far more microbial species colonizing their guts – the majority of which science has yet to identify and study because microbiota are so fragile outside the gut, you can't isolate single species and grow them as a monoculture. The ten-fold greater biodiversity of long-ago afforded people greater protection against toxins and invading pathogens, a healthier supply of trace nutrients that bacteria make available, and the execution of certain jobs within the body.

For example, certain strains of gut flora have a particular talent for capturing or neutralizing toxins such as nitrates, indoles, phenols, skatol, histamine, ksenobiotics or mercury – based on the toxin's molecular structure. Absent these rarer species, the gut loses some of its ability to protect us against unusual toxins, because each species has a key that "fits a certain lock," due to the way molecules fit together. While the immune system does have other ways to remove toxins should first options fail, no other strain has the "easy antidote" supplied by Nature. That duty then gets assigned to other mechanisms that are inferiorly-equipped for the job.

Fewer strains of microbiota also mean a more limited supply of vitamins and minerals that these microbiota either make, or help us use. For instance, some bacteria are good at making B vitamins, while some metabolize vitamins A and D well. Point is, nutrient deficiencies tend to go up as biodiversity goes down in the microbiome. And nutrient rationing makes the body employ coping mechanisms to make due with less.

Finally, narrowing of diversity means certain jobs have to be postponed or cancelled. For instance, some bacteria are good at neutralizing radioactive isotopes. Some viruses get into fat stores and chelate mercury, while others might be employed by the immune system to purposely create a fever to help fight off an infection.

What has caused this precipitous drop in diversity?

The things that corrupt the gut also narrow the microbiome's diversity, including: (1) antibiotics for humans and animals; (2) toxic chemicals and GMOs in our food supply; (3) the contraceptive pill, steroids, and long-term drug use; (4) heavy metals in dentistry, air and fish; and (5) industrial chemicals and personal care products.

To start with, a diet that lacks a variety of raw whole foods will naturally acquire fewer species of scarce soil-based bacteria, because that's primarily how we get them: the unwashed skin of naturally-grown plants, in addition to simple soil exposure, such as gardening and playing with farm animals. In simplest terms, **playing around in the dirt benefits diversity of the microbiome.** Unfortunately, it's been demonized by our culture as being uncivilized. Dogs and cats also donate their microbiota to you on a regular basis, which are beneficial, more often than not.

A microcosm of us wrecking our inner ecosystems: Sanitizing gels and repeatedly-sanitized surfaces contribute to narrowing and weakening of the microbiome, because there's very little diversity in these environments or, even worse, an inclination to host the very worst pathogens due to increasing antibiotic resistance. Ideas like this sound good to the uninitiated, but Nature always makes us pay a price.

The bottom line: There is no one-step solution to replace biodiversity in the microbiome – man-made or otherwise – besides avoiding the worst exposures, healing and sealing the gut, and letting the microbiome expand on its own through second-hand soil exposure. Some of the rarer soil-based bacteria can be challenging enough to grow outside the body. But try developing a supplement that contains trace populations of thousands of rare microbiota – most of which have never been identified, cultured or studied. See how far you get.

See the chapters "Redox Molecules and Inflammation" and "Taking Charge of Your Health" for ideas on how to revitalize microbiome diversity.

How probiotic bacteria suppress pathogens

Microorganisms use chemical warfare to keep opposing populations in check. Probiotics produce a wide variety of antibiotic, anti-viral, anti-fungal, anti-mold, anti-parasite, worm-controlling, and pest-killing substances to suppress the growth of neighbors. Pathogens do the same, only their weapons are weaker, as is their biology. Both make far more antimicrobial agents then science and industry ever will. This is how Nature encourages resiliency and continuity to the microbiome, while giving probiotics a competitive advantage.

On a side note, when drug companies search for new antimicrobial agents, they first copy the compounds made by bacteria and Co. Like the development cycle of other drugs, they observe an effect in Nature that they want to replicate. They find the molecule(s) responsible and isolate it. They synthesize it. They patent it. They promote it, and profit from it.

On the other hand, gut flora's antimicrobial agents don't decimate pathogen populations the way medicinal antibiotics do. The best they can do is gradually wear down their competitors and keep them contained. So these turf wars are closer to trench warfare than nuclear war. Neither party can overrun the other and "win" the war. Nor would we want them to, because most microbes have a place in a polite ecosystem.

Microbes just duke it out continuously – one day gaining ground due to diet, medications, or stimuli such as stress – the next day giving it back. They grow, reproduce, die, and fight with each other for control over your inner terrain. However, the microbiome resists "sea change" as a high priority for both body and mind.

Probiotics help normalize weight

Your systems that regulate hunger, digestion and metabolism work much better when good bacteria rule the microbiome. Overweight people tend to lose weight when their gut flora is normalized. Underweight people tend to gain weight when their gut flora improves. A big reason for this is that healthy gut flora help you extract maximum nutrition out of the food

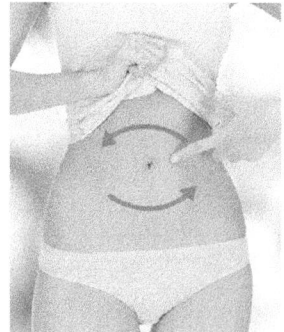

you eat, while reducing cravings for inferior foods. Those two factors tip your nutrient-to-calorie ratio in your favor. Nutrients-to-calories is far better to watch when trying to reach your ideal weight, not calories alone.

When you get the nutrients that you need, you tend to eat only as much as your body needs, without inappropriate cravings. You also tend to desire healthier types of food, and not crave those that contribute to weight gain, such as refined carbohydrates, processed foods, and convenience foods. Plus, the cleaner your system is, the less you crave sweet, salty and spicy foods. Once you and your microbial community grow accustomed to the biochemical benefits of quality food, your appetite for empty calories wanes. Junk food may taste good on a superficial level. But deep down, your body knows that convenience foods contain flavor enhancers, fillers, and minimal nutrition.

It does take some understanding and awareness to notice the subtle differences in food quality. But if you pay attention, your tongue, microflora, and gut instinct can tell the difference between real food and fake food. They sense purity and substance *vs.* foods engineered in a lab to taste good and be cheap. As a buddy of mine put it, you feel "dirty and ashamed" after gorging yourself on low-quality comfort food, like that from a late-night diner. Conversely, when you eat quality foods – like those made from scratch with naturally-grown ingredients – you feel satiated, uplifted, and you can't get enough.

Part of the reason for this is that your body knows how it processes foods. When you eat refined carbs and processed foods, your insulin level spikes. Insulin turns food into fat. High blood-sugar also keeps your body in sugar-burning mode, while suppressing ketogenic fat burning.

In summary, when pathogens compel you to eat empty foods, you absorb more calories, and fewer nutrients, which is the real goal of hunger: to get nutrients. Junk food gives you lots of calories and sparse nutrients, so your body keeps appetite and cravings turned on, hoping to get nutrients mixed in. The takeaway: Focus on nutrients more than calories when you want to lose or gain weight. The more naturally-grown and whole-food based, the better.

Probiotic bacteria are Nature's most effective chelators

Our best defense against heavy metal infiltration is a healthful balance of probiotic bacteria in your gut, because many strains of bacteria collect heavy metals in their cell walls until they leave through the bowels. To give you an idea of just how effective bacteria are at chelating heavy metals, one study showed that when you feed rats food that's high in mercury, their microbiomes chelate more than 99% of the mercury, whereas rats that have had their guts sterilized only block 10%.

Assuming gut flora works the same in humans, that means probiotic microflora capture about ten times as much heavy metal in the GI tract than a severely corrupted microbiome. This ability for probiotic bacteria to chelate heavy metals is one of the defining characteristics of a healthy gut (along with protection of enterocytes and tight junctions). Conversely, a lack of protection from heavy metals is one of the lesser-known risks of gut dysbiosis because the effects of food allergies, for example, are more evident than heavy metal exposure.

Likewise, the microbiome protects us from other toxins. Although the more unnatural the substance, the less likely it is that your microbiome has the mechanisms to deal with it efficiently at the GI level. That's because, the body comes equipped "from the factory" to deal with toxins native to our environment. But it has a harder time handling complex, man-made substances that are foreign to this earth, such as genetically modified organisms, DDT, radioactive material, bisphenol-A, and nano-size particles.

Bacteria can decontaminate pollution

You may have heard that specialized bacteria can literally eat up oil spills. But did you know that bacteria can also clean up industrial chemicals and pollutants in contaminated land? Soil microbiologist Dr. Elaine Ingham has used bacteria to remediate tracts of land contaminated by all sorts of nasty chemicals and toxins, such as petrochemicals leaked from storage tanks. And it's usually quicker, cheaper, and more effective than conventional remediation techniques that simply soak up pollution with absorbent materials and take it somewhere else.

In fact, industrial cleanup companies are frequently embarrassed to find out how much more effective a few applications of compost are at cleaning up contaminated land than their methods. The results are stunning. After a couple of applications of bacteria-rich compost are added to polluted land, new grass and vegetation can be seen growing robustly in a matter of days – even after conventional crews tried several times to recover land and failed (meaning, nothing grows because the ground is too toxic).

But, even more astounding, certain bacteria strains love to detoxify radioactive material. As Nature's crack cleanup crew, bacteria can neutralize radioactive waste from atomic bombs and nuclear power plants. They can clean up nuclear pollution from "accidents" such as Fukishima and Chernobyl. However, you won't hear anything about natural cleanup methods on the news because globalists use pollution, and the fear they created about it, to control us and profit from it. If the world knew simple strains of bacteria could clean up radioactive material, then there would be no need to bury nuclear waste and make contractors rich in the process. It could be neutralized on the spot.

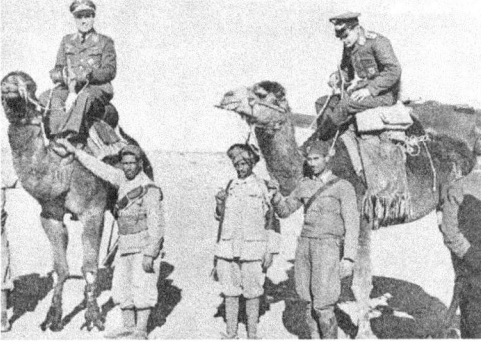

Image used courtesy of camelphotos.com

Nazi scientists were first to use probiotics therapeutically

During World War II, the Nazis were advancing into parts of North Africa. But, after drinking the local water, their troops were falling ill left and right with dysentery – a potentially life-threatening gastrointestinal infection, causing inflammation, fever, abdominal pain, vomiting and bloody diarrhea. Drinking from rivers in the area was severely disabling or killing their troops. And this threatened to stop the great German war machine from taking over Africa.

However, locals didn't have this problem. So German doctors went to work to find out why, and what they discovered mortified them: Locals would actually take the still-warm fecal matter of their cows or camels and eat it fresh. This supplied their digestive tracts with the soil-based microorganisms that killed the bacteria, viruses, parasitic worms, or protozoan that caused dysentery.

Obviously, German soldiers would be reluctant to eat steaming camel dung, to put it mildly. So the doctors identified the dysentery-killing strains of bacteria present in camel pies, cultured them, and put them in tablet form. And you know what, it worked. The probiotics they took were adept at wiping out the dysentery-causing microbes in the water supply. And through this process, Nazi doctors and scientists developed the first modern usage of therapeutic probiotics.

Similarly, water supplies in some under-developed countries still contains pathogens that cause diarrhea in visitors but not locals. Vacationers to Mexico used to call this "traveler's diarrhea" or "Montezuma's Revenge," though Mexico has modernized it water treatment facilities so it doesn't happen anymore.

Of course, drinking bottled water is one way to avoid getting sick when you're on vacation. But it's harder to avoid food that's been prepared using local water, let alone avoid it permanently when you move there. So new residents gain immunity to pathogens in local water by gradually building a tolerance to it. You have to drink local water for about a year and, eventually, your microbiome hosts enough microbes to make you immune to traveler's diarrhea.

Problems with commercial probiotic supplements

Many commercial probiotics are genetically engineered. Most probiotic supplements and foods aren't as good for us as we're told. That's because the most potent strains of probiotics are unstable outside their natural environments. Nature didn't design them to reproduce and live outside of soil, plants or the microbiome of living creatures.

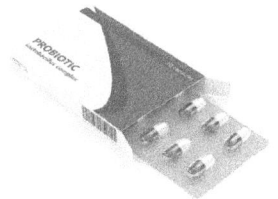

As a result, growing, transporting, and keeping probiotics in a living state are inconveniences that most manufacturers avoid if they can. They'd rather sterilize and homogenize the natural properties out of a product to make it cheaper, easier to make, and less perishable. That encourages many companies to use genetically modified strains that are easier to control.

How can you tell if the probiotics in a supplement or food are genetically modified and not naturally-occurring? Look on the label. Many GMO strains are followed by a number, such as "Bacillus coagulans GBI-30 6086," indicating the strain is proprietary and engineered. On the flip side, you can't patent a naturally-occurring microorganism.

Most commercial probiotics don't survive stomach acid well. A few probiotic brands claim they are produced or packaged in a way that enables some of them to survive the journey through the stomach's extremely acidic environment (e.g., time-release capsules). The vast majority of other brands make no claims about being acid resistant. Thus, brands that die in stomach acid, and those packaged to survive it, both highlight the weakness of their bacteria strains.

You see, the strongest probiotic bacteria strains are allowed to ferment until the pH drops well into the acid range. For example, *Inner Garden* and *Rest Easy* from Natural Plus Plus, are allowed to ferment until they reach a pH of 3.4. That's how you know the batch is done brewing. As a result, they don't mind acid environments, and survive the stomach very well. This then gives us a good metric to measure potency of probiotic supplements. Look for brands that are capable of

- surviving till consumption (e.g., drying, packaging, shipping, storage)
- making it through the stomach, to the digesting tract... alive
- suppressing pathogens
- colonizing the gut
- potent enough to protect the gut wall and nourish the body.

Until the little guys can do all five things competently, you're just wasting your money and effort.

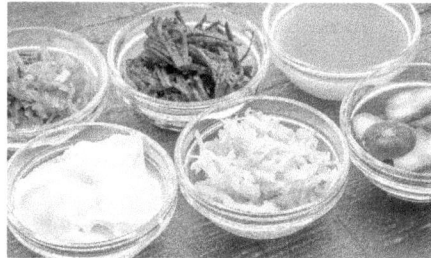

Indigenous cultures have eaten fermented foods for eons

Before refrigeration and modern preservatives, our ancestors needed a way to keep food edible beyond the few weeks of harvest. If they didn't preserve their vegetables, fish, fowl, milk, fruits or grains, those in colder climates would struggle to survive the off-season. Mankind would be limited to small groups of hunter-gatherers in equatorial zones.

But with the advent of fermentation, the practices of farming, hunting and raising livestock were able to sustain larger populations in more places, because it evened out feast and famine periods of the seasons. Fermentation also gave indigenous peoples tremendous nutritional benefits (nutritional *quality*), making the practice indispensable to their survival.

So, at some point in every indigenous culture's history, the people found out they could prepare food a certain way, let it sit for a few days or months. And some naturally-occurring process altered the food's taste and nutritional value, while greatly extending its shelf life. They knew something special was going on, but they probably didn't understand exactly what was happening biologically.

Today we call this preservation process *fermentation* or "cultured." Fermentation is the process of purposely growing probiotic microorganisms in food, without any oxygen present (whereas, oxygen just makes foods rot). Integral to various fermentation processes, the active ingredient in many "ferments" is bacteria (although many aren't added; they're naturally-occurring), while others use yeast.

Fermentation produces several foods enjoyed all over the world. There are a few that Westerners find peculiar. And still others have become popular just recently. The best-known fermented foods are yogurt, cheese, cottage cheese, sour cream, beer, wine, sauerkraut and soy sauce. Some of the more obscure ferments we think of as ethnic foods are kimchi, miso, kefir and natto. And one fermented food that's become popular in recent years is kombucha.

Why fermentation fell out of favor (for a while)

Sauerkraut used to be made and served with active cultures, but seldom is anymore because most food companies literally cook the life out of it. Today, it's made by fermenting cabbage and then cooking it, making it a "dead food." Another food that used to be fermented, but rarely is today, is pickles. They used to be prepared in bacteria culture. But manufacturers now shortcut the process by soaking cucumbers in a vinegar brine to achieve a similar taste. Most sour dough breads have vinegar added for the same reason. The notable exception to this trend is yogurt, which still contains live, active cultures today.

Another practice that undoes some of the health benefits of fermentation is the addition of ingredients to enhance their flavor. Food companies alter the flavor of fermented foods because most ferments are naturally sour-tasting. Sadly, many naturally-fermented foods taste so much different from their commercial counterparts, that modern consumers don't even know what the real food is supposed to taste like anymore. Yogurt is a sweet example. It's loaded with sugar and doesn't taste anything like unflavored yogurt, apart from the texture.

The moral of this story: Traditionally-fermented foods contain live, active probiotic cultures that do wonders for your gut health, biochemistry, and general wellness. Fermented foods, when eaten raw, are "living foods." They reward your body with a wide variety of health benefits, some of which may be described as giving their life force to you. That's why traditional cultures prized their fermented foods for their awesome ability to support life. They knew they literally could not live without them.

But today, our food system has negated these benefits (some would say blessings) by cooking the goodness right out of these foods. Heating/pasteurizing kills the probiotic microorganisms, and the health benefits they bring to your fork. In consequence, they become "dead food" – not necessarily devoid of nutrition or bad for you, but stripped of their nutritional superpowers.

Bottom line: Lack of potent probiotics in the standard American diet is a big reason why our health is in decline in the Western world. We simply cannot be optimally healthy, happy, and supported without an equally healthy, happy, and supportive microbiome feeding and protecting us from the inside-out.

The good news: Living food is making a comeback. More products are showing up on store shelves that still contain living cultures that nourish and protect the body. Flavored kimchi is one of those still-living foods that's been catching on lately. So we have ourselves to thank for both the disappearance of cultured foods prior, and their resurgence of late. The more good food we buy, the more they make.

———⸋⧫⸋———

10

HOW YOUR MICROBIOME GETS ESTABLISHED AND HOW IT GETS CORRUPTED

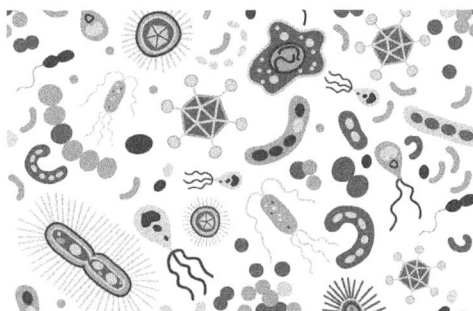

In sickness or in health, all roads lead to gut flora

The microbiome is a nexus point for virtually everything that happens in the body. Your DNA establishes the foundation for your physiology. But it's your gut flora that determines your relative health or sickness, family traits, and a large percent of your personality. Your gut flora plays a key role in making you the individual that you are, as well as your family lineage.

This chapter explains how genetics, gut flora, diet, toxins, and environmental exposures coalesce to cause ADD and GAPS conditions. It's the story of how sickness or health transpires in the human body.

GAPS is inherited primarily through the microbiome, not DNA

Practitioners who study GAPS say nearly all the patients they see for autism have gut dysbiosis. Almost all the mothers of children with learning, behavior and cognitive disabilities have deeply disturbed gut flora, as do most of the grandmothers, and many of the fathers. In fact, Dr. Natasha Campbell-McBride and Donna Gates (pioneers in gut-brain health) have never seen an autistic child who did not have a corrupted microbiome. To a lesser extent, the same holds true for attention deficit disorder, although the dysbiosis and resulting symptoms aren't as bad. So more than 9 times out of 10, behavioral, learning and attention problems are deeply rooted in GI dysfunction.

A troubled gut manifests itself in a variety of ways depending on constitution, environmental conditions and genetic factors. But just because you don't see obvious signs of gut dysbiosis does not mean you don't suffer from it in silence. Remember, the human body has incredible ability to adapt to imbalances, without ever letting you know how close you are to overt disorder. Sometimes you have to be a medical detective to read the signs of gut corruption and nutrient deficiency.

To illustrate, a friend of mine seems to have no problem digesting food. But he has large energy level swings (possibly caused by too many refined carbs, leaky gut, general nutrient deficiency, heavy metal toxicity). He has narrowing of the maxilla bone (nutrient deficiency). He

The research of Dr. Weston A. Price showed that a nutrient-deficient Western diet caused narrowing of facial structures, particularly across the cheekbones and teeth.

has periodic spells where he bruises easily (iron deficiency). He displays obsessive/compulsive/anxious behaviors (signs of mercury poisoning through glutamate dysfunction). And he notices a big difference taking drugs that alter neurotransmitter levels (whereas people with balanced biochemistry don't notice as much difference). These clues point to gut dysbiosis as a reason for ADD behaviors and brain dysfunction.

How the microbiome gets established

Medical science used to think babies were born with a sterile digestive tract. But we now know that baby's GI tract gets lightly populated with limited microbiota species in–utero as a primer. The real colonists arrive shortly thereafter through the birthing process and the feeding of colostrum and breastmilk.

As baby travels through the birth canal, it swallows its first mouthfuls of full–spectrum bacteria and other microbiota. This inoculates baby with microbial starter cultures that colonize its entire intestinal tract and body, over its first month or two. So whatever microflora lives in the mother's vagina will become the bulk of the baby's microbiome. Other sources in baby's environment, such as pacifiers, pets and floors, make up the rest.

Breast feeding is the next biggest contributor to the establishment of baby's new microbiome. In the course of breastfeeding, baby touches and suckles mom. And microbes are taken in from the environment. What's interesting is, some native populations have used the breastfeeding process to help establish a healthy microbiome. Mothers spread a thin layer of yogurt or other probiotic cultures on the nipples to suppress yeast growth and inoculate baby with probiotic organisms that it needs.

And, even before that, mothers to-be applied yogurt or cultures to the crotch, and under the arms, to increase probiotic populations, and decrease pathogens like yeast when the immune system is suppressed in pregnancy. Further aiding the process, breast milk, with its high sugar, cholesterol, and nutrient content feeds microflora as they colonize the nooks and crannies of baby's digestive tract. Milk also stimulates the production of mucus, which coats and protects the microbiome in development.

Breastfeeding lays the foundation for baby's immune system

Breastmilk is basically a mother's whole blood, without the red blood cells. Mother's milk consists mostly of: (1) cholesterol and other fats that supply the building blocks for a rapidly developing brain and nervous system, (2) white blood cells, (3) nutritional components, and (4) immune factors. These components give baby an external source of antibodies that protect it from infection and disease while nursing. This is one reason that learning and behavior problems often don't show up until after a child is weaned.

The big a-ha is that microbiota in mom's digestive tract migrates to and colonizes her birth canal, which she passes on to baby at the time of birth. So mommy's microflora becomes the vast majority of baby's microbiome. And, with it, health or imbalance is passed from generation to generation. Dads aren't exempt from the process either. His gut flora migrates to the groin area, which is shared with mommy on a regular basis. So daddy's gut flora has an indirect effect on baby's gut flora profile too. Caretakers and baby's surroundings also contribute to the baby's microflora when baby feeds, bathes, or touches anything.

This is how a person's microbiome gets established in the first twenty days of life. And it's the mechanism by which gut flora is transferred from generation to generation. **It sets the tone for a person's mental, physical, and immunological health or sickness for the rest of their life.**

Crucially, the first bacteria that colonize the gut inform the immune system which species are your own friendly flora that need to be favored and protected for the rest of your life. This establishes who is welcome in your gut by receiving virtual paperwork signifying that they are natural-born citizens of that microbiome. Or, through their absence, this establishes who is a foreigner, and needs to be deported by the immune system. Obviously, this works in your favor when you get the right microbiota from the start. On the other hand, getting started on the wrong foot with unfriendly flora puts you at a disadvantage in correcting your microbiome, and keeping it in balance.

Probiotics are the higher-successional life form

Having co-evolved and cooperated with their hosts for ages, probiotic microbes support the health of their host, and are supposed to make up the bulk of its microbiome – both man or animal. Probiotics are higher up the evolutionary scale and are stronger than pathogens. Nature designed it this way, and enforces its rule through better weaponry. That is, each microbial class – probiotics and pathogens – make and use pesticides against each other. But probiotics are supposed to have the upper hand.

Historically, they always had a stronger "offense" in the form of enemy-fighting chemicals, so they didn't need great defense in the form of chemical resistance. Probiotics could basically get the pathogens, before the pathogens got them. Probiotics are also more resistant to oxidation than pathogens because they hold on to their electrons more tightly due to higher electrical charge. This is Nature's way of protecting probiotic organisms when the body uses free radicals and inflammation to clean up an area. Oxidation does harms probiotic cells, but pathogens are hurt more, giving probiotics a competitive advantage.

Oxidation: The process of stealing electrons with free radicals to destroy things.

Point is, good bacteria are supposed to rule the inner terrain of the gut. But when they're assaulted by forces with bigger guns (antibiotics), they're defenseless. They get wiped out, leaving vast stretches of untended space in the gut for pathogens to set up shop.

How the gut gets corrupted
C-section and bottle feeding can help corrupt the microbiome

Not inevitably. Instead, they setup a neutral situation that favors neither good bacteria nor bad (as natural childbirth and breastfeeding is meant to). You see, Nature intended the holiest of holies, your microbiome, to be setup by the transfer of microbiota from mother to baby during birthing and breastfeeding. But C-section and bottle feeding allow *the environment* to dictate which starter cultures get into baby's gut and colonize it.

With all that fertile ground waiting to be colonized, baby's microbiome is going to get populated with something, one way or another. But modern rearing practices have circumvented the natural seeding of the microbiome. So any random microbes that baby is exposed to in their first twenty days of life become the majority of their microbiome – including those in the maternity ward, on healthcare workers hands, in baby's food, and anything baby touches or puts in its mouth.

Unfortunately, repeated sanitizing of surfaces tends to produce particularly nasty strains of drug-resistant organisms. Not only do microbial survivors develop drug resistance through frequent exposure and regrowth. But repeated sanitizing lets pathogens dominate relative to probiotic strains. That's important: good to bad ratios, not total populations, because probiotics are meant to suppress pathogens. However, when the good guys are worn down, pathogens take over. Once again, man has stuck his nose into Nature's business, and now we're paying the price.

Modern weaning can corrupt the gut

Early in the second half of the 20th Century, pediatric associations tried to convince mothers that breastfeeding was not as healthy for infants as formula and commercial baby food. Isn't that a laugh! Food companies actually had the gall to claim that the formula and mush they make was healthier for baby than Nature's own. Today, that idea has been debunked by insurmountable evidence that mother's milk is perfect and cannot be improved upon. But it does go to show you how ridiculous their claims have been through the years. Indeed, nothing has changed.

Here's what Nature says: Until baby has teeth to chew, and they want it, you shouldn't force them to eat solid food – even if you blend solids into mush. Their digestive systems are not ready for it. We're talking teeth, chewing and swallowing coordination, maturation of digestive organs, and a mature microbiome. Sure, if you force food into their mouth and they're hungry, eventually you can get them to swallow it. But Nature designed teeth and solid food to go together. For example, the production of enzymes that digest solid food is supposed to precede the introduction of solid food. So mother's milk is best, until baby's whole body is ready to chew, swallow, digest, metabolize, detoxify, and eliminate solid food.

The real damage is done by ingredients and contaminants in food

Instead of all the precious stuff in mother's milk – including cholesterol, saturated fat, immune factors, balanced nutrients, and foundational microflora – commercial manufacturers add substances that are harmful to babies. Commercial baby food has too much sugar, salt, carbohydrates, grains, GMOs, glutamate-based flavor enhancers, and fluoride. All of which baby's immature digestive system is ill-equipped to handle. Sugar and refined carbs over-activate baby's pancreas and insulin system. Grains start them down the path to leaky gut and gluten sensitivity. GMOs are bad for the body all around. And glutamate-based flavor enhancers contribute to brain cell death through excitotoxicity.

These reactions are bad enough for adults, but babies are far more susceptible to insults, considering their weight, immature immunity, rapid development, and heighten sensitivity. When the gut is healthy and balanced, baby *might* escape unharmed. But when a gut is corrupted from the get-go, the damage may deepen due to premature introduction of solid food – particularly these food stressors.

Gut flora are under constant attack from these offenders and more

- antibiotics
- chlorine/chloramine in water
- herbicides, insecticides, GMOs
- vaccines
- birth control pills, medications, steroids
- heavy metals in dental work
- hormone mimics
- plasticizers
- chemicals found in personal care products.

The problem is, this damage accumulates, so each generation inherits more deeply-disturbed gut flora than the one before. We're slipping further and further into gut dysbiosis, which is not only rising, it's accelerating. We're seeing it in our families, friends, relatives and neighbors. We're seeing it in our communities, social services and healthcare systems. And we're seeing it in disease rates that are almost beyond comprehension.

Antibiotics

The birth of medicinal antibiotics

September 3, 1928: Upon returning to his lab from vacation, scientist Alexander Fleming noticed something unusual happening in one of his petri dishes. One of his assistants had left a window open, allowing fungal spores from a neighboring lab to land in a culture of staphylococcus bacteria. What he saw changed medicine forever: The fungus was growing in the dish and killing the bacteria in a radial pattern around it.

From his previous work, Fleming recognized that the fungus was secreting a substance that broke down the bacterium's cell walls, which caused the cells to burst. This prevented the bacteria from reproducing. Knowing what this could mean for the treatment of infection, Fleming fashioned a way to make the mysterious substance that inhibited the growth of bacteria. This was the first time people were able to exploit the chemical warfare that happens everywhere in nature, from soil to our microbiomes.

The fungus was called penicillium. And the substance he isolated he called "penicillin." Penicillin is famous for being the first manufactured substance that selectively kills a broad array of bacteria. Fleming himself was never able to produce penicillin in sufficient quantity to turn it into a commercial drug. But, in the early 1940s, pharmacologist Howard Florey and biochemist Ernst Boris Chain led a team of scientists from the University of Oxford to develop mass production techniques for penicillin. And, in doing so, broad-spectrum antibiotics were born.

Penicillin went on to save millions of lives in World War II at a time when infection claimed more lives than battlefield injuries. And, in the decades since, penicillin has saved millions of lives from scarlet fever, pneumonia, meningitis and diphtheria. Antibiotics are now used throughout medicine and animal husbandry. In 1945, Alexander Fleming shared the Nobel Prize in Medicine or Physiology with Florey and Chain for their discovery of penicillin and the relief it offered from infectious diseases.

Broad spectrum antibiotics kill more good bugs than bad

When you take antibiotics, more good bacteria die than bad, because good bugs have less resistance to antibiotics. And beneficial bacteria are slower to develop resistance than do bad bugs. Today, pathogens are developing increased resistance to broad spectrum antibiotics through decades of over-use by medicine and commercial animal farming. Pathogens also tend to repopulate faster, because they're used to surviving repeated attack.

So with each course of antibiotics that you take, the balance tips further toward pathogen domination, as a disproportionate number of good bugs are killed, and they grow back slower. The difference used to be slight, but appears to be increasing, along with the variety and virulence of drug-resistant pathogens – particularly when antibiotics are taken by mouth.

The microbiome can recover undamaged from one or two courses of antibiotics in a lifetime, but no more

When you take a course of antibiotics by mouth, it indiscriminately wipes out large populations of bacteria. They do grow back in two weeks to two months, depending on species. However, pathogens tend to grow back faster, develop resistance over time, and crowd out the good guys. For example, bacteria may die and be replaced by candida (yeast). This means the good guys have got a fight on their hands. They slowly recover over time, but with each course of antibiotics to the next, the damage gets deeper, and is harder to reverse.

Unless you're one of the rare individuals lucky enough to have received two or fewer courses of medicinal antibiotics by adulthood, and your parents did as well, antibiotics have taken a toll on your microbiome, and possibly your mental health. Whether you realize it or not, antibiotics have corrupted your gut a little to a lot – including pretty much everyone who grew up in the care of Western medicine.

The digestive tract can handle one or two courses of antibiotics in a lifetime and recover just fine, because it's built to withstand a limited number of heavy-duty assaults such as cholera or dysentery. But any more than that and gut flora does not bounce back to its original state. Add to that: (1) antibiotics are used in the production of animal products, (2) their waste fertilizes organic food crops, and (3) antibiotics persist in soil for many years. Considering all this, it's not too hard to see where antibiotic exposure and microbiome injury comes from.

So even if you've never taken a single course of medicinal antibiotics, or eaten meat, it's virtually impossible to avoid antibiotic exposure entirely. You ingest antibiotics all the time, no matter how hard you try to avoid them. And, let's not forget, once the bad guys claim territory in the gut, they fight to the death to defend it. So you have to methodically drive them out. What's more, that damage gets passed to your child, and to their children, as your family's new genetic inheritance.

In summary, you're supposed to have thousands of different strains of microorganisms living in a balanced microbiome – some good guys, some bad guys, and some bad guys that occasionally use their superpowers for good, when the need arises. But taking repeated courses of antibiotics ravages some populations of microbes more than others. Unfortunately for us, many have gone extinct due to use and abuse of antibiotics, antibiotic practices, preservatives in food, toxins and medications.

Note to self: Shifting the balance of power away from good guys toward the bad guys changes the behavior of the microbiome from helpful to harmful – just as if you were to repeatedly round up and kill all the good people in the world, while encouraging all the sociopaths to breed like crazy. Pretty soon, you'd have a thoroughly corrupted population, rampant anti-social behavior, and wrecked neighborhoods (starting to sound familiar?).

Antibiotics kill mitochondria

The latest research shows that medicinal antibiotics, besides being good at killing bacteria, are also poisonous to our mitochondria. Bacteria-killing antibiotics reduce our mitochondrial populations by triggering an overproduction of reactive oxygen species. Increased oxidative stress then kills mitochondria, which cuts down our supply of ATP (cellular energy).

This recent finding should come as no surprise, since bacteria and mitochondria are thought to come from common ancestry. It also lines up well with the observation that most GAPS individuals have taken multiple courses of oral antibiotics in their childhood, causing systemic energy deficits, which affect psychology and detoxification.

Antibiotics fatten up farm animals by destroying pituitary function and corrupting the gut

It's standard practice in commercial animal farming to give chicken, cattle, fish, and other animals antibiotics in their feed. Ranchers will tell you this protects against the spread of germs and disease, which it does. But that's only half of the story. Their sneaky shortcut: Continuous low doses of antibiotics wreck pituitary function and corrupt gut flora – both of which cause some animals to put on weight about twice as fast as naturally-raised livestock. This technique of using antibiotics as a fattening agent is common knowledge throughout the industry. It's the dark side of antibiotics – a trick of the trade they'd rather keep secret.

Do antibiotics do the same in humans? Excellent question. Antibiotics certainly wipe out our beneficial microflora, causing a virtual train wreck of adversity to ensue. But do antibiotics also destroy pituitary function and cause endocrine system disruption, resulting in weight gain? Do they encourage pathogen growth that results in extra pounds? Science is answering 'yes' over and over in the literature.

Antibiotics are proven to cause depression and anxiety disorders

A major study evaluated 202,974 patients with clinical depression, alongside 803,961 control individuals. What they discovered: one course of antibiotics in a year increased the occurrence of major depression by 23%, and anxiety by 17%. Even more striking, two or more courses of antibiotics in a year increased risk for depression to 56%, and anxiety disorder to 44%. The study showed increased risk for other psychological disorders like psychosis and schizophrenia as well.

Man is smart and determined. But Nature is inconceivably experienced

Nature has had limitless opportunity to test and evaluate different systems and strategies to run things throughout the universe. It's had the opportunity try out an endless variety of potential configurations before arriving at the most elegant solutions possible that are altogether simple, effective, efficient, repeatable and resilient. So, in most cases, the way that biological or ecological systems are setup today is the most efficient and effective way in which they can possibly done, all things considered.

Key point: all things considered. Science and commerce can invent new substances, approaches, or ways to subvert Nature. But, lacking ability or willingness to see a situation from all angles, man almost inevitably encounters unwanted side effects that come back to bite him down the road… and with interest. He suffers backlash as a result of his bravado… his intellectual arrogance. More and more, man thinks he knows best. But Nature, again and again, has the last laugh, as we're forced to concede: "Oh, there are other factors we failed to consider. We made mistakes in judgment. And we're not as smart as we thought we were."

Prime examples are indiscriminate antibiotic use, sanitizing hand gels, campaign to demonize germs, fattening farm animals with antibiotics, and efforts to sterilize everything we eat, drink and touch – call these "antibiotic practices." Now, to be sure, these ideas have merit. But they come with risks that Industry sweeps under the rug, until their very sanctity or security is threatened by these existential oversights. They keep chugging along, business as usual, until their methods are called into question, and their reputation is on the line. Consequences are something for others to worry about, it seems. They'll keep doing what they're doing until their innately risky tactics become nightmares, such as MRSA, C. diff, mad cow disease, and other drug-resistant superbugs now dumbfounding medical science.

Admission from the front-lines: September 2016, FDA bans about 2,100 antibacterial hand soaps and body washes, representing about 40% of products in this market, saying they are no more effective than soap and water, and could cause long-term harm. This ruling confirms what many observers believe: the very premise of antibacterial products is flawed from the start. The idea that all germs are bad and need to be wiped out is not only unwise, but also deceptive and dangerous. The truth is, we need the good bugs to keep the bad ones in check, so balance is more important than the mere presence or absence of pathogens.

HOW ANTIBIOTIC RESISTANCE HAPPENS

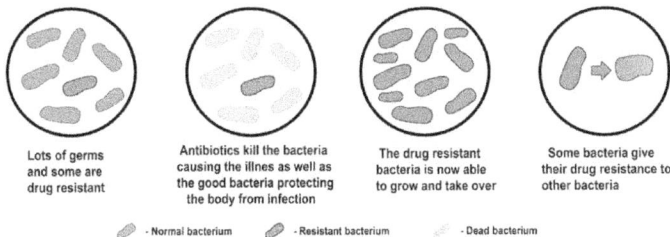

Lots of germs and some are drug resistant

Antibiotics kill the bacteria causing the illness as well as the good bacteria protecting the body from infection

The drug resistant bacteria is now able to grow and take over

Some bacteria give their drug resistance to other bacteria

- Normal bacterium   - Resistant bacterium   - Dead bacterium

Use antibiotics wisely

Without a doubt, antibiotics are a potent tool in the medical professional's arsenal. When you have a serious, life-threatening infection, antibiotics can save your life. So you shouldn't be afraid of them. You just have to respect their killing power, and use them responsibly… even cautiously. Understand that they are literally the weapon of mass destruction on a microbial level. Never use them thoughtlessly or preventively, without good reason. Remember, there's a price to pay when you use them repeatedly.

To put it more potently, **you are playing with fire when you mess with your friends in small places.** It's like playing with a loaded gun that's not only capable of injuring *you* for life, it's capable of maiming *your children* and *your children's children*, because microbiota play critical functions in your mental and physical well-being. There can be serious consequences that go on your permanent record if you mess with the balance of power in your microbiome – potentially for generations to come. So consider taking a quality probiotic supplement before and after a course of antibiotics, or any serious assault to the microbiome (e.g., C. diff). It's not a perfect replacement for probiotic populations, but it's cheap insurance.

We've corrupted our water

The water that most people drink is a persistent, lower-grade threat to gut flora and mental health. That's because tap water in many/most cities is disinfected with chlorine. Chlorine is used as both an active disinfectant at the water treatment plant, and a passive suppressant of microbial growth as the water travels through pipes, or sits in pipes as it waits to be used. The problem is, if chlorine kills microorganisms in water, wouldn't it do the same in your gut? Indeed, it does.

Chlorine gas is one of the most toxic chemicals ever used as a weapon. Its health effects were so horrendous its was banned by the Geneva Convention – even for war.

It's nowhere near as destructive to gut flora as antibiotics. But you're exposed to tap water dozens of times a day, from a variety of sources. In fact, every country in history that chlorinated its water experienced an epidemic of appendicitis (which stores good bacteria) shortly after its introduction because something very important was eliminated: living soil bacteria. It's been recorded in Russia, Britain, Europe, Singapore and China.

And drinking chlorine is only half the threat. Don't forget, much of the food you eat from around the country (and world) is grown, washed, and cooked in chlorinated water. Plus, some swimming pools are disinfected with chlorine. You can also absorb nearly a pound of water when you bathe or shower, because your skin absorbs whatever you put on it in seconds – especially when your pores are open from warm water. So whatever chemicals are present in water quickly enter the bloodstream, without going through the liver. This doesn't harm gut flora directly. But it does give your overburdened detox pathways one more job to do.

Even more damaging, a large percentage of municipalities have switched to chloramine disinfectants. Many superbugs have become chlorine resistant, so many municipalities have switched to disinfection with chloramines, which are a chemical cousin of chlorine. Unfortunately, it can be difficult to remove chloramines. You need an advanced filtering system to remove chloramines, and maintain that effectiveness for more than a few weeks.

More than 73.9% of cities in the US fluoridate their water

They say it's to prevent cavities, but that's simply not true. **There is no evidence whatsoever that fluoride prevents, or even inhibits, cavities.** No study has ever demonstrated that. In fact, our health organizations such as the American Dental Association even admit fluoride does nothing to decrease cavities (as shown by a National Science Foundation study). What's more, fluoride undeniably weakens tooth enamel in a dose-dependent manner (called fluorosis), making teeth more susceptible to cavities. Fluoride also makes bones brittle and rough, leading to broken hips, knee problems and damaged joints.

Even worse, the less toxic form of fluoride used decades ago, sodium fluoride (from the aluminum industry), has largely been replaced by hydrofluorosilicic acid, which is an <u>extremely</u> toxic by-product of the phosphate fertilizer mining industry. Hydrofluorosilicic acid is so corrosive it will eat through concrete, steel, titanium, brick, and even glass. Globalists have pressured, tricked, and defrauded lawmakers into forcing municipalities to add this super toxin to city water supplies, because it's incredibly expensive to dispose of any other way… and they have a lot of it to get rid of. So they get cities to buy it from them.

But to show you common sense still prevails in some places, China, Austria, France, Germany, Italy, Denmark, Belgium, Finland, Norway, Sweden, Northern Ireland, Scotland, Iceland, The Netherlands, Hungary, Switzerland, Luxembourg and Japan have either never fluoridated their water, or they stopped it once they found out how harmful it is to us. They all agree, there is no evidence that fluoridation prevents cavities. On the contrary, there's overwhelming evidence fluoride is toxic to all life.

Fluoride seriously affects the central nervous system

A 1995, Dr. Phyllis Mullenix (Forsyth Dental Center) proved that fluoride profoundly harms brain function. She showed that **when you feed fluoride to pregnant rats, the offspring become hyperactive.** On the other hand, **when you feed baby rats fluoride** *after birth*, **they become lethargic.** She also discovered fluoride accumulates in areas of the brain that control behavior (hippocampus and limbic areas).

After completing the study, she was asked to present her findings to The National Institute of Dental Research. Beforehand, Mullenix accidently overheard the panel being instructed not to turn the discourse into an "inquisition." However, they couldn't help themselves. They proceeded to grill her in an attempt to find fault with her research. But her methodology and conclusions were airtight – and quite innovative, as she was one of the first to use computer pattern recognition in a study of this nature.

Shortly after the meeting, her critics asked where she intended to publish the study. She refused to tell them, much their dismay. After going through an extra review process (because the subject was so controversial), *Neurotoxicology and Teratology* published the paper. In short order, she was fired from her job at Forsyth Dental Center, and never received another federal grant, despite being brought in specifically to head up the Toxicology Department at Forsyth as one of the top researchers in toxicology at the time. Conversely, her critics received several large grants from NIDH and an industrial consortium to fund research at Forsyth.

Not long after that, in 1996, Dr. Mullenix was shown declassified documents by investigative reporters Joel Griffiths and Cliff Honicker indicating one of the men overseeing her work at Forsyth, Harold Hodge, worked on the Manhattan Project decades earlier (which was created to both build the atomic bomb and study health and toxicity).

To her surprise, she found out Hodge had clinical evidence back then (circa 1943) that fluoride severely upsets the central nervous system, causing confusion, drowsiness and lassitude (lack of energy). At the time, the leaders of the project were afraid that workers exposed to the uranium hexafluoride would become a danger to themselves and others. So they asked the military for funding to study the effects, which they got. The study was halted in-progress and never resumed.

Fluoride slowly but surely dumbs you down and makes you sick

- It: accumulates in the thyroid, causing hypothyroidism, which leads to lethargy, apathy, and weakness (for decades, fluoride was the treatment of choice to slow down an overactive thyroid)
- lowers IQ of babies exposed in pregnancy
- substantially increases cancer risk and tumors
- increases fractures across all age groups
- increases arthritis
- contributes to dementia
- "calcifies" in the pineal gland, which is thought to interfere with connection to spirit
- damages sperm, increases infertility
- impairs melatonin production and sleep
- inactivates 62 enzymes.

Basically, fluoride bio-accumulates and causes problems with behavior, intelligence, learning, fertility and chronic disease. So, to make sure we get enough of it, fluoride is an active (but undeclared) ingredient in many antidepressant medications (SSRIs). Thanks Big Pharma.

Putting water quality into perspective

Our ancestors used to drink water directly from streams and lakes. These fresh, clean waters were alive with microorganisms that built up our inner ecosystem. Living water fed us and contributed to our health and vitality. But, today, we do the opposite: We remove all the life we can from it. We treat water with chemicals and processes that throw out beneficial microorganisms, trace minerals and energetic properties.

In fact, today's water is often so devoid of minerals, some call it "hungry water" because, instead of donating minerals as water is supposed to, today's water actually grabs minerals from body fluids. So this is one more instance of modern civilization taking what was once a source of nourishment – our water – and turned it into a persistent, low-dose poison that threatens our mental and physical integrity.

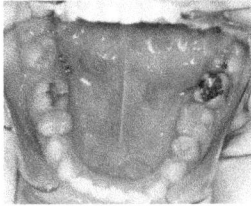

Mercury amalgam fillings

After more than fifty years of denial, avoidance and delay, dental associations in the US have only recently started to admit mercury in dental amalgam fillings *may* be harmful to human health. None have "gone on the record" as an organization and admitted mercury injury causes neurological and systemic problems. But "the dam" that's been holding back a flood of factuality for nearly a century is finally beginning to crack and the truth is trickling out.

As discussed in Chapter 15: "Detoxification and Elimination," dental amalgams emit mercury vapor (as elemental mercury) that you inhale 24/7 – especially when chewing hot food. This destroys nerve cells and interrupts a variety of biochemical processes. Mercury amalgam fillings also corrode, which you swallow as inorganic mercury. This inflames the gut's enterocytes, dysregulates the immune system (GALT), and interferes with the production of transport proteins that detox heavy metals.

According to Dr. Christopher Shade (mercury toxicity expert), mercury amalgam fillings are our #1 or 2 source of mercury exposure, depending on how much big fish you eat (the other major source). His numbers say mercury from vaccines and coal-burning power plants are a distant third and fourth. How much mercury does a person accumulate from dental amalgams? Try 1,000 to 10,000 times that of a person that has none.

Watch undeniable proof of amalgam fillings emitting mercury vapor in YouTube video "What's in your mouth... Mercury Fillings Smoking Teeth." (youtu.be/o2VCe n1vCMY).

Dr. Shade did a small, informal test in his clinic using cysteine as a provocation agent. He had people swish their mouths with a cysteine solution. Using his extremely sensitive test equipment, he found that the "rinsate" contained 1,000 to 10,000 times the mercury of those who didn't have mercury amalgams. Repeating the procedure a second time yielded even more mercury in the rinsate. These results are typical.

This goes to show that the body is capable of tucking away enormous amounts of heavy metals, while appearing only mildly dysfunctional to the untrained observer. Reaching a lethal dose of heavy metal poisoning is extremely difficult to do, and therefore rare, barring long–term occupational exposure such as hat making or intentional poisoning.

Instead, mercury fillings disrupt your body's biochemical systems, and harm you in subtle, yet noticeable ways – often leading to diseases and dysfunction that can be hard to trace back to their source due to cumulative and delayed effects. Bottom line: When your detox systems are working well, a small number of mercury fillings aren't a problem. But most people are so far beyond that point, it would truly shock them at the volume of toxins they're taking in, and the amount they're holding on to.

Mercury filling use is declining

Mankind has known for thousands of years that mercury is highly toxic in extremely minute quantities. Despite that, dental associations have trivialize the risks for decades, saying mercury occurs naturally in the environment, amalgams don't release that much mercury, or the body removes it by itself. But, after 60+ years of pressure from all directions to stop denying and starting helping, dental associations and dentists couldn't avoid the truth any longer. They're finally, if slowly, beginning to change their tune and switch to composite fillings. It may take several decades to remove mercury from dentistry entirely, but we are making progress.

Watch real footage of mercury eating away nerve fibers in video titled "How Mercury Causes Brain Neuron Damage - Uni. of Calgary." (youtu.be/XU8n Sn5Ezd8).

How other insults affect the gut, mind and body

Long–term medication use

- **Increases mineral consumption.** Many drugs crank up bodily processes to produce their effect. Forcing the body to work harder increases consumption of minerals and building blocks to facilitate these processes. The problem is, most ADD/GAPS individuals are mineral deficient, even before extra demand is placed on their diet and metabolism. This wrecks a person's neurotransmitter and hormone availability, energy level, immunity and detoxification. It depletes the body of nutrients it needs elsewhere.

- **Taxes detox organ.** Many drugs severely stress detox organs as they are eliminated, thus requiring liver testing. Virtually every drug on the market is yet one more toxin that the liver needs to deal with.

- **Kills good microbes.** Friendly flora make B vitamins. They help transport nutrients through the gut wall. So taking meds long–term can contribute to corruption of the gut and nutrient deficiencies.

- **Overworks vital organs.** Stimulants, as a class, can overwork the adrenals and exhaust the entire body. Proton pump inhibitors decrease stomach acid, which inhibits digestion and makes the rest of the GI tract work that much harder.

- **Upsets your biochemistry.** Cholesterol-lowering medications inhibit the production of essential hormones and building blocks, such as cortisol, testosterone and estrogen. In doing so, statins wreak havoc on brain function, mood and blood vessel repair. The Pill upsets the body's delicate balance of hormones. And women will often take it for many years before trying to start a family. Pain killers, anti-inflammatories, and anti-psychotics manipulate the body's biochemistry for an isolated, and often short-term, gain.

In short, all drugs are toxic. Long-term medication use disrupts, steals from, delays or suppresses essential processes. And those assaults on the body show up as behavioral problems, nutrient deficiencies, hormonal imbalances, gut dysbiosis, organ failure and toxicity issues. Conclusion: Many drugs have a net positive effect. A few can be life-saving. But there's a price to pay when you take synthetic drugs long-term (as opposed to substances Nature makes). So make sure you understand the potential downsides when subjecting your body to any substance long-term. Do your own research. And don't blindly believe what you're told.

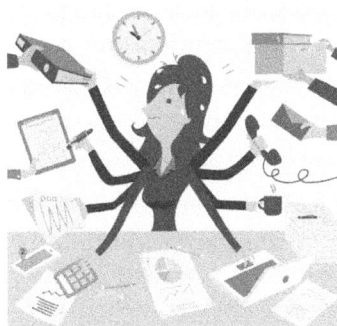

Stress

All forms of stress – be they mental, emotional, physical or chemical – cause the body to release the stress chemicals cortisol, adrenaline, norepinephrine and calcium. Adrenaline and norepinephrine are known to help you concentrate. But excessive amounts can overtax the adrenal glands, keep you up at night, suppress appetite, and wear out the body. They also slow down healing and recovery, because living in a stressed state not only creates more wear and tear on your body, but you also don't get as much deeply restorative sleep to reset your systems. Plus, about half the adrenaline that the body releases goes straight to the gut, which massively stimulates pathogen growth such as E. coli by 10,000 times. Over time, this contributes substantially to pathogen overgrowth and corruption of the gut.

Stress also shuts down routine energy production and consumption, switching the body's energy usage to the stress hormones cortisol and adrenaline. Meaning, you're not digesting food and making energy to fuel your brain and body, as you normally would. Instead, you're storing that food as belly fat. Lacking normal fat and glucose metabolism, you then feel more physically drained, emotionally spent, and mentally cloudy than you would in an unstressed state. All of which accentuate ADD symptoms.

Interestingly enough, stress hormones are made from cholesterol. So cholesterol-lowering drugs interfere with your body's ability to make the hormones that help you manage stress. As a result, you tend to have less patience and anger more easily. You become mean and difficult to live with. Mentally, stress is able to increase brain function. It sharpens your mind and helps your body overcome challenges. But if you rely on stress too much – as people do using stimulants, drama, and social media to enhance focus – it becomes harmful and eventually counter-productive.

Old age

As we age, every system in the body works just a little less efficiently – which means it works harder accomplishing the same task, or its performance degrades over time. No surprise. But there are several downstream effects when organs and processes lose functionality.

For one, imbalances and impairments increase as the body runs out of places to put toxins. Detoxing is one of the most important things that the body must do – perhaps its most underrated. Yet general practitioners are taught very little about detoxification in medical school, so they don't recognize its effects, treat, or even pay much attention to it. As a result, our toxin load steadily increases, unbeknownst to the individual, until the body runs out of places to put the stuff that it can't eliminate. Extreme example: An individual undergoing a heavy detox program noticed his bowels reeked of chlorine that was likely stored away decades earlier when he swam competitively.

At the same time, most people decrease their physical activity over time. This slows the release of toxins, because the squeezing action of muscles is the main way that lymph vessels pump toxins through the system. Movement mobilizes toxins. But when toxins stagnate in the lymph, or anywhere in the body, they interfere with a variety of biochemical processes that lead to degeneration. For instance, when heavy metals enter the brain, they don't leave easily, which can lead to Alzheimer's or dementia in increasingly younger populations. When heavy metals land on receptor sites in the nervous system that are designed to hold trace minerals, metabolism, cell reproduction, and energy production are disrupted.

As we age, liver function also slows due to a decrease in the production of transport proteins, among hundreds of things that the liver does for us. Our cell walls also lose permeability, which impairs hydration, nutrient uptake, and elimination on a cellular level. Plus, our bowels tend to get clogged and have a harder time passing digested food, respiratory waste products, and toxins that need to go.

The entire digestive system declines, because our stomach doesn't produce as much acid. The pancreas doesn't make enzymes like it used to. Our liver doesn't release as much bile that breaks down fat. And our gut flora tends to shift toward pathogen-dominance as the years go by. These things lead to fewer nutrients being produced, circulated, used and eliminated. It means the body has to work harder to compensate for these vitamin and mineral deficiencies. And it means the body has to do without some of the activities that once kept it healthy.

So, to recap, the body does an amazing job of getting rid of toxins on a daily and lifelong basis. It does an equally incredible job of storing toxins that it can't get rid of in silos around the body. But, as we age, our detox system runs out of places to put the trash. And the garbage spills into sensitive, mission critical workspaces. Blockages happen. That's when slowdowns and breakdowns in old age start presenting symptoms that we call disorder and disease.

Alcohol

Having alcohol in your system is called "intoxicated" for a reason: Ethyl alcohol (ethanol) is a poison that your liver and detox organs need to remove as quickly as possible before it damages cells. Specifically, alcohol dissolves the membranes that keep the inside of cells separate from the outside. It denatures proteins, which literally dissolves cell walls that hold organs and tissues together. That's important in GAPS individuals, because alcohol also does the same thing to bacteria and microbiota in your gut: it kills them and contributes to corruption of the gut.

As a result, alcohol decreases executive function and coordination while you're under the influence. Meanwhile, it increases your animal instincts due to lack of inhibition. And it erodes the structure and function of the brain through chronic exposure. It also gives your liver more work to do on an emergent basis, thereby slowing its ability to detoxify other poisons from the body.

Nuclear radiation poisoning

Radioactive contamination messes with cellular function directly by interfering with protein production. It disturbs cell replication by creating DNA mutations. And it injures, mutates, and kills gut flora.

Radioactivity is a much more serious threat than most people realize – particularly in children, and in regions where nuclear weapons were (intentionally) tested, such as New Mexico and the Pacific islands. Equally bad are "accidents," such as Fukushima and Chernobyl. Incidences like these threaten life all over the world from radiation riding atmospheric and ocean currents. Unfortunately, radioactivity can take hundreds of thousands of years to degrade on its own.

One of the primarily ways that radioactive isotopes ravage the body is through destruction of thyroid function. The thyroid requires iodine to run its delicate hormonal activities. Iodine is so desperately needed for the thyroid to work properly that it's been added to refined salt for decades. However, the thyroid can't tell the difference between radioactive iodine and non-radioactive. So it absorbs every bit of either that it can get. The right kind helps the thyroid regulate the body's idle speed. The radioactive variety destroys the thyroid, leading to underactive thyroid or overactive, as well as a litany of problems related to each.

The best defense against this type of radiation exposure is to take potassium iodide before the exposure or immediately after. (Iodide is the ionic version of iodine that's bonded to potassium.) Potassium iodide is the most effective prevention/treatment against radiation poisoning. It protects you by saturating the thyroid with non-radioactive iodide/iodine so that radioactive potassium iodine 131 can't get into the thyroid (as well as blood cells and other organs) and cause any damage. Talk to your health practitioner if you experience a sudden onset of acute pain in the gut area that you suspect may be caused by radiation exposure.

See Recommended Resources section at back for products to detox from radiation poisoning.

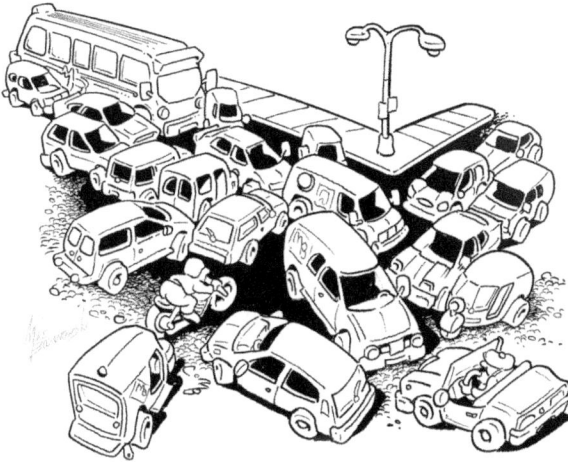

11

IS A CORRUPTED GUT CAUSING THESE PROBLEMS IN YOU?

Visible signs of ADD and GAPS conditions
Facial bones can display signs of nutrient deficiencies in ADD/GAPS

One of the first places in the body to show visible signs of nutrient deficiency, and susceptibility to ADD, is in the bones of the face. The first to be affected is the maxilla, then the lower jaw, then the hip bones. The maxilla, which forms the upper jaw and middle-third of the face (cheekbones), is one of the first bones to suffer from underdevelopment when the body lacks the nutrition it needs in childhood to grow to its full genetic potential.

When you're undernourished, the maxilla grows narrower, shorter, and smaller than it's genetically programmed to, making the middle third of the face, from the eyes to the upper jaw, appear less robustly constructed than it's designed to be – in some cases like they're hanging off an enlarged skull (picture starving African children). This causes the upper palate of the mouth to be smaller than it should be. Teeth come in crooked. And wisdom teeth usually have to be pulled due to overcrowding. Cleft palate and cleft lip are likely caused by the same thing: select nutrient deficiencies (as suggested by Dr. Francis Pottenger's cat studies).

Images on pp. 189–190 are the copyrighted property of the Price-Pottenger Nutrition Foundation, Inc. All rights reserved. Used with permission.

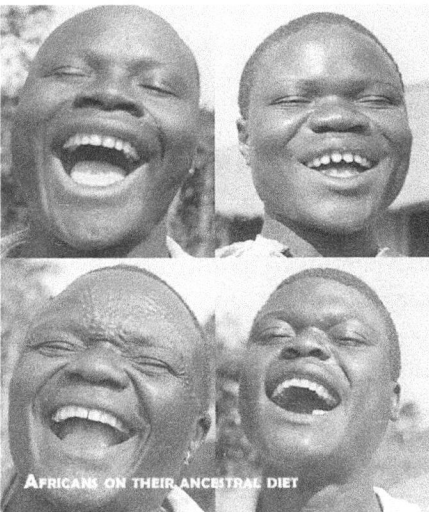

Conversely, when you're properly nourished, the maxilla grows to its full size. All the teeth come in straight, and you don't need braces. There's even room for the wisdom teeth without overcrowding. That's the way our bone structure is genetically designed to be. Dr. Weston A. Price documented all this when he studied nutrition and physical degeneration in the 1920s and '30s (now largely ignored by mainstream medicine). He spent over ten years studying native populations around the world that were born and raised eating their traditional diets, as well as the first generation to eat a Western diet of processed foods.

He found that native populations eating whole foods from the land and sea did not suffer from

AFRICANS ON THEIR ANCESTRAL DIET

cavities, degenerative diseases, or difficult childbirth. Cancer, diabetes, and arthritis were practically non–existent. Their babies didn't cry inconsolably. They were happy and content. The people had broad faces and pleasant dispositions. The men in a village all looked like brothers, and the women sisters, because they received the nutrients they needed in childhood to reach their genetic potential – including vitamins A, D, E and K, plus minerals.

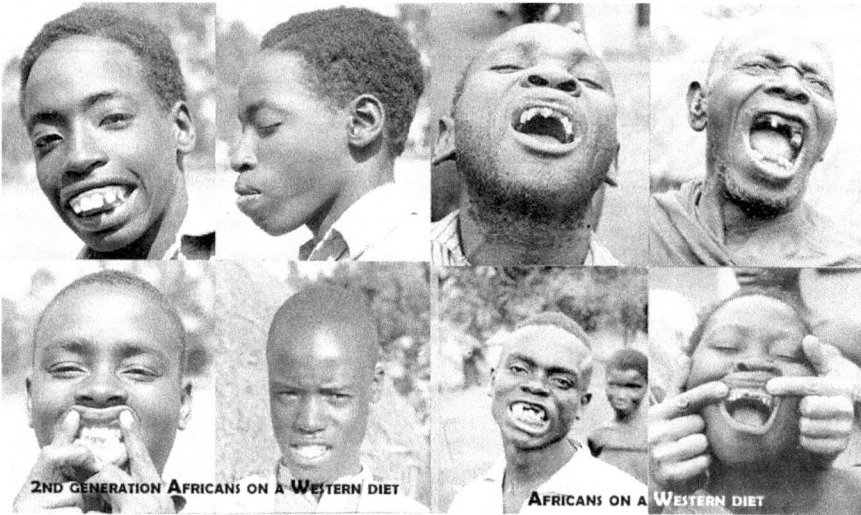

2ND GENERATION AFRICANS ON A WESTERN DIET   AFRICANS ON A WESTERN DIET

On the other hand, the first generation born and raised on foods made from white flour, sugar, vegetable oils, and processed ingredients developed dental deformities, including narrow palate, crooked teeth, cleft palate, overbites and underbites. Women had more pain and difficulty in childbirth due to narrowing of hip bones. Babies cried regularly. They all developed the degenerative diseases we accept as normal today. And they lost some of their positive outlook.

Dr. Price saw the difference in people's faces and documented in pictures what happens when you switch from a diet of natural, whole foods to a diet of processed, unhealthy foods made by commercial food companies. He showed that nutrient-sparse foods clearly changed facial features for the worse. But what pained him the most was seeing the immense suffering that tooth decay caused before the native populations had dentists to fix the damage caused by cavity-causing foods. He saw previously healthy populations stricken with diabetes, obesity and modern diseases.

Today, narrowing of the face is so common, we think nothing of it. However, the eye still reveres high cheekbones and a symmetrical face indicative of proper nutrition and underlying good health. Terrific bone structure is still coveted in the modeling industry. If you want to track

Please visit price-pottenger.org and/or read Dr. Price's book, Nutrition and Physical Degeneration, *to learn more about how the nutrients that Nature puts into food give people beautiful skeletal structure and robust health, whereas commercial food production and processing depletes "food" of nutrients, predisposing you to the diseases of civilization.*

this phenomenon happening over generations, examine old photos from several generations ago – those most likely to have eaten pastured-raised animal products and whole foods from nature. You'll see most of them had broad faces and high cheekbones that we still consider attractive today. Look at old family photos of multiple generations side by side and you might see an increasingly narrow face from one generation to the next.

Conclusion: Although you can't say for sure that a person who has a narrow face definitely has ADD. And you also can't say that a person who has a broad face and naturally straight teeth does not have ADD. But there is a strong correlation between the two, because gut dysbiosis does cause both ADD and nutrient deficiencies that lead to underdevelopment of facial bones. They're frequently seen together.

Autistic facial features can normalize when malnutrition is corrected

Think autistic facial features are set in stone and can never be reversed? Think again. As Dr. Zach Bush explains, autistic facial features are not hard-wired into an individual at birth. Rather, they're caused by nutrient deficiencies and resulting epigenetic alterations, in which the genetic expression of autistics give them facial features as much like each other as siblings or parents. The effect is not quite as dramatic as Down's syndrome. But autistics do tend to have a pathologically absent expression – like they're not intellectually present in the moment. It alters physical features noticeably, but almost indescribably. And it often produces dark circles around the eyes, which is a tell-tale sign of nutrient deficiency.

What may come as a surprise to you and the medical community is that these deviations from your genetic design can be reversed. It doesn't happen quickly or easily. But when you correct nutrient deficiencies, and fix underlying problems that cause autism, you can normalize a person's "look about them," eliminate dark circles under the eyes, and remodel bones of the face over a course of years – especially when started in their formative years.

Fidgeting, knee bouncing, pen twiddling and finger drumming

Many ADD individuals repetitively bounce their leg up and down when sitting, in order to stimulate brain function. They say it feels good. More accurately, it feels satisfying because the activation of muscles releases neurotransmitters in the brain which also fuel cognition. Like a natural biohack, fidgeting or any movement calms the discomforting feelings that come from an underactive prefrontal cortex by increasing activity in the brain centers responsible for movement, coordination and cognition. This increases the availability of neurotransmitter "juice" for the entire brain to use – particularly cognitive function. Very similar is the salesmen's saying 'motion creates emotion,' in that movement stimulates brain function.

Thus, chronic leg bouncing is a tell-tale sign of ADD. It comes from stimulation-seeking behavior by a nervous system that's uncomfortable in an underactive state. The ADD brain needs the increased physical activity to raise its mental function. So it compels the body to move in any way that's socially-acceptable at the time (or not). It would be fair to call this sort of ADD compulsion a more controlled/controllable version of autistic "stimming" in that they're doing it to make their nervous system feel more comfortable. However, ADD'ers have greater conscious control over it.

On the other hand, neurotypical people don't feel that same urge to consume "nervous energy." Their cognitive function operates in a comfortable range the vast majority of the time, so they feel fine in a completely relaxed neuromuscular state. Until they get tired, nervous or otherwise depleted, non-GAPS people are content just being still.

Uncontrolled blinking, facial tics, neck twitching, shoulder shrugging

Some GAPS individuals experience facial tics or forceful, involuntary blinking. Less common are neck twitching or shoulder shrugging. While these kinds of muscle spasms are not connected to cognitive function, they certainly don't do you any favors in terms of first impressions or social cues.

To observers, it's a dead giveaway that something is short-circuiting in the brain, causing the person to lose muscle control for a split second. That's probably why rapid, uncontrolled movements like these are unsettling to observe – especially for women: there's a brief loss of motor control indicative of a potential psychological disorder. Presumably, our subconscious suspects that tics and twitches are caused by the same mechanisms of action that cause brain disorders.

Instinct tells us that inappropriate firing of nerve cells (i.e., lack of neuronal inhibition), and miscommunication in the brain, causes these macro movements to occur without intent or restraint. That flips a switch in people's awareness, telling them something's not quite right here, so watch out. This caution/fear is hardwired into humans in response to those lacking mental or physical control over themselves.

Whatever the case may be, unregulated movements such as these may be caused or worsened by magnesium deficiency. Recall that magnesium lets cells, muscles, and blood vessels relax by inhibiting inappropriate or excessive firing of nerves. According to recent reports, some 80% of Americans are magnesium deficient. And it's no wonder. Here are a few ways that we get to be magnesium deficient:

- high sugar/carb diet depletes magnesium levels
- low dietary intake of magnesium
- mal-absorption due to a corrupted gut
- increased magnesium consumption from medications
- nnEMF exposure, such as cell phones and Wi-Fi.

Another circumstance that causes/contributes to facial tics is neurotransmitter imbalances messing up communications between brain centers. Ordinarily, the prefrontal cortex (PFC) quashes erroneous signals before they're passed around the brain and out to the body. Without proper neurotransmitter levels to excite or inhibit brain function – especially when lacking PFC gatekeeper function – false excitatory signals escape uncorrected, resulting in twitches. This enables "micro seizures" to occur.

Corruption of the gut
When your gut flora turn on you, the gut wall loses competence

Friendly gut flora are a major source of nourishment and protection for cells lining the digestive tract. However, beneficial bacteria have to nourish themselves first, before they can feed cells of the gut wall and the rest of the body. So there's a few mouths to feed before organs and tissues get any nourishment. Cells of the gut lining are in the middle of it.

It's estimated that the gut wall (epithelium) gets 60–70% of its energy directly from bacterial activity. So when the microbiome is overrun by pathogens, epithelial cells don't eat well, and their ability to make, digest, and pass nutrients to the body dwindles. Unable to stay fit, the cells of the gut wall weaken. The gut wall becomes more vulnerable to attack from gluten and glyphosate in wheat. Too much zonulin gets made. The gut wall fails to provide a tight-knit defensive barrier for the rest of the body. And toxins enter the bloodstream, driving the immune system crazy.

There's a river of toxicity flowing from a leaky gut. When a person's gut becomes porous, a river of toxicity slips through the gut wall and flows into the bloodstream. Heavy metals, toxins produced by pathogens, chemicals such as glyphosate, undigested food particles, and unfriendly microbes get past your probiotic and enterocyte defenses and run free in the body. Most damaging to cognition are the hundreds of metabolic waste products that unfriendly microbes produce that pollute the chemistry and functioning of the brain.

Image used under Creative Commons 4.0 license. Author: BallenaBlanca.

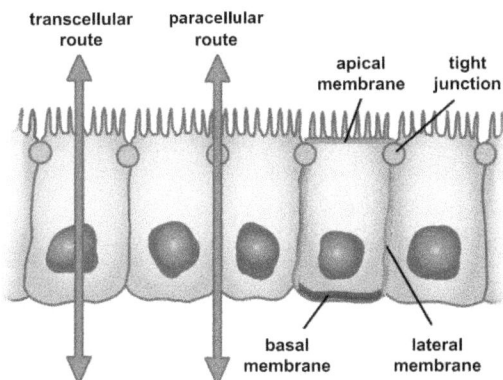

transcellular route | paracellular route | apical membrane | tight junction | basal membrane | lateral membrane

How leaky gut happens

Pathogenic microbes living in your digestive tract excrete waste products that dissolve the tight junctions that hold enterocytes tightly together. When tight junctions are intact, nothing can get through the gut wall because (smaller) micronutrients are transported <u>through</u> enterocytes to reach the bloodstream, while (larger) macronutrients enter the bloodstream by going <u>in between</u> enterocytes. That's when the gut is healthy.

But, when there are too many pathogens of a certain type living in the gut (particularly candida), their toxins eat holes in the gut lining, which lets all sorts of undesirable substances into the bloodstream. This condition is lovingly called "leaky gut" by natural healers, referring to the fact that a healthy gut blocks almost every substance that's harmful to the body. Equally bad, those microbial toxins and zonulin can then circulate in the bloodstream and break down protective membranes throughout the body, causing leaky blood vessels, leaky kidney tubules and, instrumental to GAPS, a leaky blood-brain barrier.

Leaky membranes are so new to medical science that they haven't even gotten around to inventing fancier names than "leaky blood-brain barrier, leaky kidney tubules, and leaky blood vessels." Leaky membranes – first at the gut, then throughout the body – conspire to form a river of toxicity that pollutes the bloodstream and every organ, especially the brain. What happens then is disastrous because of how upsetting chemicals are to the mental state of millions.

To put the danger of leaky gut into perspective, the intestinal wall in a healthy person is so impenetrable to inappropriate substances that drug companies used to have trouble getting medications into the bloodstream via the digestive tract. With some drugs, medicated skin patches had to be used to get chemicals into the bloodstream through transdermal absorption.

200+ autoimmune conditions originate in the gut

While mainstream medicine sees no evil, hears no evil, and speaks no evil when it comes to explaining autoimmune conditions, Dr. Natasha, Dr. Alessio Fasano, and fellow gut-brain pioneers figured it out long ago: a corrupted gut is the root cause of 200+ autoimmune diseases.

Gut dysbiosis initiates autoimmune disorders such as

- **Arthritis.** When toxins attach themselves to collagen in your joints, the immune system can mistake one for the other, causing arthritis.
- **Type 1 diabetes.** When toxins get into the pancreas, pancreatic beta cells can be damaged so they can't produce insulin.
- **Multiple sclerosis.** When toxins get into the myelin nerve sheath, the immune system can attack, causing multiple sclerosis.
- **Inflammatory bowel disease, Chron's disease and celiac disease.** When the walls of the GI tract become overloaded with toxins, serious autoimmune-related digestive disorders often show up.
- **Psoriasis and Eczema.** When toxins accumulate in the skin, psoriasis or eczema can result.
- **Lupus.** When the immune system is hyperactivated, a wide variety of lupus symptoms can show up all over the body.

How autoimmunity develops

Toxic substances swim around in the bloodstream, until they come into contact with a type of tissue that has an affinity for that toxin due to compatible molecular shapes and unoccupied binding sites. They then stick together like sweethearts who have found their soulmate. This can happen anywhere in the body: joints (arthritis), pancreas (diabetes type 1), nerve insulation (MS), kidneys (renal failure), heart valves (heart disease), or skin (psoriasis, eczema).

The body's immune system, constantly on the lookout for threats, then looks at the new shape of the tissue, with toxin(s) attached. It doesn't have its shape "on file" as something friendly or innocuous. Meaning, it doesn't recognize the structure as belonging to you anymore. And it doesn't think it's food either. The immune system basically decides *that's not me*. It assumes the toxin-human tissue combination is a foreign invader and assaults it with intent to kill (through TH_2 cells). This continues unless/until the gut lining is healed and sealed.

While all this is happening, your body's repair mechanisms are trying to rebuild tissues maimed through these attacks. It's like trench warfare where one side gains ground one day, and the other side wins it back the next. This conflict can go on for years or decades. And, eventually, this mistaken identity-friendly fire situation, and subsequent attempts to fix the damage, can turn into chronic disease in almost any tissue of the body. This is the chain of events by which autoimmunity develops. In simpler terms, **all autoimmune disease is born in the gut. At its core, autoimmunity is a digestive disorder.**

The truth about food intolerances

Many people have raised a fuss about "allergies" that affected individuals have to milk, wheat, nuts, soy, eggs and shellfish. Meanwhile, the Feingold crowd believes that behavior problems are caused by artificial colors, flavors, sweeteners and preservatives. While autism associations have made the "Gluten-free, casein-free" diet their unofficial diet of choice for autism.

But, the truth of the matter is, it's not the foods we need to focus on. It's the corrupted gut itself. As long as the gut wall lets food pass into the bloodstream partially digested, you're going to react to pretty much anything that you eat frequently, because you're going to react to more and more foods in your diet, until you hardly have anything left to eat. As you eliminate one food after another, the increased exposure to those remaining in your diet irritate the immune system and raise your sensitivity to those foods. The solution: heal and seal the gut lining.

True food allergies are rare

A real food allergy is when the *adaptive immune system*, after prolonged exposure to an inappropriate substance, targets that product with antibodies for many months to years – even after removing the offending substance from your diet.

But what happens in most cases of food sensitivity is that a leaky gut lets partially digested food into the bloodstream. This chronically over-activates the *innate* immune system, which is non-selective. Using a shotgun approach, it attacks everything it thinks is harmful. This subjects your own cells to collateral damage. Fortunately, as soon as offending substances are removed from the diet, the innate immune system turns off, and adverse reactions go away in a couple of days to months.

Humans are not naturally prone to gluten sensitivity
Normally, CXCR3 receptors that bind to gliadin and release zonulin are very poorly expressed in intestinal cells without some sort of provocation. They're scarce on our small intestine and colon cells, in a healthy state. But, within hours of glyphosate exposure, expression of CXCR3 receptors explodes, dramatically increasing your vulnerability to tight junction injury from gluten. At that point, any gluten that you eat triggers a massive release of zonulin, which breaks down tight junctions, causing leaky gut. Unfortunately, the standard American diet now routinely doses us with both glyphosate and gluten in each bite. So, over time, that makes us far more sensitive to gluten, as well as alkaloid-containing nightshade vegetables, proteins, and many foods you eat frequently.

Food sensitivities can cause any symptom under the sun
When partially-digested food particles get into the bloodstream and cause a food intolerance, sensitivity or allergy (however you define it), this can trigger a wide variety of symptoms, such as headache, rash, hypoglycemia, drop in energy, mood swing, panic attack, eczema or psoriasis. These can happen minutes, hours, days, or even weeks later. So, at any given moment, a person has no idea what they're reacting to because symptoms can be delayed, and overlap with each other. This can make it difficult to pinpoint the source of annoyances. For this reason, elimination diets are losing utility, in favor of gut healing protocols.

Expressions of poor digestion

Acid reflux
Candida produce a waste product that the liver converts into acetaldehyde – a potent toxin that can paralyze the stomach valve leading into the esophagus, called the "esophageal sphincter." When this valve malfunctions, stomach contents can leak into the esophagus when you lie down, causing acid reflux, heartburn, and sometimes vomiting in babies.

Acid reflux: Acid leaking into the lower throat/windpipe.

This is another situation in which modern medicine causes unintended consequences with their drugs. When you reduce stomach acid production with proton pump inhibitors, your stomach can't do its job of breaking down food properly. The less acidic environment allows bacteria to grow in the stomach, which is supposed to be virtually devoid of bacteria. Decreased stomach acid also means less digestion takes place before food passes into the GI tract, thus contributing to food intolerances, auto-immune reactions, and small intestine bacterial overgrowth (SIBO).

Making matters worse, drinking too much water with meals dilutes stomach acid further. Instead, you want to drink the majority of your water forty-five minutes to an hour before a meal, or an hour to an hour-and-a-half after eating a meal. Thankfully, acid reflux tends to clear up more quickly and easily than other manifestations of a corrupted gut. It's been known to go away in a few weeks to months by taking steps to reduce candida overgrowth.

Low stomach acid

Low stomach acid production inhibits digestion. Contrary to what Big Pharma tell us, excess stomach acid does not cause heartburn, indigestion, gas, bloating or acid reflux. Instead, digestive juices in the stomach need to be as acidic as possible to break down food properly – particularly proteins. Otherwise, the burden of digestion shifts further down the GI tract onto organs and microorganisms that are ill-equipped for the job. Poor digestion and mal-absorption then stress the GI tract and microbiome, leading to nutrient deficiencies, leaky gut, inflammation and autoimmunity.

The most common cause of low stomach acid is an overgrowth of pathogens releasing their toxic waste products around the stomach valve and lower esophagus, causing a failure of the mechanism that regulates stomach acid production. Fortunately, most cases of stomach acid deficiency sort themselves out when the microbiome and gut are healed. In the meantime, your functional medicine practitioner may recommend a stomach acid enhancer like Betaine HCL. In any case, low stomach acidity can undermine your progress, if it's weak and you fail to notice it.

Small intestinal bacterial overgrowth (SIBO)

Contrary to what people think, pathogenic bacteria that cause SIBO in the small intestine don't migrate up from the colon. Rather, they travel down from the nasal sinuses pathologically. SIBO is a result of glyphosate and other toxins breaking down the barrier protecting the sinus cavity from pollen, dander, dust and mold spores.

Intrusions like these irritate the immune system, left vulnerable behind the tight junctions of the nasal sinus barrier. To defend itself, the immune system in the sinuses chronically produces mucus to capture and carry away irritants such as pollen that overwork the immune system. This "post-nasal drainage" has become as common as allergies.

How it happens: Overnight, when we sleep, our stomach is supposed to rest with us. Not expecting to get any food to digest, stomach acid production drops. Lower acidity in the stomach weakens the stomach's ability to kill bacteria coming from the sinuses that are supposed to live in the sinuses, not the small intestine. This happens in addition to any low-acid conditions in the stomach due to a corrupted microbiome, and/or any drugs that block stomach acid production.

So all night long, post-nasal drainage is leaking bacteria into the stomach. When enough of them survive the trip through the stomach, and overgrow in the small intestine, you get SIBO. The fix then is two-fold: rebuild the two defensive lines – the sinus barrier and stomach acid – and SIBO can't survive. Protect the tight junctions, nasal sinus barrier, and immune system in the nose with ION Sinus Support, and correct the low stomach acid condition with a product such as HCL with betaine.

Many GAPS people can't digest fats properly

Bile flow is one of the main highways of detoxification. In a healthy system, the liver cleanses itself by releasing toxins into the flow of bile made by the liver. Bile flow breaks down fat, and transports toxins into the digestive system to be neutralized, chelated, or otherwise removed by the GI tract and microbiota. The toxic soup then joins other waste products, aggregates into stools as fluid is removed, and then leaves through the colon.

So, normally, digesting fats encourages the liver to release chemicals, toxins, and pathogens into bile, and on to the digestive tract. That means **fats in the diet regulate how fast or slowly bile carries toxins out of the body.** However, the whole process gets derailed when you eat a low-fat diet, which is common in vegans, vegetarians, anorexia, autistics, and other GAPS conditions. That sets off a series of unfortunate events.

For example, when the liver can't excrete toxins in a timely manner, it imprisons them. It coats the foreign invaders in a layer of bile, forming a soft clump. As bile flow slows further, the clumps calcify into stones, they roughen and get stuck in the bile ducts. At the same time, corrupted gut flora can't do their job of cleaning house in the intestines either. So toxins, pathogens, and worms get stuck in the bile ducts, halting their flow.

When that happens, the liver can't release bile, toxins lose mobility through the body, fat is not broken down, and essential fats cannot be distributed to the brain, nervous system, hair, skin, nails, bones, and glands, which need fats for maintenance. This is a serious problem for vital organs and processes that use fat as a building material, process facilitator, energy source, or transportation medium.

Hormone imbalances

The hormonal system is a chemical means of communication by which endocrine glands such as adrenals, pancreas and ovaries, regulate bodily function at a distance by secreting hormones into the bloodstream.

Hormones tell organs throughout the body what controller glands such as the pituitary, thyroid, adrenal, and pineal want to have done. Some of the more important functions that hormones regulate are: energy level, metabolism, sleep, growth and development, sexual function and mood.

A hormone, when released into the blood by an endocrine gland, floats inertly throughout the body, until it lands on a receptor site of its destination organ. When that connection is made, several bodily processes are typically activated. Insulin is one of these hormones that trigger actions in the body through its presence in the blood.

But, most important, hormones tell organs what to do using infinitesimal volumes – we're talking trillionths of a liter, in some cases – to relay a signal. So not only are hormones incredibly important in making the body run properly, they're also extremely sensitive to deviation. The slightest variation, no matter how minute, produces operational anomalies. So it's not hard to see why hormone imbalances create health disturbances ranging from annoying to devastating.

Toxins interfere with endocrine function

Toxins enter the picture and mess up delicate processes of hormone production and interaction. They can clog receptor sites so hormones can't do their job. The result being, multi-factorial processes such as sugar metabolism, energy production or disordered sleep. Individual organs become glitchy. And organ systems diverge from "the program."

Dr. Natasha

"All our hormones in the body work as a team. They control each other. They talk to each other. And they regulate each other's levels – like through the circadian rhythm. They're different at night, during the day, and by lunchtime – they're all different. And these toxins interfere in that very delicate balance. And as a result, because hormones rule our whole metabolism, they are extremely powerful. If they're abnormal, so many things go wrong in the body."

PART 3

---❧---

The Science and Mystery of ADD

I2

VACCINES

Know the risks before you vaccinate

Nearly everyone that receives the standard vaccine schedule today is being harmed chronically. In fact, **over half of our children today have at least one chronic disease, if not many (not including obesity); 21% are developmentally delayed.** There is a reason, and vaccines are a big part of it. You can thank vaccines for laying a lot of the foundation for modern disease to occur in much of our population. At the root of the problem is repeated vaccination leaves people susceptible to genetic and environmental vulnerabilities that would otherwise remain dormant, given appropriate immune response and healing capacity to spare. Three categories of injury:

1. **Lowered immunity.** Almost everyone receiving the CDC's full vaccine schedule will experience lowered immunity to all infections for many years to come.
2. **Degradation of brain function.** The majority will suffer not-so-obvious, ongoing damage to brain cells from the release of neuro-destructive chemicals such as cytokines and glutamate, along with prolonged inflammation of the brain's special immune cells: microglia.
3. **Serious complications.** A tiny minority will suffer serious reactions to the viral/bacteria agent in the vaccines (antigen), substances added to stimulate the immune system (adjuvants), and/or contaminants such as campylobacter bacteria in the growth medium.

These effects are caused by multiple circumstances aligning to cause over-activation of the immune system and prolonged hypersensitivity. Guillain-Barré Syndrome is one such extreme outcome. In short, virtually everyone that gets the recommended shots, at the recommended times, **will be dumbed down a little to a lot. Most will be hit harder, and more frequently, by illnesses throughout their lifetime. An unfortunate few will be left dead, permanently disabled, or dysfunctional in some way.** And a small minority will escape unharmed.

History of modern vaccination

Before the modern era of vaccination, ancient Egyptians, Chinese, Arabs and Danish were believed to have used various methods of inoculating people to give them immunity against disease. More recently, Polish, Scottish and English healers are said to have done the same. One such technique is blowing the dried powder of a "pock" into a person's nose in an attempt to stimulate an immune response.

Then, in 1791–1796, Edward Jenner, an English apothecary barber/surgeon, is generally credited with inventing modern vaccination. As the story goes, he heard rumors amongst dairy maids that people who contracted *cow pox* somehow were protected against getting *smallpox* (a potentially fatal disease). To test his theory, he took fluid from a cow pox pustule and injected it into the arm of James Phipps, a healthy 8-year-old boy.

Phipps contracted cow pox as expected and got over it. Eight weeks later, Jenner injected Phipps with smallpox fluid. When Phipps did not come down with smallpox, Jenner proclaimed his theory correct: *immunity can be induced through inoculation with an agent related to the disease* (in this case, to a similar disease). Jenner vaccinated his own son multiple times, and re-vaccinated Phipps twenty times. Sadly, Phipps and Jenner's son both died from tuberculosis, age 20 and 21, respectively. Researchers today suspect there's a link between the smallpox vaccine and tuberculosis.

Fast forward almost a century to Leicester, England, around 1885: 95–100% of the town's population were vaccinated against smallpox, yet the town suffered terrible epidemics of smallpox anyway. Outraged, 80,000 residents protested the town's mandatory vaccination laws, which persuaded town leaders to stop vaccinating. Instead, they cleaned up their dairies. They cleaned up their streets. They installed plumbing. They focused on nutrition. And within several years, smallpox outbreaks had gone down by 80%.

Conclusion: Jenner's theory is the entire premise upon which the paradigm of vaccination rests. However, no convincing evidence has ever been proffered to support the notion that vaccination gives you immunity that's anywhere near as strong, or as long-lasting, as naturally-acquired immunity. Vaccine experts agree on this.

Did vaccines really eradicate diseases?

Health experts claim that vaccines wiped out many serious diseases that used to cause major epidemics. But, when you look at statistics honestly from the first half of the 20th Century, you see mortality rates had been dropping well before vaccines were ever introduced. Mortality from measles, scarlet fever, typhoid, whooping cough, and diphtheria all decreased between 60%–95% before vaccines for them were ever introduced.

How did that happen? Improvements in nutrition, sanitation such as purifying water and pasteurizing milk, education, and public healthcare were the real reasons that infection and mortality rates went down. And that was pre-1950. We've made even greater strides since the 1950s improving environmental conditions that cause health problems. And we find even more proof, looking further back in history.

Hundreds of years ago, lots of people died of scurvy, bubonic plague, tuberculosis, scarlet fever and yellow fever. In fact, populations throughout history have been hit with run-of-the-mill epidemics to biblical-style plagues in city ghettos, confined ships and even hospitals. But infection and mortality from these diseases largely vanished before vaccines were ever created. However, when you massage the reporting of historical events, you can make it seem like vaccines deserve the credit where no credit is due.

Remember, prior to the second half of the 1800s – before Pasteur came up with his germ theory – doctors knew nothing about germs, and they didn't wash their hands before doing medical procedures (after shoveling shit and milking cows). They didn't have clean, running water. They used outhouses (or worse). They lived in crowded quarters. And most people ate poorly, when they ate at all.

Bottom line: Plagues of old, including bubonic plague, scarlet fever, and yellow fever went away not through vaccination, but by reducing exposure to infectious agents, and by creating more healthful conditions that strengthened the body's ability to fight disease. In fact, government statistics show death from disease declined steadily from 1900 to the early '70s. They bottomed out between 1976 and 1986. Then, after 1986, mortality rates started to climb as vaccination programs ramped up. The trend continues to this day, with countries promoting the most bloated vaccine schedules suffering the worst infant mortality rates and chronic diseases in adults.

How naturally acquired immunity works

When you come down with a disease "organically," two sides of your immune system get activated: your "innate" immune system, which is non-specific, and your "adaptive" immune system (aka "acquired" immune system), which is specific.

Your **innate immune system** is like a shot gun in its approach to extinguishing infections. It has no intelligence built into it. It doesn't remember past infections. And it doesn't selectively go after certain invaders and not others. It just attacks and kills everything that it deems to be foreign to the body. Most important in understanding the innate immune system, it behaves exactly this way for all future infections and threats. So it doesn't learn, and it doesn't adapt, as its regular process. However, it does have one special talent: It's very good at distinguishing your own cells from ones that don't belong to you. For this reason, your innate immunity is not primarily responsible for autoimmune reactions.

On the other side, your **adaptive immune system,** works like a rifle in its approach to targeting pathogens. The first time your immune system encounters an enemy that it doesn't recognize, it learns which microbes are the bad guys, and it tags them with "antibodies." The

B-cell activation

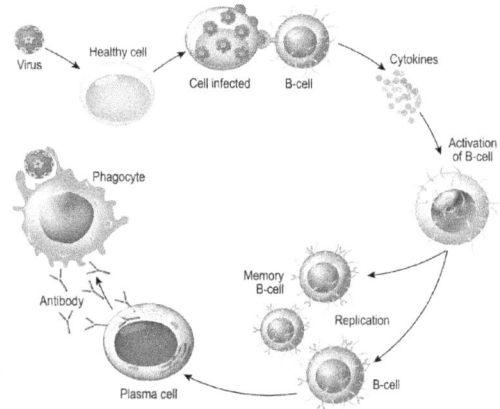

adaptive immune system then clones an army of fighter "B-cells" (called "Effector" cells), specifically made to seek out and destroy just that pathogen. B-cells produce antibodies that help the immune system kill pathogens in three ways:

1. **Tagging.** B-cells pump out masses of tagging molecules called antibodies that stick to pathogens, identifying them as the enemy for immune cells to attack.
2. **Receptor site clogging.** Antibodies swarm the virus particle and block its receptor sites so the virus can't bind to your cells.
3. **Clumping.** Antibodies cause viral particles to clump together, limiting their mobility so they're sitting ducks for your immune cells.

The immune system response reaches full strength after a few days. The invasion is suppressed. Or you die. Then, after the invasion is defeated, your active fighter cells commit suicide, leaving only a skeleton crew of "Memory" B-cells behind to call the immune system into action, should the pathogen ever return.

Secondary response: Any time your immune system encounters that pest in the future, the recognition, replication and eradication processes are shortcutted by the secondary response. This allows it to respond faster and stronger than the first time – most of the time wiping it out before you even notice you were exposed. This is called *acquired immunity*.

Now, problems arise when B-cells don't mature properly. When things are working well, B-cells are good at recognizing friendly cells from foes. But when things go haywire, mistakes are made in the recognition, replication, and/or eradication processes. Autoimmune conditions, hypersensitivities, and vulnerabilities happen as a result of B-cells mistaking your own cells for foreign ones. The immune system is far more complicated than that, but you get the point.

Vaccination circumvents the body's natural defenses

Your skin, digestive tract, and immune system are supposed to serve as front-line defenders against invading microbes and pathogens. But when you inject substances such as vaccines directly into the bloodstream, you bypass your body's primary defense systems, including skin, stomach acid, gut flora, gut lining and GALT (Gut Associated Lymphoid Tissue).

Once inside, bacteria, viruses, foreign DNA, adjuvants, preservatives and gross stuff in vaccines then have unhindered access to organs and tissues *before* the immune system has a chance to respond. Like a Trojan horse scenario, when foreign material is injected directly into the bloodstream, it doesn't have to fight its way through multiple defensive lines. Rather, it gains immediate access to almost anywhere in the body that it wants to go (e.g., the wrong side of the blood-brain barrier is a big one for GAPS people). And it does so at full strength, without being weakened in battle, or reduced in numbers. To Average Joes, that means vaccines present much greater danger to organs, tissues, and the immune system than through environmental exposure.

Vaccines contain seriously toxic substances

Public health agencies admit: both active ingredients and additives are highly toxic. Yet they say the doses aren't high enough to cause most people injury, unless they're allergic. The data says otherwise. Most vaccines contain four categories of material:

1. **Viral or bacterial agent, called an "antigen."** The active ingredient in vaccines (supposedly) is the viral or bacterial agent.
2. **Adjuvant.** Additional substances are added to amplify the immune system response.
3. **Preservatives.** Substances are added to inhibit microorganism growth.
4. **Contaminants.** Most vaccines have accidental or objectional substances in them, such as DNA from chickens or monkeys, viral fragments, and even aborted human fetal cells.

Antigens

The whole idea of vaccination is based on the assumption that weakened, disabled, or otherwise inactive (called "attenuated") viruses or bacteria will create nearly the same immune reaction and immunity as a live virus, without having to suffer through the full-blown disease itself. The viral or bacterial agent that prompts the immune system to produce antibodies is called an antigen. Chemicals, heavy metals, cancer cells, or anything else that triggers an immune response is also loosely viewed to be an antigen, in that each helps to produce an "antibody generator" effect.

Getting a vaccine shot containing an attenuated virus supposedly activates the immune system into releasing antibodies that fight the viral agent. Since the infectious agent is either non-living, or not at full strength, the body should be able to fight it off with ease. The immune system then keeps a record of that virus on file for future reference. It records that infectious agent's genetic "signature" in its database so that it knows how to kill it before it multiplies with the help of antibodies. At the same time, the immune system keeps a few B-cells in circulation – patrolling for a return of the virus.

The immune system then has the knowledge, weaponry, and rapid response capabilities to quickly defeat future invasions before they gain traction. Basically, secondary exposures to an infectious agent cause the immune system to rapidly ramp up antibody production, making the pathogenic microbe easy for the immune system to spot and exterminate.

That's the theory of how vaccines are supposed to give you immunity to an infectious disease. However, it's a leap of logic (some would say leap of faith) to assume that the *vaccine way* of acquiring immunity happens the same as the natural way. For one, vaccine formulation is highly questionable. They can't test the formula to any reasonable degree. And the manufacturing process is crude to say the least. Furthermore, the immune system is extremely complex. Scientists cannot know exactly how the immune system is going to respond to a threat. So manufacturers are just guessing when they proclaim to know what a vaccine's effects and side effects will be. Real-world results bear this out.

Adjuvants

A weakened virus means less protection for you – in both strength and longevity. Viral/bacterial agents, by themselves, often don't stimulate the immune system enough to produce a robust reaction. So a trick that vaccine makers play to increase overall effectiveness is they add substances to make the immune system react more strongly. The goal is to agitate the immune system in the hope of increasing its reaction, antibody production, and future immunity. These substances are called "adjuvants."

Adjuvants stimulate the immune system with irritants such as mercury and aluminum, monosodium glutamate (MSG), formaldehyde (cancer-causing preservative), polysorbate 80 (used as a spermicide), viral and mycoplasmal contaminants, live viruses (MMR and polio), viral and bacterial fragments, protein additives and contaminants (chicken and monkey DNA), polysaccharides, or insect repellant (2 phenoxyethanol).

Proponents claim these adjuvants improve the vaccine's overall effectiveness. But here's the risk: In the same way that halting an asthma attack or a fever stops the body's natural healing process, vaccination probably does the same: it interferes with the immunity-building process by shortcutting the progression of disease. Full immunity is never achieved because your body didn't go through the whole disease and recovery process. Thus, whatever protection you gain is shorter and weaker.

So what do vaccine makers do? They add more adjuvants to each shot, make the adjuvants stronger, put more than one antigen in some shots, give a child more shots in each office visit, and space the shots closer together in the first 18 months of life. A sensible person would think that would traumatize the immune system and cause unpredictable adverse effects. But that's classic Big Pharma thinking for you: more has got to be better. And they make money from your chronic diseases, while taking no responsibility. Nice business model, if you're psychopathic and greedy.

Preservatives

Vaccines need to have preservatives added so microorganisms won't grow in them. The most common preservatives are aluminum or mercury-based, because they're lethal to a wide variety of cells in extremely small doses. These heavy metals also have the advantage (from a vaccine perspective) of stimulating a response from the immune system. So they act as both a preservative and an adjuvant.

A few years ago, mercury was widely used in vaccines. But many parents and advocacy groups believed it caused autism, ADD and GAPS conditions. So they protested loudly in the court of public opinion and took legal action. As a result, drug makers have steadily pulled it out of vaccines and replaced it with aluminum, which is frankly no better, just different. As of 2018, a few vaccines (such as the flu) still contain mercury as their primary preservative. Most others now use aluminum, with a mere trace of mercury.

Formulating vaccines is a gross manipulation of Nature

First, you take a virus or bacteria and weaken it so that it's strong enough to create an immune response, yet weak enough to not cause the full-blown disease. The pathogen must be weakened, incapacitated, or otherwise altered to the point that the immune system produces antibodies, but can still keep the pathogen under control. The sweet spot is somewhere in the middle.

The secret potency standard that vaccine manufacturers target is 20%. If greater than 20% of vaccinated children have nasty side effects after getting a shot, they'll make it weaker. Less than that, and the formulation is considered safe enough to use on people. Unfortunately, it's hard to test formulations or batches on real people, because they can't exactly inject kids with live, potent viruses just to see what happens. So they must release it first (sans liability) and keep their fingers crossed.

To formulate a viral "starter culture" from which vaccine batches are mass-produced, you have to first find and grow a "virus" in the lab. Then you weaken it (called "attenuation") – usually by growing the culture in foreign host tissue, like that from another species. At that point, it's referred to as a "viral agent" due to the fact that it's been altered. That viral/bacterial agent can then be added to a growth medium such as chicken embryos or bovine serum (derived from cow's blood) to make starter cultures for mass production.

Mass manufacturing of vaccines is even more gross

The way vaccines are made is a clumsy process that's highly susceptible to contamination. Experts say contamination is unavoidable. I think we can all agree: it's disgusting. Reader discretion is advised:

They take raw chicken eggs and fertilize them. They let the embryos grow in an incubator for a few days. Then they kill the embryo. They mash it up to form the growth medium. They add the viral agent(s) from the process described above. They let the "soup" culture grow. They manually suck the fluid from underneath the cell culture into a laboratory syringe called a pipette. Then the unwanted substances larger than a virus are filtered out. What's left is the minimally purified viral agent, called a "substrate." Other ingredients are added to provoke an immune response (e.g., formaldehyde), preserve it (e.g., aluminum), and so forth. That's basically how vaccines are made.

Problems with these techniques

First, any biological products that can reproduce are greatly amplified by the culturing process. Second, there's no way to remove or neutralize the toxic, non-biological substances that find their way into the finished vaccine. Cellular debris from chicken embryos or monkey kidneys are two of the more unpleasant contaminants often found in vaccines. In fact, many experts say there's no way for vaccine makers to remove or disable viral contaminants from their vaccines because it would neutralize the viral agent being grown. They can't test for DNA contamination either. Both can't be done with current technology.

One example of bacterial contamination is uncomfortably common: Some eggs are contaminated with campylobacter jejuni (a fairly common bacteria infecting chickens and causing food poisoning in humans). Some experts strongly suspect that campylobacter contamination in the chicken egg growth medium is what causes Guillain-Barré Syndrome in rare cases of vaccination injury. That's because campylobacter infection is known to cause Guillain-Barré on occasion. That's where your immune system is unable to distinguish between the insulation around your nerves and campylobacter cells. It attacks them both and causes varying degrees of nerve destruction, paralysis, and even death.

Fueling the quality control debate further, many vaccines are made in China, with essentially no regulatory oversight or enforcement capabilities by the USFDA. Talk about a national security threat. If an evildoer wanted to sneak extremely harmful substances into vaccines that were impossible to get rid of, and hard to trace potentially years after the fact, this is one way it could be done. Moreover, the USFDA is only able to "inspect" Chinese manufacturing plants once every 13 years. However, they're not allowed in the building. They can only visit their offices and inspect their paperwork. In contrast, vaccine makers in the US may get a visit from the USFDA every couple of years.

Weakened vaccines can mutate back to potency

Restored virulence: We know that viruses and bacteria, attenuated or not, can mutate over time. Their genetic code can revert from an attenuated (inactivated) form into a fully virulent (active) one. Sometimes they mutate in vaccine form as the starter culture morphs its DNA over time. Other times, they mutate after entering the body as the virus lingers, fights the immune system, and interacts with subsequent vaccinations. In simplest terms, they can mutate back to nearly full strength.

Incremental virulence: Many vaccines are given as a multi-dose series. And we know that vaccines lower your immunity for quite some time. So, from the first shot to the second to the third, the likelihood increases that a vaccine will cause the active disease, due to progressive weakening of the immune system. This is what we're actually seeing take place.

We also know that combination vaccines mutate. Putting multiple viral/bacterial agents into one shot is asking for trouble because they interact with each other and mutate when comingled. Whether the antigen is completely alive, attenuated or dead, it will continue to interact, adapt and change. In other words, all life forms, pseudo-life forms like viruses, and pre-life forms are endowed with a survival instinct. They mutate and evolve. And they will use every means at their disposal to survive and replicate.

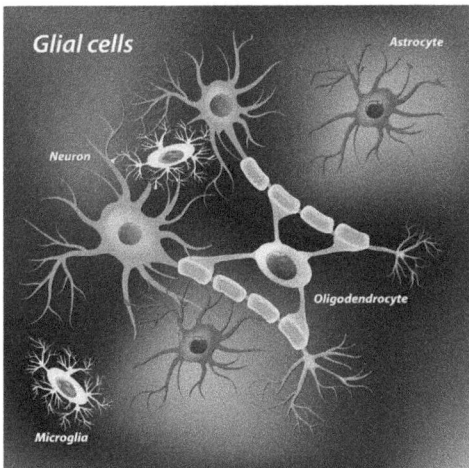

Glial cells — Astrocyte, Neuron, Oligodendrocyte, Microglia

Excitotoxicity

Nerves in the brain and body carry communications using chemical messenger molecules called neurotransmitters. When activated electrically, nerve cells (called a pre-synaptic "terminal") release a neurotransmitter such as dopamine, serotonin or glutamate. Neighboring (but not touching) cells receive it on their receptor sites. This is repeated along a chain of nerve cells to form a nerve impulse. This is how neurons transmit signals electro-chemically along a nerve pathway. It's how thoughts are transmitted in the brain, muscles are instructed to contract or relax, and nerves communicate the sensations of touch/heat/cold to the brain. Neurotransmitters are the electro-chemical "juice" that transmits nerve impulses.

Excitotoxicity is the process by which excessive neurotransmitter levels make brain cells over-fire, which damages or kills them. Whether a neurotransmitter surplus comes from inside the body or from food, excitotoxicity makes nerves fire too easily, too often, or too strongly. This basically excites nerve cells to death.

The two best-known excitotoxins are glutamate (e.g., MSG) and aspartame (artificial sweetener). Glutamate is the most abundant neurotransmitter in the brain. It's responsible for sending impulses of excitation, or stimulation, as opposed to inhibitory. However, it's destructive when present outside of astrocytes, which are supposed to contain it. Glutamate transporter proteins are very important in keeping excitotoxicity down because they move glutamate into astrocytes where it's harmless.

But how do we know excitotoxicity does such damage? Studies have shown, you can block injury to the brain in sub-acute cases of mercury exposure by blocking the effect of excitotoxins, thus reducing mercury toxicity, without changing exposure level.

Immunoexcitotoxicity is the synergistic toxicity between an excitotoxin and an over-activated immune system

Coined by Dr. Russell Blaylock (retired brain surgeon and leading researcher in the field of brain toxicology), "immunoexcitotoxicity" is the synergistic toxic reaction between *an overactivated immune system* and *excitotoxicity*. Specifically, immunoexcitotoxicity is the magnified toxic effect when excess glutamate (the excitotoxin) mixes with pro-inflammatory cytokines (the immune system chemicals *interleukin 1 beta* and *tumor necrosis factor alpha*) to cause a much more intense reaction and damage than either would alone.

The following is an overview of how immunoexcitotoxicity works: When the immune system is stimulated for any reason, three things happen in the brain: (1) microglia get activated, (2) pro-inflammatory cytokines are released, and (3) glutamate is released. What makes immunoexcitotoxicity so damaging is it sets off a toxic reactionary cascade that has synergistic ability to damage or kill brain cells.

In other words, glutamate causes inflammation, which triggers the release of pro-inflammatory cytokines, which increase glutamate levels further by blocking the transport proteins that take glutamate into the astrocytes. Both of them are caused by stimulating the immune system anywhere in the body. It's a vicious cycle now affecting nearly everyone getting the recommended vaccine schedule.

Over-activation of microglia causes chronic injury of brain cells

According to Dr. Blaylock, it's not primarily the mercury, aluminum, protein adjuvants, viral and bacterial fragments, or contaminants that do the most damage to brain cells. Rather, it's the fact that adjuvants in the vaccines activate the microglia, which are the brain's special immune cells that use a specialized form of inflammation to defend the brain against injury.

When activated, microglia release pro-inflammatory substances called cytokines, that are designed to fight pathogens. However, they end up killing your own brain cells over time when inflammation doesn't stop. Accentuating that process, each subsequent adjuvant exposure significantly increases the duration and intensity of microglia activation in a process called "priming." Once primed, the brain and immune system can live in a perpetual state of neuro-destructive inflammation and hypersensitivity to toxins and pathogens for a few years to many decades. Your immune system then overreacts to every poison or pathogen you're exposed to.

This chronic state of inflammation and hypersensitivity over many years is what causes increased vulnerability to infections, toxins, and any attack on the immune system. It causes destruction of brain cells which leads to GAPS conditions. It's as if priming the microglia causes the immune system to use a machine gun to kill infections, when a pistol is all that's needed. From that point forward, routine infections like an ear infection or the common cold can kill brain cells thanks to microglia gone wild. This has been proven through numerous studies: Brain damage occurs when the microglia are activated, even when there is no virus or bacteria present.

To add insult to injury, vaccines typically contain three or more adjuvants per shot. An infant will typically receive around five or six shots per office visit (totaling about 23 adjuvants per office visit). As of 2018, the standard vaccination schedule calls for a round of shots at birth, at 2 months, at 4 months, at 6 months, and at one year. That means there's a lot of microglial activation going on in almost all our over-vaccinated children today. That means ADD, autism, and GAPS conditions will continue to rise as long as we continue to abuse our children's immune systems and brains.

Important in GAPS treatments, anything that lowers mitochondrial function greatly magnifies excitotoxicity and cell death

The brain needs energy to protect itself against glutamate excitotoxicity (whether made by the body, or consumed in food as a flavor enhancer). So much so, that even normal levels of glutamate in the brain become neurotoxic when mitochondria are unable to manufacture enough ATP to protect brain cells. This can tip the balance so that damage to brain cells happens faster than repair can take place.

It's one very important reason that energy – every bit of it you can get – is so crucial to getting all the improvement you can from a healing effort, and why mitochondria need to be supported. Unfortunately, virtually all GAPS individuals, and especially autistics, suffer from frail mitochondria. It's one of the more influential, but lesser-known, mechanisms by which brain function becomes impaired in autistics and ADD individuals.

A baby's brain grows extra cells in its first two years and trims the excess

A child's brain is always developing rapidly. But there's a period of extra-rapid development, from the third trimester in pregnancy to about two years of age, where baby's brain grows far more brain cells (neurons) and connections (synapses) than it needs. It then prunes back the excess, to configure the brain perfectly, according to plan and demand.

This is a crucial period in the architectural development of a baby's brain, because if the building and pruning process gets messed up, the physical structure of the brain is built with flaws in its foundation. Brain function then suffers. Similar to the way a gardener prunes branches from a rose bush to give remaining ones more resources, there's a programmed rise and fall of glutamate and pro-inflammatory cytokine levels, in which innate, intentional immune-excitotoxicity sheds excess brain cells.

As we just talked about, these two substances, glutamate and pro-inflammatory cytokines, are extra toxic to brain cells when they're present together – so much so that even normal levels of glutamate become toxic (and glutamate in food is not helping). This appears to be Nature's way of fine tuning the brain's development, based on a combination of genetic blueprint and the demands placed on it by learning and stimulation.

To phrase it differently, Nature builds redundancy into the brain's formation because early development is so important, yet so delicate. Unfortunately for those being raised in our medical system, problems occur when this process gets activated and doesn't shut off, as is the case when multiple vaccines are given close together.

Conclusion: In some individuals, the brain's development slips into chronic degradation over time. While in others, it slowly improves, depending on which side is winning: addition or subtraction. Either way, one thing is for sure: almost every substance found in vaccines increases the length and severity of inflammation and hypersensitivity. Vaccines given according the CDC schedule can activate microglia for four decades or more. This is what's happening to a large percentage of our children today. Or, to say it another way, only a small percentage of people escape unharmed due to their particularly strong combination of genes, diet, toxin load, microbiome and environment.

The problems with vaccines
The immunity that mother gives to baby is lowered by vaccines

Before mass vaccination, a mother would pass her own potent, naturally-acquired antibodies through to baby while she was pregnant, and again through breastfeeding. This immunity continued for some time until the protection offered by mother's antibodies ran out around the same time that baby's own immune system started to gain competence (another miracle of Nature). But now, with the introduction of vaccines, mother's antibodies are weaker and shorter-lived. So baby's immunity is substantially reduced from birth onward.

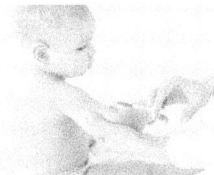

The industry's definition of "effective" is seriously flawed

When people hear industry reps say that vaccines are "effective" they assume that means a vaccine will prevent them from getting the full-blown disease. The average person thinks that they can't get the disease or spread it. But that's not at all what "effective" means in their book.

Their definition: Health officials from the FDA, CDC, and NIH call a vaccine "effective" when the immune system produces antibodies. That's it. However, an antibody response does not at all mean that you're protected against that disease. It does not mean you won't come down with the disease, or even that you have increased resistance to it. It simply means the immune system is doing something, anything, in response to the vaccine. Antibodies are their measurement of success when they talk about "effectiveness" in public statements, literature and legislation.

When challenged on this issue, they say it's unethical to expose people to live diseases, so they can't study it in a direct, meaningful way, such as placebo controls. In any case, we do know that studies show you can vaccinate an animal, their immune system will make antibodies, yet they can still contract the disease when exposed to it. So, no, there are no studies that show the presence of antibodies will protect you in the real world from acquiring a disease. Furthermore, some elderly or immune-compromised people will not even generate antibodies because their immune systems are so weak. So vaccines make them worse off than before.

Will a flu vaccine truly protect you?

There are many strains of influenza. And you only gain immunity to the 1–3 particular strains of flu that are in any one shot. If you're exposed to any other strain, the shot is not only totally worthless, it's a health risk. So health authorities are basically guessing, months ahead of each flu season, as to which strains will go around in the coming months. But how could they possibly know? As a rough guesstimate, they have at-best a 16% chance of choosing correctly. And vaccines never work 100% of the time. So it's really hit-or-miss as to how much protection the vaccine really offers you. Heaven forbid you would actually rely on it to "keep you covered," because the odds aren't good. And don't forget, as of 2018, most flu vaccines still contain a big dose of mercury.

So, instead, do you think it would be better to proactively take steps to strengthen your immune system, rather than putting a vaccine in your body that inflames the brain's microglia, lowers your immunity to all infections, and potentially causes long-term damage to brain cells?

Health authorities exaggerate safety claims

Vaccine advocates shift their position on the safety of vaccines between two different contentions, depending on context, and their role in the industry. Sometimes they'll say or suggest that vaccines are completely safe and effective when making general statements to the public – implying that no one ever gets hurt from vaccines.

Other times, when they need to cover their butts legally, they'll say (admit) that vaccines cannot be made 100% free of side effects. They'll concede that there will always be some percentage of the population that will be harmed through vaccination, and there's nothing anyone can do to prevent it. They admit that vaccines are "unavoidably <u>unsafe</u>."

They're very non-committal in taking an official stance and sticking by it, because they paint the rosiest picture they can when putting on their dog and pony show for the public. While privately, they know vaccines have high failure rates in terms of protection, duration, adverse events, lingering problems, increased sensitivities/susceptibilities, and the occasional severe reaction. Thus, they need to avoid language that incurs legal liability.

Most notably, behind closed doors, most industry insiders realize there's a strong connection between vaccines and autism, ADD and other GAPS conditions. Most of the people in power know that the scientific literature, group statistics, and real-world observations of practitioners and parents all show that vaccines cause a variety of unintended consequences that cannot reasonably be ignored. However, they're ignoring and deny the facts as long as they can to continue raking in big profits from the only division in their companies that's growing rapidly… and to avoid admitting that they've been lying for years.

What they do admit to – the FDA, CDC and American Association of Pharmaceutical Scientists – is that 90–99% of adverse events are never reported to databases like VAERS, DMED or CMS. So the actual number of people harmed by vaccines is around 10–100 times greater than those reported. That means between 5 and 20% of people who take a vaccine suffer serious side effects, depending on which one(s) you're getting, where you are in the schedule, and your personal constitution.

Adjuvants cause more problems than any other vaccine ingredient, including the viral/bacterial agent itself

There is ample evidence that provoking the immune system with adjuvants does boost immune response. But at what cost? Along with that stimulatory effect, there's a mountain of evidence proving that adjuvants trigger inflammation that persists for two years to several decades, depending on which ones are given, how many are given, and when.

In other words, the more adjuvants you give, and the closer you space them, the more you hyperactivate the immune system, and the longer the effects last. Study after study shows that adjuvants are the root cause of chronic inflammation, brain cell destruction, and degeneration of brain function. And they do this by over-stimulating microglia cells so that they don't shut off for quite a long time.

As we discussed, inflammation is the process by which the immune system destroys invading organisms, toxins, heavy metals, and your own worn out/damaged cells… before the healing phase can begin. Specifically, inflammation in the *body* uses free radicals to oxidize harmful things, while inflammation in the *brain* uses inflammatory cytokines and glutamate as "disinfecting" agents. So inflammation can be good or bad, depending on how long it's switched on.

Important in understanding inflammation, your immune system can't avoid killing your own healthy cells in the process of obliterating harmful things, because it increases the destructiveness of its attack to whatever level is necessary to wipe out a threat, regardless of how many of your own healthy cells it sacrifices in the process. So the immune system will harm or even kill *you* in the process of killing pathogens, if that's what it takes.

For this reason, giving multiple adjuvants, in multiple shots, repeatedly over a baby's first few months of life causes the destruction process to rage on for an extended period. This is how virtually every young person's brain is being compromised through today's vaccine schedule. This shows itself as increased vulnerability to sickness and disease throughout of person's life. It might become slow degradation of brain function, or a GAPS condition. Or a person might escape side effects altogether, depending on genes, lifestyle and environmental exposures.

Mass vaccination often increases risk of infection and adverse effects

This has been demonstrated repeatedly in measles, polio, HPV and pertussis.

Measles. Measles was not a severe or deadly disease before a vaccine was introduced. Almost all children got it and recovered without any problems. But, in the 1970s and '80s, measles outbreaks occurred in fully vaccinated populations. Even more damning, the few that hadn't been vaccinated did not come down with it. Then, in the 1990s (30 years after the measles vaccine was introduced), 24% of cases happened in infants, which can be life-threatening at that age. The uncomfortable truth: **You're more likely to contract measles if you <u>have</u> been vaccinated, than if you hadn't. And it's more likely to cause lasting damage.**

Mumps. In an outbreak of mumps a few years ago in Ohio, 67% of those infected had been vaccinated one, two or three times with the MMR vaccine (measles, mumps, rubella vaccine).

Polio. Before vaccines, 95% of people acquired polio from water sources and experienced no symptoms. They didn't even know they had it. Five percent experienced mild symptoms and got over them without incidence. A small percentage of that 5% had serious complications such as stunted growth of limbs, varying forms of paralysis and death.

But several decades after the introduction of polio vaccines, nearly all cases of polio in the US were in vaccinated populations, which can only be caused by live polio virus. For this reason, we no longer use the live polio vaccine in Western countries. However, it's cheaper to make, so drug companies still use the live polio vaccine in Third World countries – sometimes on purpose, and sometimes by "accident."

Case in point, before 2012, about a dozen people died, or were paralyzed, by the wild-type polio per year in India. Then, in 2012, a few years into large-scale vaccination, a claim was made that no one came down with wild-type polio infection. Seems like a win for vaccines – except for the fact that about 47,500 people suffered paralysis which was likely caused by the polio vaccine – reclassified as acute flaccid paralysis to hide the connection.

So, in a two-year span, India went from about twelve serious cases of polio to almost 50,000 cases. Does it make sense to cause 50,000 cases of paralysis or death to eliminate twelve cases of wild polio? It does if you profit from the sale and distribution of vaccines.

Pertussis. We see para-pertussis colonizing in the throats of people vaccinated against pertussis, which turns them into carriers for the disease. Meaning, the pertussis vaccine actually facilitates the spread of para-pertussis. Whereas, naturally-infected and recovered people do not spread either. In other words, vaccinated people are spreading disease, not the unvaccinated.

Vaccines turn trivial childhood ailments into serious diseases

Prior to the 1990s, most childhood diseases were trivial. They came and went without incident. Virtually everyone got them, and it was no big deal. You got infected, you felt crummy for a week or two, and you got over it with no lasting effects. Your reward was lifetime immunity. You couldn't catch it again, and you couldn't spread it.

Chicken pox is the ultimate example. Chicken pox was so common and harmless to children, that neighborhoods actually had chicken pox parties, where parents would purposely expose their children to an infected child, just so they could get it over with while they're young and it was extremely unlikely to cause problems. On the other hand, chicken pox can be far more harmful to get as an adult. It's not uncommon for adults to need hospitalization. Plus, you're much more likely to contract real chicken pox when you're older using the vaccine approach, because vaccine-acquired immunity is weaker and temporary.

By their own admission, health authorities claim most vaccines "work" for about five years, and you need booster shots periodically to maintain that immunity. Some vaccines "work" for 10 years. A few, as much as 15 years. And there are many newer ones that are believed to work for two years or less. In contrast, naturally-acquired immunity lasts a lifetime for a good many diseases. So, to our disservice, vaccines create health risks and health problems than didn't exist before. For instance, the incidence of shingles is rising sharply because people's immune systems are not being periodically boosted by re-exposure to children who have the natural form of chicken pox, thus preventing shingles. Bottom line: The chicken pox vaccine offers moderate-to-high risk for miniscule benefit.

Robert Mendelsohn, MD pediatrician, warned us in the 1970s that vaccines were a medical time bomb

"We're trading the benefit of a life-long immunity from normal childhood illnesses, for a life-long suffering of chronic diseases."

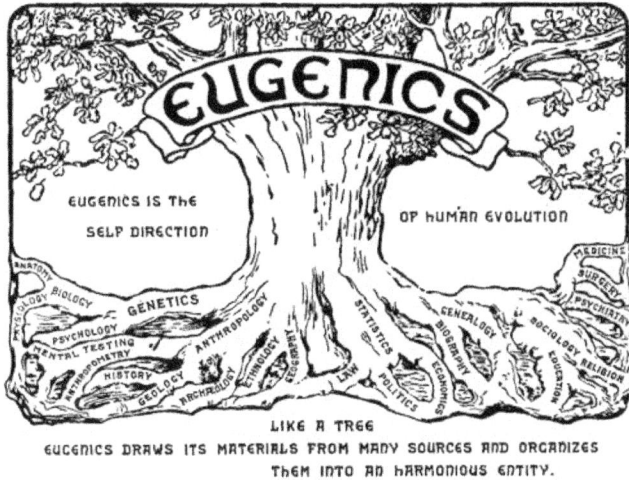

EUGENICS

EUGENICS IS THE
SELF DIRECTION

OF HUMAN EVOLUTION

LIKE A TREE
EUGENICS DRAWS ITS MATERIALS FROM MANY SOURCES AND ORGANIZES
THEM INTO AN HARMONIOUS ENTITY.

Logo of the Second International Congress of Eugenics, 1921, by Harry H. Laughlin. Image used under Creative Commons as public domain.

The agenda to wipe out the "useless eaters"

In the early part of the 20th Century (circa 1910), John D. Rockefeller, Andrew Carnegie, and their elitist friends believed society had too many undesirable people – including "feeble-minded" people, those suffering physical defects and diseases, and commoners who behaved in a vulgar manner. So, drawing on elitist ideals of the past, they decided to redesign man according to their image of what they thought man should be. They called it "eugenics."

The purpose of eugenics was the "self-direction of human evolution" to eliminate bad genes from the gene pool and create a more evolved being. In other words, reduce the population of "undesirables" so the elite could enjoy the fruits of the land and labor of the people, basically. Drawing on many disciplines, eugenics operates primarily through genetics, psychology/psychiatry, sociology, physiology/anatomy, ethnology/genealogy, biology, history, geography, law, statistics, politics, economics, education, medicine and religion.

Or, more simply, the philosophy and practice of eugenics incorporates every means possible to promote desirable traits in humans, while shunning undesirable traits. Naturally, that means killing off people that don't measure up to their standards, or at least keeping them from breeding. Methods include disease, infertility, chemical/lifestyle/electronic pacification, all sorts of control, and dumbing people down as levers in their plan.

What's interesting is, in the early days, they made no secret about their beliefs and intentions. Led by the Rockefeller Foundation's "Science of Man Project," Ford Foundation and Carnegie Foundation, they talked openly about their contempt for the common man. They wrote extensively about it. They set up labs and institutions to research methods to carry out their plans. And they practiced it out in the open. They were proud of it.

However, they didn't know about DNA in the early 20th Century, so they thought in terms of crude genetics, including the notion of survival of the fittest, genealogy, anatomy (such as measuring skull dimensions), and human behavior. And the tools they had to carry out their plans were selective breeding, systematic suppression and forced sterilization.

In those early days, Rockefeller and Carnegie got together and poured money into Caltech, Harvard, Johns Hopkins, Columbia, and the University of Chicago to study how to meld man more to their liking. They actively pursued their agendas in full public view for a couple of decades (albeit in more innocent-appearing forms than what's going on today).

Hitler showed the eugenicists how it's done

Representatives of Rockefeller travelled to Germany to meet with Hitler in the 1930s before he came to power, so they could trade notes with him. The elites knew he was going places, because they were secretly financing, training and supporting him. At the time they got together, the US side was far more advanced than the Germans. So most of Hitler's techniques and directions for research came from the Rockefeller camp.

But Hitler was even more fanatical than they realized, and he took eugenics to the extreme. He and his henchmen practiced eugenics so viciously that he made the US camp jealous at how inhumanely he was able to carry out the craft that they, and their ancestors, had invented. They admired his cruelty, and his latitude to practice eugenics as he wished – having many of the world's top scientists, and being a ruthless dictator and all (the United States was too conservative for experimentation to go on out in the open).

Unfortunately for the eugenics movement, which had a world-wide following, WWII didn't go so well for Germany. So when the horrors of the eugenics program came to light – revealing concentration camps, Dr. Mengele's barbaric research, and The Holocaust – most of the original programs were abandoned. The Rockefeller Foundation told its followers to stop using the term "eugenics," and instead use the terms "social engineering," "New Science of Man," and "behavioralism."

The term *eugenics* was tarnished forever, so they had to re-brand it (standard procedure in secret programs: simply change the names when their ideas get a bad reputation). Point being, it's the same product in a new package: redesigning man, and his behavior, as well as controlling people through elitist ideas and tactics. And they would do it through new science.

After the war, the US group wanted to keep the good times rolling, so they covertly scooped up all the German scientists that wanted to continue working on advanced Nazi technologies. The US government brought over the scientists that didn't want to join the Soviet Union's program, gave them new identities, and put them to work in secret government programs such as MK Ultra mind control, under the auspices of Project Paperclip. Top-Secret programs like these enabled the work to continue uninterrupted.

On the public side, the elite used money from their tax-exempt mega foundations to fund institutions, programs, people, research, and media to increase their control over every aspect of society – including medical schools, government health policy, non-profit foundations, and public opinion. Using the persuasion/coercion that unlimited funding buys you, Rockefeller and his cronies appointed professors, funded scientists and research, and supported companies that had similar thinking to his: that man should be redesigned, but that they should do it using more sophisticated methods than the eugenics of old.

They've continued to refine their technologies and tactics over the last 80+ years. And their elitist ideas have evolved into a fairly straightforward aspiration today: Depopulate the earth on a massive scale… or at least suck the life and liberty out of the peons until The Elite can make it happen. Simply put, they want to eliminate 80% of the world's population – or about 6 billion people – so they can rape and pillage the earth unencumbered by morality, conscience or opposition.

Of course, most of them talk about their beliefs using more politically-correct terminology. They say "population control" when they really mean depopulation. They talk in terms of "proposed areas of study" and "future aspirations," while they assemble the pieces of depopulation plans that their parents and grandparents started generations ago. In any case, their actions reveal their true intentions. Through their private (meaning, secret and accountable to no one), multi-billion-dollar (some might be worth trillions, but we'll never know) tax-free foundations, these plans are well underway today (some under the guise of "transhumanism").

Interesting to note: This entire section, virtually unaltered, was written around 2015–2018. How well do you think the arguments have held up in 2022?

That means weakening the constitution of the masses through vaccination. That means testing various methods of sterilizing people by sneaking "contaminants" into vaccines (like the tens of thousands of women "accidentally" sterilized in Africa). It means dumbing people down through prolonged brain inflammation and lowering the immune system after vaccination (e.g., autism and GAPS conditions). It means making money from mass sickness (we're talking chronic diseases you need drugs to fight). And it means knowing how to permanently disable or kill people through vaccination, when they so choose (e.g., live polio vaccine).

But don't worry; the most unconscionable acts are being carried out on Third World populations for now. People in the First World are just getting the health sucked out of them slowly so no one notices. Basically, if a group of people wanted to harm the life-long health of masses of people, and they wanted to keep it secret as to how they did it, mandatory childhood vaccines would be a perfect delivery vehicle.

The Powers That Be want to force everyone to be vaccinated

Vaccine companies want to take away your right to choose what's right for you and your family. Big Pharma is getting desperate because faith in vaccines is collapsing. They're worried one of their biggest cash cows is gaining a bad reputation, so they're taking steps to force people into it. People are waking up to the fact that the vaccine industry's products and programs do not stand on their own merit. Vaccines are not as "safe and effective" as they're claimed to be. As a result, people are refusing to vaccinate their children in ever-greater numbers. So The Powers That Be are applying pressure to influencers in an effort to cajole or intimidate families into getting vaccinated.

Family doctors, school administrators, health officials, and employers with government contracts are being threatened with getting their government funding yanked, or even being fined personally, if compliance rates of their constituency falls below a certain level. At the same time, vaccine makers are lobbying hard to eliminate all exemptions, such as religious reasons, in the present system. They want to make it illegal for families to refuse. They want to make noncompliance punishable by exclusion from school, denial of treatment, denial of employment, fines, imprisonment, or seizing your children via Child Protective Services.

Vaccine makers even want to mandate vaccines for which the risks are practically non-existent. They want to forcibly vaccinate your children for diseases not seen in many decades, or were never serious to begin with. For example, they want to force all young boys to get HPV shots – supposedly so they can't become a carrier and pass it to future sexual partners.

They say mass vaccination creates "herd immunity"

Vaccine experts claim that when at least 95% of a population is immunized against a disease, the whole group is protected. They need that many people to be vaccinated in order to protect us all. But, to their embarrassment, many recent outbreaks prove exactly the opposite. In many outbreaks of recent decades, most of the people that got the disease had been vaccinated one, two or three times. Often, 60–95% of those afflicted had been vaccinated and still got the disease.

Meanwhile, the few that hadn't been vaccinated, none of them got sick. The official explanation usually sounds something like the following: 'The large percentage that supposedly were immune to the disease were providing the unvaccinated with protection via herd immunity.' Make any sense to you? If you believe their way of thinking, those who are vaccinated are providing protection for everyone. They can't get it and they can't spread it.

On the other side of their argument, they say that if you don't vaccinate your children, you're accepting the risks that they can get the disease and spread it. However, real world experience shows that vaccines make you more likely to get the disease. And to throw one more monkey wrench into the theory of herd immunity, naturally-acquired immunity to some diseases wears off after a few decades, so tens of millions of adults are running around with no immunity (i.e., low percentage of "herd immunity"). And, yet, we see infection rates declining in unvaccinated populations anyway. So "herd immunity" just doesn't translate from theory into practice.

Vaccines are big business

The pharmaceutical industry is one of the biggest in the world. And vaccines are the fastest-growing division in many of these drug companies (while other divisions struggle to grow). In 2005, world-wide vaccine

I couldn't find combined sales figures, but sales of COVID-19 vaccines, by themselves, totaled about $60 billion in 2021. So total sales are probably in excess of $100 billion.

sales were *$10 billion* USD. In 2009, they were *$23 billion*. And, in 2015, worldwide vaccine sales were *$41 billion* USD. For those who love numbers, their sales quadrupled in just ten years. Looks like a lot of motivation to manipulate people and policy, as well as success at doing it, as evidenced by the hundreds of new vaccines in the development pipeline.

The profit motive behind the vaccine agenda

Imagine selling a drug that: (1) everyone is required to take, (2) is far cheaper to develop than others (no clinical trials), (3) has fat profit margins, (4) lower marketing costs, and (5) zero liability expenses (insurance premiums). Seeing these kinds of dollar signs blind vaccine makers to any harm or wrongdoing they have to commit to get their vaccines forced on to the American people in the name of "public good."

Do you honestly think drug companies want to mandate vaccines out of altruism? Or are they thinking they've hit pay dirt using trickery and manipulation, disguised as benevolence? Fact: They've shown no interest in curing diseases before. What makes anyone think they would start now?

For many drug companies, laws were meant to be broken

Here are the twenty largest civil and criminal settlements reached between the US Department of Justice and pharmaceutical companies. (Imagine how often they *didn't* get caught, compared to this list.)

Source: Wikipedia.

Year	Company	Settlement	Violation(s)
2012	GlaxoSmithKline	$3 billion ($1B criminal, $2B civil)	Criminal: Off-label promotion, failure to disclose safety data. Civil: kickbacks to physicians, false and misleading statements, reporting false best prices, underpaying rebates.
2009	Pfizer	$2.3 billion	Off-label promotion, kickbacks
2013	Johnson & Johnson	$2.2 billion	Off-label promotion, kickbacks
2012	Abbott Laboratories	$1.5 billion	Off-label promotion
2009	Eli Lilly	$1.4 billion	Off-label promotion
2001	TAP Pharmaceutical	$875 million	Medicare fraud, kickbacks
2012	Amgen	$762 million	Off-label promotion, kickbacks
2010	GlaxoSmithKline	$750 million	Poor manufacturing practices
2005	Serono	$704 million	Off-label promotion, kickbacks, monopolistic practices
2008	Merck	$650 million	Medicare fraud, kickbacks
2007	Purdue Pharma	$601 million	Off-label promotion
2010	Allergan	$600 million	Off-label promotion
2010	AstraZeneca	$520 million	Off-label promotion, kickbacks
2007	Bristol-Myers Squibb	$515 million	Off-label promotion, kickbacks, Medicare fraud
2002	Schering-Plough	$500 million	Poor manufacturing practices
2006	Mylan	$465 million	Misclassification under the Medicaid Drug Rebate Program
2006	Schering-Plough	$435 million	Off-label promotion, kickbacks, Medicare fraud
2004	Pfizer	$430 million	Off-label promotion
2008	Cephalon	$425 million	Off-label promotion
2010	Novartis	$423 million	Off-label promotion, kickbacks
2003	AstraZeneca	$355 million	Medicare fraud
2004	Schering-Plough	$345 million	Medicare fraud, kickbacks

At the same time, these companies are excused from all liability for vaccines on the childhood schedule. You can't sue them when your child is hurt by a vaccine. Most important, no one goes to jail when their illegal activity is uncovered. Basically, they have a free pass, because government agencies have got their back legally and financially. Large criminal fines are strictly business to them. The net effect: Vaccine companies have no incentive to make their vaccines safe. Just as bad, they have very little incentive to make sure their vaccines are effective. So they can do pretty much whatever they want and get away with it.

The US Centers for Disease Control and Prevention (CDC) act as an unofficial marketing and distribution arm for the vaccine makers
The CDC has a vested financial interest in promoting vaccines. The agency buys and distributes $4.4 billion worth of vaccines a year (pre-COVID). So they stand to lose billions of dollars in funding, inventory, and credibility if people see vaccines for what they really are. For health consumers, this means that the CDC has a multi-billion-dollar incentive to deceive and defraud the public about the risks and theoretical rewards of vaccination, which become cover-ups such as data manipulation and illegal document shredding when facts emerge that they don't like.

A documented case, based on CDC's own records: A study that the CDC was looking at prior to its publication showed the occurrence of autism drops by 75% when you give a vaccine after the age of three, rather than before. This information was very damaging to their claim that vaccines don't cause autism or ADD. So what did the CDC do? CDC administrators and scientists conspired through multiple rounds of data manipulation to reduce the statistical association, until the link was reduced to a negligible effect. They basically removed certain data points, and changed the way they analyzed the data, to cloud the association. This is one way that fake science is fabricated by people who have mastered the fine art of fraud and corruption.

Vaccine makers routinely exchange top executives with government agencies like the FDA and CDC
Dozens of these industry prostitutes have done special favors for vaccine companies while working in high government posts, then just happen to find their way into high-paying jobs at these companies, after their work in the agency is completed.

Here's how it happens: Either through subversion or promotion, vaccine companies find a malleable person inside an agency or out who's willing to sell out their morals and conscience for a buck. Those willing to play ball are promoted or appointed in the agency, and promised a lot of money to come work for the vaccine maker, after they

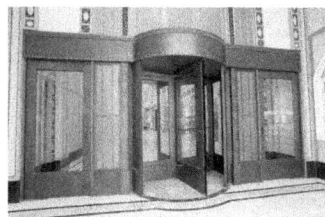

leave the agency. On the other hand, those who stand in the way are removed or silenced, one way or another. After the insider agent helps establish a crucial policy, program, or precedence that supports the vaccine industry's agenda, that agent joins the vaccine company to continue promoting vaccines from the other side of the fence. There, they cash in for the favors they did for Big Pharma. Sometimes, these sell-outs go back to the agency on another mission.

This is how billions of dollars of influence, and a lot of questionable intentions, turn into pro-vaccine policies, programs, and precedences that do not make the slightest bit of sense from a health perspective. This is the mechanism of undue influence by which our vaccine schedule came into being. It's a major building block in causing the epidemics of autism, ADD, mental health disorders, and most modern diseases. And it's why the health of our nation is collapsing faster than all efforts to prop it up.

In 1986, The National Vaccine Injury Compensation Program was established to compensate people injured by vaccines

Sounds benevolent, right? Sure it does… if you believe the official story and fail to see the hidden agenda. You see, cases are heard and decided upon not by judges and juries, but by Special Masters who are not health professionals, nor scientists. Rather, they're lawyers appointed to The Court.

Unfortunately for those injured, standard rules of civil procedure do not apply, such as "discovery" (the finding of evidence) and admission of evidence into the court records. Normal rights of appeal do not apply. Just as bad, awards are paid out by the government, not by vaccine manufacturers. Indeed, no one can sue the vaccine manufacturers directly. You must go through The Program to seek compensation when your child is injured or dies from a vaccine.

So if your child suffers mild to moderate injuries, you're not going to consider bringing the case before The Program because convincing the Special Masters is not easy – even if you could find an attorney to take your case. And the risk-to-reward ratio sucks. To illustrate, an obvious "open and shut" case may take seven years to be decided. But, although it is very difficult to win your case (about 20% prevail), The Program has paid out over $2.5 billion dollars to about 3,200 families in its 30 years of existence.

Conclusion: The Program gave vaccine makers something even better than a "get out of jail free" card: it gave them blanket immunity and a license to make their vaccines as harmful and deadly as they can get away with. Dr. Jonas Salk, developer of the polio vaccine, said as much. He warned congress that The Program would take away the incentive for vaccine manufacturers to make vaccines safer and more effective.

In any case, the very existence of The Program proves the pro-vaccine camp *knows* that vaccines are dangerous, and has taken steps to reduce their risk exposure. Indeed, it's their strategy to shield themselves from any damages. Not only are vaccine companies shielded from financial liability through The Program. But they also avoid the discovery processes of depositions and document searches to expose their misdeeds.

Mary Holland, Esq., Professor NYU

Mary Holland, JD, currently serves as President and general counsel of Children's Health Defense.

"It boggles my mind that we could imagine, somehow, that **the pharmaceutical industry, who routinely get hit with the world's largest-ever civil and criminal fines, would behave in completely illegal and immoral ways with respect to prescription drugs. But they would be boy scouts when it comes to vaccines.** That is a level of cognitive dissonance [inability to see the truth that's right in front of your face] that I cannot understand. It's crazy.

They've hidden the science. They've withheld information they were required to give the FDA. They've suppressed information that shows what great harm their drugs do [e.g., at least 100,000 confirmed deaths from Vioxx]. They've made false claims in their marketing… illegally marketing drugs for off-label uses. I don't see why we would think the same things aren't going on with vaccines. That level of malfeasance… that level of disregard for human life. To imagine that those are the same companies… predators… who are producing vaccines… I find extraordinary."

Dr. Russell Blaylock sums up the risks of the vaccine program

Quote from his 2011 Vaccine Safety Conference presentation: "We are sequentially vaccinating these children with powerful immune adjuvants in a manner which, if you repeated in animals – and this has been done many times – produces activation of the brain's microglia, and initiates chronic neuro-degeneration. The degree of that neuro-degeneration depends on a lot of factors: your antioxidants, your genetics, your glutathione levels.

All these things make a difference. Some are going to be impacted more than others. All are going to suffer damage. And I contend with this vaccine schedule that we use in the United States, we are damaging virtually everyone's brain. It's the degree to which we're damaging [that's important to understand]. So if you just lowered IQ ten points, they might not be quite as bright. But if you test them, you're not going to find a big difference.

We're going to look at their attention… their ability to pay attention. We know it's going to be impaired – severe in some, very mildly in others. You do the usual tests they do, you're not going to pick it up. But mom will notice it. The teacher will notice it. And the child will not be able to compete in the school as well as they should be. So it's a dumbing down process. We won't have as many high IQ children as we had in previous generations because of this process. When we looked at the studies of Vargas and the autistic brain, the microglia were activated for four decades."

Do vaccines cause autism? What about mercury?

A few years ago, there was a storm of controversy in the autistic community that blamed vaccines with causing autism – particularly those containing mercury. Backers of the idea based their theory on the observation that many once-healthy, normal young children suddenly developed autistic symptoms hours to weeks after receiving one or more vaccines.

Dr. Natasha's conclusion, based on her clinical experience: Vaccines are not the cause of autism. They can be a cause of autism, as a powerful contributor. They can be the straw that breaks the camel's back in a person already susceptible due to a weakened immune system – particularly those affected by a corrupted gut. And the "smoking gun" that disproves the 1-to-1 vaccine-autism connection is this: Despite the all-too-common observation that vaccines have been known to trigger autistic symptoms, Dr. Natasha has also seen a growing number of autistic children in her clinic who did not receive any vaccines.

Similarly, evidence shows mercury specifically does not cause autism, because makers have steadily been removing it from vaccines (the flu vaccine being the most glaring holdout) with no corresponding decline in autism rates. But we're not going to remove vaccines or mercury from our suspect list just yet. Here are a few reasons why: There's evidence to suggest that the blood-brain barrier breaks down after getting the MMR vaccine. This unprotected border lets any toxins in the bloodstream get into the brain. When you combine a leaky gut with a leaky blood-brain barrier, both defensive walls are breeched so nothing is stopping toxins from entering the body and reaching places that cause psychological disorders. Conversely, a healthy microbiome captures 99% of the mercury you eat, while a severely corrupted one blocks only 10%.

Dr. Blaylock also does not believe mercury alone causes autism

He actually warned the community beforehand, that removing mercury from vaccines would not cause autism rates to go down appreciably. And they didn't. The reason is, it isn't the mercury, or any antigens in particular, that cause autism. Rather, it's a combination of all the adjuvants, antigens, preservatives, contaminants, multiple doses in a single shot, multiple shots in one office visits, and frequency of the vaccine schedule, that are weakening the immune system in almost everyone, while causing autism in an unfortunate minority.

To illustrate the insanity, aluminum, which took mercury's place as the vaccine makers' preservative of choice, is at least as destructive to the brain as mercury due to its ability to activate microglia. So mental health disorders will continue to rise as long as vaccines contain neuro-toxic adjuvants. So, no, mercury or any single vaccine alone do not cause autism. Instead, it's all the immune system irritants we're exposed to in both vaccines and the environment that "dog pile" one on top of another to cause autism – not one single agent. Vaccines just happen to be the clearest, most present danger in their potency and frequency, because they each hyperactivate the brain's microglia that much more.

Why lie about the risks of vaccination?

The CDC refuses to admit that vaccines carry substantial risk, while offering minimal reward because 'fessing up' at this point tells people they have been lying all along. It opens them up to liability. As a result, CDC continues to plead ignorance about the link between vaccines and autism. They say they don't know what causes autism. They hypothesize that there 'appears to be a genetic component.' All they know is, they are sure that vaccines have nothing to do with it. Meanwhile, mainstream media refuses to hold public debates about the risks of vaccines because, in non-election years, about 75% of advertising revenue comes from drug companies.

What we do know for sure

1. **Combo shots.** There are no studies to show that multiple viral/bacterial antigens in a single shot is safe.
2. **Multiple shots at once.** There are no studies to show that multiple vaccine shots in a single office visit is safe.
3. **Adjuvant safety questionable.** There are no studies to show adjuvants are safe – either alone or in combination.
4. **Vaccine schedule.** There's no evidence the vaccine schedule is safe.
5. **Vaccinated *vs.* unvaccinated.** There are no studies of vaccinated populations *vs.* unvaccinated. In fact, public health agencies in charge of such things refuse to fund such clearly relevant studies.
6. **Short studies.** Studies that the vaccine industry relies upon to claim vaccines are "safe" usually last about 2–5 weeks. But autoimmune diseases typically develop over several weeks to many months. So they wouldn't catch most autoimmune and inflammatory injuries.
7. **Aluminum overdose.** The average vaccine shot given to a baby contains about 20–50 times the toxic daily dose of aluminum for a full-grown adult, according to the EPA.
8. **No independently-funded studies.** It's very hard to find any vaccine study done in the US that was not funded by a vaccine maker.

In summary: It appears many vaccines offer at least a little protection against disease. It appears that protection does not last as long as people would like, so more boosters may be necessary to achieve immunity. And the large majority who get vaccinated experience no serious side effects that are obvious to the untrained observer.

However, no one can predict exactly how your son or daughter will react to a vaccine with any certainty. And it appears the risk-to-benefit ratio is tilted far more toward the 'risk' side than many parents would feel comfortable with, were they to know the truth. It's the subtle changes and progressive deterioration to keep an eye out for.

At the very least, the CDC needs to rethink its vaccine schedule

We need to take a good, long look at how and when we administer vaccines to children today – particularly newborns and infants – because the side effects appear to be unacceptably common and considerable, compared to the benefits promised. As of 2013, the CDC recommends vaccination against at least fourteen diseases. Before age six, children in the US receive as many as 49 vaccine doses… up to five shots or more during one office visit, and several in consecutive months. So if a person adheres to the CDC schedule, they will receive 100–150 vaccines in their lifetime!

Does that make the least bit of sense, considering what a vaccine does in the body? It does if you believe vaccines only do what they claim to do, always work, and never do any harm. It does if you believe all immune systems are strong enough to handle the attacks – regardless of age, genetics, or state of health/disease. Key point: Vaccines are designed for healthy people with competent, mature immune systems, which babies, very young children and some seniors simply do not possess.

Certainly, most vaccinations don't produce observable side effects. But maybe we should think about evaluating babies first to make sure their immune systems are healthy enough to fight off an infection? Perhaps we should screen young children for preexisting conditions or predispositions that may counter-indicate vaccines until the situation clears (like finding the immune system over-activated due to a leaky gut)? Maybe we should not give three different immunizations in a single shot, like MMR and DTP do. Maybe we should spread them out to give the immune system more time to recover between shots? Maybe we should stop using preservatives made from extremely potent neurotoxins, like mercury and aluminum?

Yes, there are risks to not getting vaccinated. But it's becoming abundantly clear that the risks of getting vaccinated outweigh the risks of not. Unfortunately for the health of our young ones, discussion of vaccine safety and efficacy is being suppressed by public health agencies as if side effects are rare and insignificant. Try convincing the parent of a severely autistic child that autism is rare and no big deal.

Conclusion

Carefully consider which vaccines you choose to give your child, and when. Learn the dangers before blindly agreeing to the ever-increasing vaccination schedule being promoted by the drug companies and health agencies. Keep in mind that babies are born with an immature immune system that needs to be educated. It needs to build its strength up over time. Does it make any sense to overload a newborn baby's immune system in ways that would never occur in nature? Consider getting vaccines later, when the immune system is stronger. Consider spreading them out. You may consider forgoing them altogether. Do your research. And remember, you do have choice (for the moment). Don't give up control over your family's health to anyone.

2022 update: Proof that vaccines cause chronic illness

A pediatrician with a large practice had data analyzed that was collected from thousands of vaccinated and unvaccinated children. This was the first study comparing vaccinated to unvaccinated populations ever done.

He found convincing evidence that vaccines increase the occurrence of dozens of diseases. In other words, **unvaccinated children are demonstrably healthier than those who have been vaccinated.** A growing number of clinicians are seeing the same pattern in their practices: unvaccinated children just don't get sick nearly as often as the vaccinated. On the other hand, **the data clearly showed that chronic, degenerative diseases occur much more frequently in vaccinated children.**

The study was published in a peer-reviewed medical journal, and subsequently retracted. Shortly thereafter, the doctor's medical license was suspended, pending review by his medical board.

13

ANSWERS TO THE ADD ENIGMA

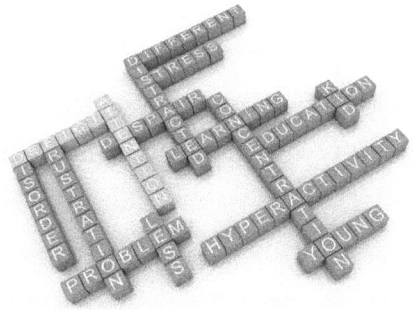

ADD: The biggest mystery in the field of psychology

Attention deficit disorder has been a hotly debated subject among parents, teachers, practitioners, and those impacted. Everyone and their favorite expert seem to have their own opinion about what causes ADD, why so many people seem to have it these days, and how to handle it.

Confusion and disagreement concerning its sources and solutions are so widespread that many skeptics say ADD/ADHD does not even exist. They say it's a just kids being kids. The rise in cases is simply increased awareness and improvements in diagnosis. Still others say it's just a label invented to sell more drugs. Experienced clinicians and researchers even contend that it's a discipline problem, personality defect, by-product of over-stimulation, or genetic disorder. Perhaps it's just a fad diagnosis that will one day fall out of fashion?

Examine ADD casually or obsessively and we can all agree: ADD is the biggest mystery in all of psychology and human behavior. And, considering ADD's multi-factorial origin in the human body, who can blame them? There's no way to say by testing or observation how ADD comes to affect a person because its root causes are undetectable by looking at psychology, physiology or symptoms.

Well, we're here to break through the fog of these misconceptions. We are going to shed much-needed light on the mystery that is ADD, explain its biological origins, and touch on how our beliefs about it have changed over the years, so that we can loosen the grip it has over society.

The mind is a marvelously complex, precision piece of equipment

It is designed to be both robust and sensitive, depending on which function you're talking about. Any number of things can and do go wrong to throw off its delicate balance and create dysfunction. As we'll discuss, ADD is nothing more than a few core causes, mixed with perturbations that cause "satellite" symptoms such as hyperactivity. These recent discoveries and new explanations for old ideas will advance our understanding of mental health disorders, and help define ADD for years to come.

What DOES NOT cause ADD

- sugar, foods and food additives
- genes
- bad parenting
- excessive video games and TV.

Sugar, gluten and casein don't cause ADD

Sugar, gluten and casein don't cause attention deficit – at least not in a healthy body. They can certainly contribute to highs and lows in physical energy, mental clarity and emotions. But they don't cause the underlying failure of inhibition that regulates what a person thinks, says and does. They merely make matters worse. The physical and biochemical nature of ADD comes first. That's the foundation of disorder. Adding sugar, gluten or casein on top of that just turns the volume up or down on dysfunction. Sensitivities like these are an amplification of the manifestation. At least that's how I'm choosing to define ADD.

When your digestion and sugar metabolism are working properly, your body is better-equipped to handle excessive sugar, and you don't get allergic reactions to gluten and casein. Environmental insults in a healthy state are less intense and shorter-lived. But when those insults pile up, that's when coping mechanisms fail and disease processes kick in. Same thing with bad parenting, destructive environments, video games, and TV watching: they add fuel to the fire, but can't start it.

Genes don't cause ADD (by themselves)

Clinicians and researchers widely believe that there is a genetic component to ADD because it definitely runs in families. Dr. Daniel Amen writes that if one parent has ADD, 60% of offspring will have it. If both parents have ADD, there's an 85 to 90% chance their children will have it too. The anecdotal evidence is so clear that no one doubts heredity plays a role in ADD. But how big is that role? Here's the missing information that demystifies this reasonable-sounding, but incomplete, belief:

Dr. Gabor Mate contends in his book *Scattered* that ADD is caused by social imprinting from parents, with some genetics mixed in

He contends that poor family dynamics, stress, peer pressure, substance abuse, and social conditioning rewire a child's brain to be ADD. On first blush, this explanation sounds like it could be possible, because this does happen in extreme cases of abuse and stress. It's a fact: you can break the mind and cause irreversible psychological problems that overlap with ADD. But it's becoming clear that his rationale are merely contributing factors to more tangible, physical problems in a vast majority of cases.

Overstimulation from technology and society

As the pace of life and technology accelerate, "armchair psychiatrists" and some professionals have blamed ADD on the non-stop stimulation of our "Attention Age." They think modern society, with its video games, quick-cut movies and TV, smartphones, energy drinks, Facebook, Twitter, non-stop action, instant access to information, and technology… They think the unrelenting siege of stimulation from the world around us has eroded attention spans to the point where it's changing the way the human brain is wired. But which one is cause, and which one is effect? Answer: biology and psychology set the stage. They come first and lay the foundation. Stimulation just fuels the fire. ADD provides the fundamental need/desire for stimulation, and non-stop stimulation reinforces the resulting behavior, which becomes habit/addiction.

Many people refuse to believe that ADD exists

Many skeptics think ADD is a made-up disease by the pharmaceutical companies to sell more drugs. Response: Although Big Pharma has certainly done their part to make it appear as if that were true, in this case, it's not. ADD is for real. I believe this is a rare instance where Big Pharma acted like a guilty party (i.e., with malice), but their intentions are simply commercial. I say the drug companies are innocent opportunists in the ADD phenomenon (if there is such a thing). They're willing participants that saw an opportunity to make some money on an emerging problem, and they took it and ran with it.

Conclusion: ADD is far more microbial, environmental, and observationally-acquired than it is hereditary

Like most health disorders, genes "load the gun" and create susceptibility to ADD. But it's environmental factors that actually "pull the trigger" and make ADD materialize. You need both factors for ADD to occur. The reason we know that genes don't cause ADD by themselves is that the human genome doesn't change perceptibly over one or two generations. DNA doesn't change that fast. Yet ADD has exploded in recent decades – far more than we can attribute to improved awareness and diagnosing. Therefore, genetics are a constant in the ADD equation, while environmental threats have increased dramatically in scope and severity over just one generation. Let's examine the reasons:

Multi-factorial. ADD, GAPS conditions, and most diseases are usually not caused by one thing, as we're conditioned to think. The body is too forgiving to let one threat damage it quickly or easily. Instead, it's typically a combination of risk factors, or one big, insurmountable attack that overwhelms the body's healing and defenses to cause disease.

Where your microbes come from. Father shares his gut flora with mother on a regular basis. Mother then passes her gut flora onto baby at the time of birth (vaginal birth), and/or through breastfeeding. If her microbiome is healthy, she passes healthy gut flora onto baby as a form of genetic inheritance. Unfortunately, as the list of environmental toxins grows, mothers are passing deeply disturbed, pathogen-dominated microbiota on to their children. This sets them up for GAPS conditions.

Learned behaviors. Children unconsciously pick up behavior patterns from adults they observe. They eat whatever mom or dad eats, and thus learn food and nutrition habits from their parents. Unfortunately, today that means they learn to eat lots of processed foods, white flour, white sugar, man-made seed oils, and artificial ingredients – all things that damage gut flora. Thus, many kids are picking up not food and nutrition habits, but junk food and anti-nutrient habits. Children also tend to get imprinted with, and habituated to, lifestyle choices of family and friends growing up. They tend to follow along blindly as their "normal," unless/until they make a conscious decision to change. For example:

- Girls may see mom cleaning house with certain cleaners and buy those.
- Boys may see dad spraying certain chemicals on the lawn and copy him.
- Girls may see mom using certain personal care products and imitate her.
- And both genders may see mom or dad drinking or smoking and fall into the habit like they never had a choice.

Equally influential, children may see how their family handled wellness or illness, and do the same without questioning what it's doing to their long-term health. This has led to overuse/abuse of antibiotics, pain killers, antidepressants, anti-anxiety meds, and birth control pills.

So, you see, ADD does run in families. But DNA is not the largest component of it. A person's genes are only the beginning of a long chain of events that lead to health or sickness. More and more often, it's corrupted gut flora that's growing more damaged from one generation to the next that creates neurotransmitter imbalances, nutrient deficiencies, leaky barriers, toxin damage, and degeneration of grey matter.

It's an unhealthy microbiome that leaves people with a weakened immune system and overworked detoxification pathways. And it's pathogens and their toxic waste products that are altering the way a family's genes are being expressed in successive generations (aka epigenetics). And then, after all that's established, a person's nutritional and lifestyle choices come along and push the individual's precarious biochemistry into full-blown disease.

Overstimulation. Without a doubt, the pace of stimulation bombarding everyone's brains today is eroding attention spans – especially young children and teens. But if overstimulation were the only factor at play, everyone that watches TV, uses a smartphone, is active on social media, lives in a big city, or plays video games would be attention-deficient by now. Overstimulation contributes to ADD, but cannot cause it.

Environmental. The environmental insults we subject our gut flora to are a leading cause of ADD, not genes or overstimulation. And those toxin exposures, which run in families just as much as genes do, are upsetting people's biochemistry. This is affecting the way our genes are expressed. So let us forget the idea that ADD is primarily hereditary. That argument just doesn't hold water. In fact, by some estimates, genes only play a 4–6% role in causing any disease. Blaming ADD on genes is also dismissive. It's taking the easy way out, relieving ourselves of personal responsibility. It's a disempowering way to think.

It's what we do to ourselves – what we expose ourselves to – that begets the health problems we're seeing today. That's both more influential in causing disease, and more reversible. In other words, we have new information and explanations that tell you which substances, practices, and processes cause ADD in a person. And, knowing that, you now can do something about it.

Furthermore, when quicker, easier efforts don't give you the results you are looking for, this material gives you specific things to try in the effort to beat brain dysfunction. That means you won't have to settle for being 'a little better' or 'as good as it gets' when unrestricted brain function is really what you want for you and your child. If you're willing to make the effort, now you have tools to take your recovery closer to 100% than you might have thought.

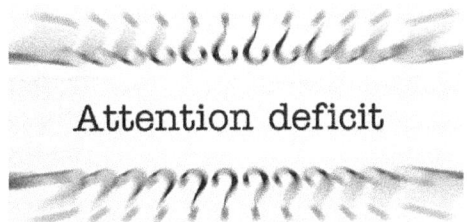

Attention deficit

Our understanding of attention deficit disorder has evolved through five (overlapping) stages, over 50+ years

1. **Pre-1980.** ADD went by a different name: "hyperkinetic impulse disorder." It was not commonly diagnosed as a mental health disorder or physiological problem. Rather, it was treated as a self-control/behavioral issue.

2. **1980 on.** Attention deficit disorder becomes a named disease in the DSM-III. In a radical move with far-reaching consequences, the medical field stops trying to explain causality of disease, and starts defining disorders based on symptoms alone. ADD starts to spread through the population.

    DSM-III: The standard diagnostic manual for mental health professionals.

3. **Late '80s through early 2010s.** ADD starts affecting families and society in earnest, while experts try explaining what the diagnostic manual DSM-III declines to discuss about why ADD occurs.

4. **Mid '90s through present.** Dr. Daniel Amen proves that the ADD brain functions differently than the unaffected brain through functional SPECT scans.
5. **Early 2000s to the present day.** Dr. Natasha Campbell-McBride and Donna Gates explain the biological basis for ADD. By understanding ADD's mechanisms of action, practitioners learn how to reverse root causes of ADD, instead of managing symptoms.

1. Pre-1980: In the old days, the mind and body were considered separate and distinct entities, and ADD was just bad behavior

Mind and body seemingly had nothing to do with one another. When the body malfunctioned, doctors treated that. And when an individual exhibited anti-social behavior, parents, teachers, therapists and law enforcement officers blamed the individual for their bad behavior, being undisciplined, and making poor choices.

The individual was reprimanded for the error of their ways – as if they were in complete control of their thoughts and actions. And, in those days, behavior problems were more likely to be products of a disturbed mind, rather than the body, as they are today. Those were the days of the psychiatrist's couch and talk therapy. ADD existed as "hyperkinetic impulse disorder," but it was rarely diagnosed as a mental health condition needing treatment, compared with today.

2. Post-1980: ADD becomes a named disease, and Big Pharma capitalizes on the rise of mental health disorders

In 1980, attention deficit disorder became an official named diagnosis when the Third Edition of the Diagnostic and Statistical Manual of Mental Disorders (DSM) changed "hyperkinetic impulse disorder" to ADD. Throughout the 1980s and '90s, ADD, autism, dyslexia, schizophrenia, depression, and eating disorder rates started to climb (along with degenerative diseases in general). The field of psychiatry took off as new drugs hit the market to treat these conditions. Research and development money poured into finding new drugs.

The third edition of the DSM also included a radical change to the way health professionals diagnose and treat mental health conditions. Unlike the two previous editions, the DSM-III was symptom-based and atheoretical – meaning it described mental disorders without reference to etiology (cause). As a result, mental health disorders became entirely defined by symptoms, with very little attention paid to root causes. In other words, the field of mental health was *descriptive* in its diagnoses and treatment ideology, not physiological as a paradigm.

Then, in 1985 and 1997, advertising restrictions were relaxed that once prohibited drug companies from advertising drugs direct to consumers. This opened the floodgates of promoting pharmaceuticals in mass media to large audiences. The mantra "ask your doctor if XYZ drug is right for you" began to fill the airwaves.

The modern era of psychiatry sprang from new definitions for disease, new drugs to treat them, and direct-to-consumer advertising
The practice of medicine has followed a similar path. It's even fair to say ADD could have served as the poster child for this new business model:

1. **New definitions:** Having no understanding of what causes ADD, public health agencies define it as the collection of symptoms you're all familiar with: can't sit still, can't pay attention, poor impulse control, lack of planning, poor judgment, and stimulation seeking.
2. **New drugs:** Dozens and dozens of stimulant, serotonin-enhancing, and psychoactive drugs have been developed to treat the many symptoms central and comorbid (occurring together) with ADD.
3. **Direct-to-consumer advertising:** ADD drugs are among the most heavily-promoted class of pharmaceutical, and most profitable.

3. Late 1980s to early 2010s: Progressive minds try to explain root causes that the "bible of psychiatry" (the DSM) ignores
Dr. Ben Feingold and his elimination diet, the Feingold diet, had the most success and supporters in this category. He blamed food dyes, artificial flavors, artificial sweeteners, preservatives, and chemical sensitivities with causing hyperactivity in ADHD. Since the late 1970s, the Feingold diet has worked for a minority of children whose parents sought solution for their child's hyperactivity. And it's true: eliminating certain chemicals in foods has been known to fix behavior problems – not necessarily problems with inhibition and executive function but, rather, lightening the load on the PFC, without fixing the source issue.

The net of it: the Feingold diet has not caught on as well as one would expect if it worked better, for more people. It doesn't look like the Feingold diet is going away anytime soon. But its popularity has declined, because it focuses on hyperactivity, when it does work.

4. Mid 1990s to present: Dr. Daniel Amen proves, once and for all, that ADD exists using functional brain SPECT scans (video)
Since 1989, Dr. Daniel Amen has studied brain function and its effects on learning, behavior and social skills. He's looked at over 100,000 brain scans of people on and off medications, head trauma, toxin exposures, birth defects, therapies/coping strategies, and diet interventions. As both a psychiatrist and brain imaging specialist, he's been able to link cognitive

function with actual brain activity. By examining functional brain SPECT scans, he sees when and where dysfunction happens *in real time*.

He was the first to do this routinely, without suspecting traumatic brain injury. And, along the way, he's lifted the field of mental health out of the dark ages of talk-therapy, and almost single-headedly given it a scientific underpinning that it didn't have before. He gave psychiatry and behavioral sciences answers to long-standing conjecture.

To give you some background, before he started scanning people's brains to see how well they work in functional situations, mental health professionals did not routinely do this when they saw patients. Health professionals that dealt with learning, behavior, social/family problems diagnosed and treated patients by asking them questions, making observations, and matching their responses to symptom clusters found in the DSM.

That was how they diagnosed and treated patients. And it was standard medical practice. They largely ignored the structure and performance of the brain itself, unless they had reason to suspect acute head trauma and brain damage. In other words, they guessed at diagnosing and treating what we now know to be primarily physical issues. That was considered normal.

Psychiatry was the only medical specialty that did not normally look at the organ and system it diagnosed and treated

Cardiologists look at the heart. Orthopedists look at bones on x-rays. Gastroenterologists look at the colon. But before Dr. Amen came along, psychiatrist did not routinely look at the brain. Almost every medical specialty inspects the organ and supporting systems in their field of practice, before they diagnose and treat anything. They could easily be sued for malpractice if they didn't. But not psychiatry. How strange.

What Dr. Amen did when he started bringing SPECT imaging into standard practice is he changed the way his patients and medical community viewed mental health disorders. For the first time, mental health conditions were understood to be both physical and psychological in nature. This was a genuine breakthrough in our understanding of mental health, and a significant advancement in how we treat learning, behavior, and social difficulties. But, like all great paradigm shifts, it wasn't easy. The establishment resisted Amen's innovations, every step of the way:

- fighting the use of imaging technologies, common in other specialties
- ridiculed by peers
- hauled in front of medical review boards to question his methods
- finding supporters to build a new *standard of care*.

We'll probably look back at the 2010s as the decade his work started the revolution of understanding that helped us look at mental health in a whole new light. It started us down a path by which we identify, understand, accept, and successfully treat brain health problems that prevent an individual from living a normal life.

With the advent of SPECT scans to show a brain's functionality, people now see their learning, behavioral and social problems as a medical issue, not a moral one. It decreased shame and guilt. It increased forgiveness and compassion from families and associates. Nothing in the field of psychiatry had done that prior. But, when tangible proof of dysfunction is staring you in the face in the form of a brain scan, it's hard to argue. Showing people how well their brain functions in actual use is undeniable. And it completely changed the mental health conversation.

Today, having done over 120,000 brain scans in his Amen Clinics, his work is widely recognized as having pioneered our understanding of how the brain shapes behavior and makes us who we are. There's more work to be done on finding the biological basis for what Dr. Amen is seeing on SPECT scans. But we have the major pieces at-hand. We can see brain dysfunction when it happens. We know a great deal about its mechanisms of action, and its root causes. And we're well on the way to being able to reverse those triggers and begin the journey of healing. We have Dr. Daniel Amen to thank for catapulting us far down the correct path.

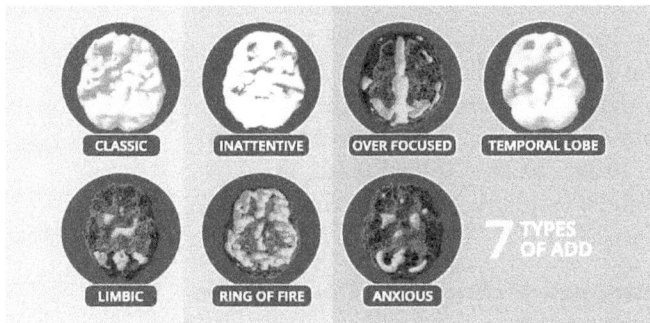

Image used courtesy of Dr. Daniel Amen

Along the way, Dr. Amen discovered 7 distinct types of ADD

The inability to put your focus where you want, when you want, is just one of them, called "Classic." "Inattentive" is another. "Over focused" is the third. "Temporal Lobe" is the fourth. "Limbic" is the fifth. "Ring of Fire" is the sixth. And "Anxious" is Amen's seventh type. Check out his book *Healing ADD* for specifics. These are all characterized by an abnormal activity level – too low or too high – in different areas of the brain, as shown on functional (SPECT) brain scans – not primarily symptoms.

Most important, all seven of them except for Ring of Fire have an underactive prefrontal cortex (PFC) – the area responsible for focus, concentration, decision-making, judgment, problem-solving, planning, and much more. The prefrontal cortex is responsible for doing so many things that it's been called the executive center of the brain. It communicates with and controls all areas of the brain related to thinking, perception, learning, behavior and social skills. It's the CEO of your brain… the director of your show. Evolutionarily speaking, it is the most sophisticated area of the brain, and the part of the body most responsible for giving people human characteristics such as intelligence, reasoning, abstract thought, and complex social dynamics.

In his books, Dr. Amen further explains the "anterior cingulate gyrus" acts as the brain's "gear shifter." The "temporal lobes" house memories and experience, as well as control a person's aggression. The "basal ganglia" produces dopamine and is involved with motor control. And the "deep limbic system" acts as the brain's mood-control center.

Of special interest to a lot of parents with unruly children, **hyperactivity is not a specific type of ADD, nor is it caused by a genetic defect.** Rather, it's a symptom. It's an effect, not a cause, which we'll discuss in a little bit. Hyperactivity is most common in Amen's Type 1 "Classic" variety. Key point: When practitioners or diagnostic manuals define ADD as a collection of symptoms such as hyperactivity, they are behind the times in understanding it and defining it, because there is a biological basis for the symptoms... a root cause.

Therefore, looking only at symptoms is a naïve way to define ADD, because whether individual symptoms present themselves or not, the underlying root cause of Attention Deficit is still there. It's chronically impacting the individual's productivity, relationships, and quality of life. That means many people grow out of hyperactivity as they mature and gain self-control. But unless/until the root cause is dealt with, the biochemical reactions and other effects, remain. They continue to affect the person's life – usually for the worse.

5. Present day: Dr. Natasha Campbell-McBride and Donna Gates explain what causes ADD in most people

Most cases of ADD are caused by a combination of overlapping mechanisms originating in the gut. On top of that, you may have symptoms that come and go due to environmental exposures such as sugar or food colorings. It's not usually a single factor that causes true biologically-based ADD (as defined below). Which is to say, a body whose constitution and resiliency is at full strength will typically have the resources to overcome imbalances, weaknesses and threats. Like fighting a war on multiple fronts, it's the spreading of the body's healing and regeneration resources thin that produces regrettable situations.

The gut controls so many biochemical processes that, when it's unable to do its many jobs correctly, the resulting malfunctions impact brain performance in many ways. Hence, ADD is not one behavior or dysfunction. It's often a "constellation" of peculiarities that come and go for no discernable rhyme or reason to the casual observer. That's one of the reasons the true causes of ADD have been so hard to pinpoint through *single cause, single treatment* thinking.

It's a big reason why ADD has defied explanation through observation, testing and analysis: It isn't just one toxin, reaction, genetic predisposition, or malfunction in the body. It's more than one thing. And as these exposures fluctuate, so do ADD symptoms. This is why lots of explanations and remedies have been proffered through the decades. Yet none of them have solved very much, despite the fact that all the solutions have been successful at helping some of the people, some of the time.

Now you know why it's been so hard for smart and well-meaning people to wrap their arms entirely around the pathology of ADD: people have approached it with tunnel vision. Until you think about ADD as (1) physiological problems emanating from a corrupted gut, (2) manifesting through multiple mechanisms of action, and (3) topped off by a variety of complications that may come and go, it will continue to defy explanation. Let's unpack the mechanisms one-by-one:

Any combination of five mechanisms can cause ADD

A corrupted gut is largely to blame for all three core mechanisms of action that cause most cases of conventional ADD. This is where most ADD comes from, so let's put them in a category called **"gut-based ADD."**

1. **Neurotransmitter imbalances.** Individual brain centers get too little, or too much, of the neurotransmitters they need to run properly, causing under-activity, over-activity or malfunctioning.
2. **Chemical intoxication (transient).** Toxic substances get into the bloodstream and affect brain function temporarily, as if you're drunk, poisoned, or allergic to the toxin.
3. **Cellular degeneration and atrophy (persistent).** Brain cells die when chronically inflamed from poison or neglect.

Numbers 1 and 2 are reversible when you heal your gut. Number 3 is residual damage to cells that has accumulated over time, causing a structural loss of grey matter. The amount of cellular degeneration a person has suffered determines how much dysfunction can be reversed *vs.* how much will remain after treatment. That is, the amount of cell death from toxicity poisoning, atrophy, and other factors determines the amount of healing that is possible through successful treatment *vs.* how much damage is more or less permanent. Exposure to toxins in the womb is included in this category.

Two more mechanisms can cause/contribute to ADD in exceptional cases. We'll call these **"rudimentary ADD"**:

4. **Structural brain damage (by irrevocable event).** These are problems with your brain's hardware (neurons and glial cells) – either from birth defect or traumatic brain injury.
5. **Emotional trauma.** These are problems with your brain's operating system, as a result of abuse or extreme psychological stress.

Number 4 "Structural" is a relatively permanent physical problem, while Number 5 "Emotional" is a deep-seated psychological one. We'll call these "rudimentary" ADD mechanisms, because the brain and psyche are far more rigidly rooted to these foundational elements than gut-based ADD tends to be. In other words, categories #4 and #5, when present, are the groundwork upon which cognitive, behavioral, and social functioning of the brain is built. For that reason, they tend to be somewhat more set in stone, once put into place, as opposed to being fluid and relatively more reversible the way gut-based ADD is.

Rudimentary ADD and gut-based ADD definitely can and do happen simultaneously. But gut-based ADD is far more common than rudimentary ADD. So we're focusing our attention on the gut and all that it does for the mind and body, rather than the less-reversible effects of head trauma, birth defects, and ritual abuse.

Neurotransmitters

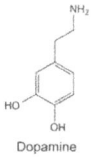

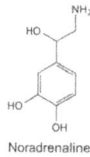

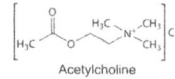

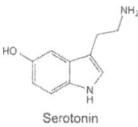

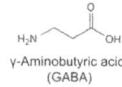

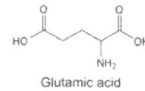

Dopamine

Noradrenaline

Acetylcholine

Serotonin

γ-Aminobutyric acid (GABA)

Glutamic acid

ADD cause #1: Neurotransmitter imbalances

Neurotransmitter imbalances are the defining characteristic of the standard-type ADD, which is gut-based. They affect brain function in four ways:

1. **Attention deficit disorder** in general is caused by low levels of the neurotransmitters dopamine and serotonin.
2. **Focus.** Brain functions involving purposeful concentration are controlled primarily by dopamine and norepinephrine.
3. **Positive emotions.** Brain activity involving happiness and feeling good are regulated by serotonin and norepinephrine.
4. **Negativity.** Brain centers dealing with mood and temper are put in their "happy place" largely through GABA and serotonin.

Neurotransmitter imbalances are the main mechanism through which ADD presents itself because neurotransmitters enable communication between brains cells, brain centers, and the rest of the body. The fidelity with which the brain operates impacts the way you think, feel, learn, create, and act around others. It makes you the person that you are.

More than anything else, the brain connects your inside world to your outside world. So when your neurotransmitter levels are out of balance, you don't have as much control over the things that your brain is supposed to run and regulate. You are not quite the same person that you're designed to be. And one of the first brain functions affecting the way you relate to other human beings is your ability to direct attention.

Raising neurotransmitter levels through *exogenous substances*

We know that neurotransmitter imbalances are responsible for attention anomalies, because when you give an attention-deficient individual stimulants to correct their neurotransmitter levels, brain function normalizes and the individual can focus. On a biological level, when you give a person psychoactive drugs like Ritalin or Adderall, you rev up their adrenal system using the so-called "fight or flight" response. This releases more dopamine, serotonin, norepinephrine, GABA, or other neurotransmitters in the body's effort to help you survive a stressful situation.

Then, when you have sufficient chemical messengers present for brain cells to communicate, the individual thinks, feels, and behaves more appropriately. So the purpose of stimulants and psychoactive drugs is to adjust neurotransmitter levels into a normal range. This allows the brain and body to function closer to 100%. Conversely, when neurotransmitter levels are off, your brain operates sub-optimally, and you're a different person cognitively, behaviorally and socially.

Raising neurotransmitter levels through *stimulation-seeking behavior*

Most ADD individuals can focus quite easily on things that interest, excite, scare, or otherwise stimulate them. In fact, many on the ADD spectrum have an abundance of focus to spend on people or passions in which they find highly engaging. Some describe this as being hyper-focused. Others call it a superpower when it helps the person, an addiction when it hurts them. It's only when the person is bored that their brain goes into "energy conservation" mode, and they lose ability to focus.

Thus, the term "attention deficit" is somewhat of a misnomer because most people that have ADD don't lack the ability to pay attention. Rather, they have less control over when and where they apply their attention, compared to unaffected people. You can say they have less attention available "in the tank" to use as they wish, so they need to use it sparingly on unexciting things. In other words, they don't have any *extra* attention to spend frivolously.

Therefore, in an effort to save your limited supply of neurotransmitters and attention span, you spend them generously on things that interest you, and sparingly on things that don't, to get maximum satisfaction out of life. You need to conserve brain chemicals that are in short supply, which makes you somewhat of a slave to your impulses and primal desires.

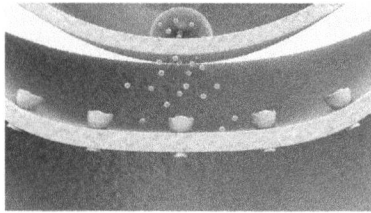

You use up neurotransmitter and biochemical supplies when you're active, and replenish them when you sleep

When you don't get enough sleep, the next day your eyes may be open, and you may look like you're awake, but your brain and body are operating in power conservation mode. You're half human-half zombie on an underfilled gas tank. You can't think, react, and be fully creative when you're sleep deprived because your body cuts back on its consumption of resources in a state of scarcity. This is why you can get seriously screwed up when deeply deprived of sleep, and can actually die when you run out.

You can drink pots of coffee to force your body into releasing its backup supplies of dopamine, cortisol and adrenaline. But you're drawing from your emergency reserves when you do that, instead of making biochemicals the natural and sustainable way: in sleep and downtime. So, it only stands to reason, if you survive too long on energy drinks and drama, something's got to give. Which is exactly what Dr. Amen has seen on functional SPECT scans: Caffeine enhances brain function short-term. But if you go the stimulant route too much and too often, you deplete your mineral stores, build a tolerance to caffeine, blood flow to the brain decreases, and the adrenals collapse, along with brain function.

Sleep is that important in keeping your brain operating at peak efficiency because the body prepares hormones and neurotransmitters while you sleep. Conversely, when neurotypical people are exhausted or sleepy, they catch a glimpse of what it's like to have underactive brain centers, like that in the ADD brain.

Psychoactive drugs can turn you into a completely different person

Anyone who's taken psychoactive drugs knows that altering brain chemistry can change the way your brain perceives the world and processes information. It can make you interact with family and friends through different filters. Clinical conditions like psychosis and paranoia aside, when your brain chemistry changes, you literally *are* a different person in the same body.

When you get your brain chemistry right, you're lucid, stable, and you feel good. But, when you get it wrong, you might experience anger, anxiety, depression, derangement, or paranoia – all the way up to suicidal or homicidal tendencies. Underappreciated by those outside the mental health profession, neurotransmitter levels are a huge part of who you are because they power your personality.

Gut-based ADD is primarily a biochemical problem, not structural, genetic, or stimulation-caused

The previous four observations are strong confirmations that there is nothing physically wrong with the ADD individual's brain. It works fine, given the right supplies and/or circumstances. Whether through external drugs or internal "Type-A" behaviors, both allow the brain to work within its proper neurotransmitter range, and thus uncompromised. Whereas, if the brain were defective or damaged – if there were something truly wrong with it – it wouldn't work properly no matter what you did to try and tweak its performance.

When neurotransmitters levels are off, you can't feel good as easily

Neurotransmitters enable a person to feel happiness and well-being. We experience emotions and physical satisfaction through dopamine, serotonin, norepinephrine (adrenaline), GABA, endorphins and others. When these levels are "within specs," you feel better all the time (on average). But when your levels are irregular, everything you feel is taken down a notch or two. You feel more depressed, less physically well, and less at ease. Your brain and body feel less comfortable and content than those that have the biochemicals to activate such signaling. **Thus, it's only a mild exaggeration to say the ADD individual's *peak experience* is the way a balanced person feels *all the time*.** This is why ADD individuals love things that stimulate their brain: they need stimulation just to feel normal.

Clinical depression

Clinical depression is associated with low neurotransmitter levels similar to those described above – although serotonin deficiency in depression presents more like a gloomy outlook on life than a feeling of discontent. To give neurotypical people an idea of what this constant state of "less than" feels like, imagine cramming all night for mid-terms. You depleted your neurotransmitters concentrating for hours on end. You're super sleepy, hungry and exhausted. You fidget to preoccupy your brain and suppress the feeling of unease throughout your body. That's what ADD feels like most of the time, until something novel, interesting, dangerous, or scary stimulates the person's brain to spike their neurotransmitter levels.

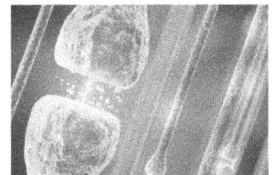

Six neurotransmitters control your most important cognitive functions

1. **Dopamine** controls the brain functions that humans and higher life forms are known for, such as attention, judgment, abstract thinking, planning, decision-making and impulse control.
2. **Serotonin** is a "sister" neurotransmitter to dopamine. As dopamine's opposite in several ways, serotonin controls brain functions having to do with emotions, social interactions and comfort. So it regulates mood, behavior, appetite, sleep, memory and learning. Serotonin also helps the brain shift from one thought to the next, and one physical movement to the next. It helps you let go of the last thing.

3. **Norepinephrine** is both a neurotransmitter and stress hormone that prepares the body and mind for stressful situations by increasing heart rate, blood pressure, respiration, and glucose level. Norepinephrine also helps regulate attention, sleep, learning and mood.

4. **GABA** is the opposite of glutamate. It's an inhibitory neurotransmitter. It quiets the firing of nerve pathways. A shortage of GABA is notorious for "heating up" the brain's temporal lobes, which control mood stability, learning and memory. So poor temporal lobe function makes you more susceptible to anger management issues, irritability and anxiety – leading to a short temper, dark thoughts, social/marital problems, violence and suicide.

5. **Glutamate** is an excitatory neurotransmitter. It encourages nerve cells to fire, and nerve impulses to propagate along nerve pathways.

6. **Acetylcholine** is involved in muscle movement, arousal, motivation, learning, memory, verbal/logical reasoning, attention and concentration.

Of the six, imbalances in dopamine, serotonin, norepinephrine, and GABA are most responsible for causing Dr. Amen's 7 types of ADD. Amen's Type 1 (loosely equivalent to classic AD(H)D) is caused mostly by dopamine and serotonin deficiencies under-activating the PFC. Dopamine and serotonin dysregulation cause more psychological disorders than any other neurotransmitters because the PFC is the command-and-control center of the brain. It combines the activity of individual brain centers into a cohesive whole. Amen's 6 other ADD varieties result from serotonin, norepinephrine, and GABA imbalances impacting the cingulate system, temporal lobes, limbic system, and basal ganglia.

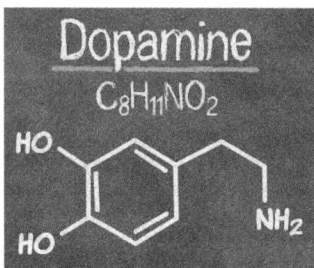

Dopamine

As one of the brain's primary reward chemicals, dopamine's claim to fame is that it activates the prefrontal cortex (PFC). Integral to advanced brain function, the PFC controls concentration and executive function by using dopamine as a reward chemical to promote certain behaviors. When you do something stimulating, whether that be hanging out with friends, posting on social media, playing video games, or even creating drama in your life, your brain releases dopamine to make you feel good and, by consequence, encourage more of that activity. When you need to concentrate on a task for any length of time, dopamine is the primary neurotransmitter that engages the PFC and enables you to maintain focus on that one thing by giving your brain the fuel to feel satisfied.

Conversely, when you're running low on dopamine, the PFC can't keep you focused on boring tasks because they feel tedious, tiring, or even annoying to you. In other words, it's mildly torturous to concentrate for some length of time when dopamine is low and the PFC is disengaged. Without reward chemicals, executive function of the brain takes a break and attention wanders.

When this happens, you do have attention available to allocate, but its supply is limited. Thus, the PFC can't always direct your attention where you want it to be, and you're less capable of controlling your thoughts, feelings, and actions. So you lose interest, become more impulsive, and seek out things that excite the brain into releasing reward chemicals. Stimulants such as Ritalin (methylphenidate), Adderall, and caffeine are the most popular chemical approaches to increasing dopamine availability.

The PFC: The brain center most responsible for our human-ness

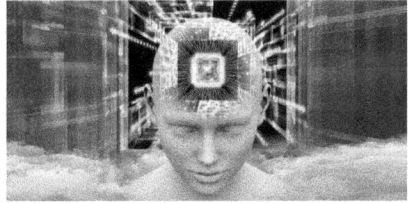

The prefrontal cortex controls complex thought, decision-making, analysis, predicting future outcomes, planning and directing attention. It's the one thing, more than any other, that gives you human thinking and reasoning ability, because when your PFC is underactive, you lose higher brain functions used toward abstract thought and goal-directed behavior.

In effect, you're a little less human in self-direction and self-control, and you're more animalistic in your behavior patterns. As PFC activity drops, you become more irrational and impulsive in your thoughts and behaviors. While at the same time, the primitive parts of your brain assert more control over you, including stimulation-seeking behavior and instant gratification. When you can't concentrate, your intellect and reason are subdued, and your primal instincts surface.

This does not mean your brain has no ability to pay attention. It does not mean ADD makes you stupid. It does not typically mean that your brain is permanently damaged. It simply means you cannot direct your concentration where you want, as long as you want, when you lack the biochemicals that promote focused attention, which are primarily dopamine, norepinephrine (adrenaline), and serotonin.

Why ADD individuals get more "turned on" by stimulation

Anything that stimulates the brain has the effect of raising dopamine. And when dopamine levels approach a normal range, the attention span of a neurotypical person emerges, if only temporarily. So the hardware that controls attention span in the ADD brain works just fine in most people. It's the messenger molecules powering these processes that is upset.

Up high, when your brain is intensely stimulated and dopamine is plentiful, that's when some ADD individuals over-focus their attention. They fixate on things that turn them on and make them feel good, because peak experiences release a flood of reward chemicals that potentiate attention. Feeling that rush, the person can get addicted to stimulation-seeking behaviors. Obsessing over your favorite celebrity crush, hobby, TV show, or action in general are good examples.

Whatever that activity or thought may be, stimulation makes the ADD brain feel better than it usually does, so they continue doing it. Unfortunately, the ADD brain needs extra stimulation to bring it up to the comfort level of a neurotypical person. Without it, they feel perpetually bored or frustrated, when under-stimulated. On the other hand, when they experience a high level of stimulation, they're doubly turned on escaping their usual "stimulation starvation."

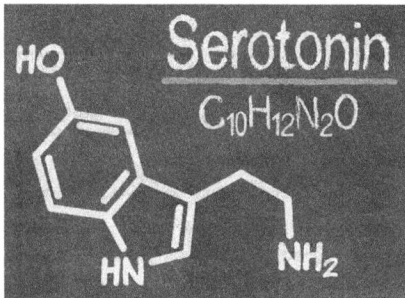

Serotonin

Serotonin calms you down and gives you a sense of well-being. It helps relay messages from one area of the brain to another. It controls mood, social behavior, appetite, digestion, sleep, sexual desire, memory and learning. So it's the body's primary "feel good and relaxed" chemical.

Conversely, when you're low on serotonin, you can feel depressed, anxious, unable to sleep, un-centered, and less than 100% in how you experience life. When your nervous system doesn't have an adequate supply of serotonin to make you feel happy and whole, you're unable to enjoy life to the fullest. Serotonin imbalance is one of the most common mental health challenges facing Westerners today… and not just in cases of ADD. Due to widespread gut dysbiosis, and the number of jobs that it does, disordered serotonin cycling plays a role in most GAPS conditions. Hundreds of millions of people around the world now suffer from depression and anxiety as a result of serotonin deficiency.

According to a 2012 study, 1 in 8 Americans (the majority being women) is taking some form of prescription SSRI medication (serotonin selective re-uptake inhibitor) to enhance their serotonin availability. In fact, so many people are taking antidepressants such as Prozac, Zoloft, and Paxil today that ecologists are finding trace amounts of these drugs in our drinking water, soil, plants and wildlife. That's scary.

Norepinephrine

Norepinephrine's main mission in life is to speed up the mind and body to help you handle stressful situations. It makes you more mentally awake, aware, and focused by raising blood pressure, heart rate, respiratory rate and blood-glucose levels. In doing these things,

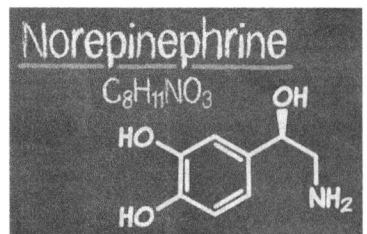

norepinephrine gets you ready to fight, fight or flee through adrenal function and the stress response.

Norepinephrine also helps regulate day-to-day activity of the limbic system through its ability to control cognitive arousal. You see, low norepinephrine partners with low serotonin to cause major depression. That's because the limbic system helps set your emotional tone – particularly toward the dark, depressive side of the spectrum. It's the "party pooper" of the brain, because the limbic system skews your perception of events toward the negative, when running in high gear.

Countering this effect, norepinephrine quiets the limbic system. When norepinephrine dips due to circumstance or shortage, the limbic system heats up, producing feelings of helplessness, negativity, lethargy, trouble focusing and brain fog. Conversely, when norepinephrine is elevated, the limbic system calms down, making you feel more positive – as if norepinephrine (the "bliss booster") were quenching the limbic system fire and inducing mild elation.

Armed with this knowledge, drug makers have been promoting the ability of newer drugs such as tricyclic antidepressants to upregulate norepinephrine in order to boost attention span and motivation in a round-about way (stimulants being the direct route).

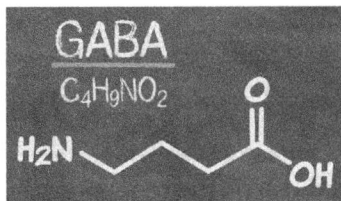

GABA

GABA deficiency is entwined with anger and irritability traits in several ADD types – particularly "Type 4: Temporal Lobe" and "Type 6: Ring of Fire" varieties. Intimately involved in inhibiting excessive firing of brain cells, GABA powers the temporal lobes.

The temporal lobes suppress anger impulses by helping to extinguish angry and aggressive thoughts before they enter your stream of consciousness. When GABA is low, a person's temporal lobes go to sleep, bringing about anger management issues such as road rage and oppositional defiant disorder. It can cause anxiety, epilepsy or PMS, as examples.

Classes of drugs known to enhance GABA are hypnotics, sedatives, tranquillizers and anticonvulsants. In this category, benzodiazepines such as Valium became the most commonly prescribed class of drug in the 1970s – even achieving cult-like status among high society. However, dependency and withdrawal difficulties became hard to ignore in the 1980s, and they fell out of favor. Today, anticonvulsants such as Neurontin, Depakote and Lamictal are very popular in calming anger, aggression, seizures, and emotional instability in the GAPS population – often through normalizing temporal lobe function.

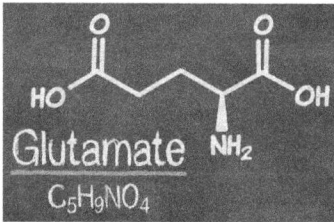

Glutamate

Glutamate is the most abundant neurotransmitter by far. It's also the most neuro-destructive at high levels. Over half of all nerve impulses in the brain (over 90% in the cortex) use glutamate as a signaling molecule – far exceeding all other neurotransmitters put together. Glutamate also regulates the use of other neurotransmitters. So it's both plentiful and essential. However, high levels of glutamate outside of brain cells damages or kills them, which is easy to do nowadays for a variety of reasons:

- Normally, 1,000 times more glutamate is inside brain cells than out.
- Any time the immune system is provoked (e.g., viral infection), glutamate is released into the extracellular space between brain cells.
- Any time that microglia (the brain's special immune cells) are activated for any reason (e.g., adjuvants in vaccines), pro-inflammatory cytokines are released, which greatly amplify glutamate toxicity.
- The glutamate in MSG (and all derivatives), increases glutamate levels in the brain.

This is where glutamate transport proteins are designed to protect against glutamate toxicity. They are supposed to take glutamate found outside cells and transport them inside, where it's harmless. Unfortunately, glutamate transport proteins are easily oxidized (broken down) by free radicals through the inflammation process. Inflammation releases inflammatory cytokines that powerfully inhibit the transport proteins. So when transportation of glutamate into the cells slows to a crawl, extracellular (outside/between) glutamate rises to toxic levels.

Glutamate, in all its forms, contributes to injury of brain cells

Hidden in thousands of food products, and going by dozens of innocent-sounding names such as "spices" or "natural flavoring," glutamate is added to most salty/savory processed foods in order to give the brain an explosion of flavor when eaten. Glutamate flavorings have become so pervasive since Big Food took over our food supply that it's getting hard to find packaged foods that don't contain glutamate-based flavor enhancers.

But, while our taste buds rejoice in decadent flavor, glutamate derivatives overexcite and kill brain cells the same way that glutamate made by the brain does. MSG, and its offshoots, encourage brain cells to fire as motivation to eat certain foods. The problem is, the brain doesn't have a "rev limiter" to limit brain cell activation to a safe level. Thus, high levels of MSG in food make brain cells fire excessively and inappropriately, until injured or killed.

And that's exactly what's happening when you eat too much glutamate in foods: externally-sourced glutamate piles onto that produced by the brain, to produce toxic levels to astrocytes. As a result, chronic over-stimulation of brain cells from glutamate – whatever the source – is a primary mechanism by which brain degradation occurs in GAPS individuals. It's a major mechanism by which brain dysfunction takes place – chronic over-activation of the brain's immune system, and resulting inflammation, being the other "dance partner" in brain cell destruction.

In summary, glutamate has the dubious distinction of causing the majority of excitotoxicity (brain cell death due to over-stimulation) in people. Excitotoxicity spells neuron damage and degradation of brain function. However, practitioners don't usually target glutamate dysregulation to fix ADD issues. It's only the enlightened ones that work on reducing glutamate levels to prevent erosion of cognition in autistics.

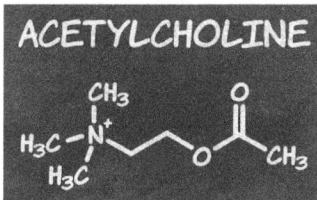

Acetylcholine

Acetylcholine is the forgotten stepchild among the six neurotransmitters most responsible for causing ADD symptoms. Apart from its leading role in the expression of Alzheimer's, acetylcholine is blamed for a variety of peripheral challenges in GAPS conditions. It's important enough to mention, because it does have something to do with cognitive deficits in GAPS individuals. However, practitioners, researchers, and drug companies don't focus on correcting acetylcholine levels in ADD. And no drugs currently target acetylcholine. So we'll leave it alone at this time too.

Underneath biochemical imbalances, and resulting dysfunctions, the ADD individual's full faculties hibernate

It never ceases to amaze parents, friends, teachers and practitioners who know the affected individual: When you normalize neurotransmitter levels, a person's real brain power is unshackled. Like getting a complete engine overhaul on a car that seemed destined for the scrap heap, you're then able to see what their cognitive ability is really like, as it was meant to be. Elevating neurotransmitter levels in a previously dopamine- or serotonin-deficient person reveals the intelligence, self-control and empathy that they've had all along, but were unable to exhibit because those qualities were hidden beneath biochemical imbalances.

Unfortunately, reaching a high functional level is easier said than done because environmental threats abound, and the prefrontal cortex is hyper-

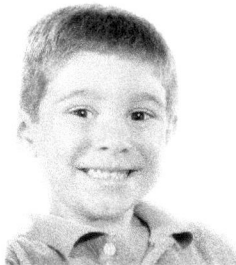

sensitive to operational defects. Indeed, the PFC is one of the first areas of the brain to be affected by slight neurotransmitter imbalances. Similarly, the "poster child" for mild-to-moderate brain dysfunction, ADD, is considered by many practitioners to be near the beginning of the Gut and Psychology Syndrome spectrum in severity (autism and schizophrenia being near the deep end). That's why ADD is so common today: the causes seem endless, and it doesn't take much to upset brain function.

To summarize, most ADD behaviors are the brain's effort to make up for dopamine, serotonin and norepinephrine deficiencies. Consequently, a good portion of the ADD individual's life is spent in search of people, things, and activities that stimulate their brain into releasing reward chemicals in order to experience the same pleasure for life that neurotypical people take for granted.

How we know that the brain still works (and has since birth)
Brain function sometimes improves suddenly and dramatically when you

1. eat nutritious foods and avoid junk food
2. have good bacteria to digest, make nutrients and protect the gut wall
3. get plenty of restorative sleep
4. dial in your medication regimen
5. stimulate the mind
6. stop toxin flow from the gut, like enemas often do.

If you notice, all of these enhance the biochemistry of the brain and body. In particular, **by stopping the flow toxins coming from the bowels, practitioners have seen enemas radically improve brain function into a normal range.** Unfortunately, those improvements are usually temporary, not a permanent reversal… that is unless/until you fix the underlying problem, which is a corrupted gut.

Now, medical experts say that the brain can't repair itself after suffering true anatomical damage. But I believe the brain is more plastic than they think. When practitioners show that the brain can, and does, function at a high level through simple interventions like an enema, it likely never lost that capacity since birth. Which means these individuals were born with perfectly normal brains.

What hinders neurotransmitter availability
Neurotransmitter cycling is a sensitive process. Many things can go wrong in the production, usage and recycling of neurotransmitters. Leaky gut, food sensitivities, heavy metals and toxins, hormones, medications, stress, lack of sleep, aging, and epigenetic/gene abnormalities can all impair brain chemistry and function.

Leaky gut and food sensitivities. The most common glitch in neurotransmitter production is having too many pathogens, and not enough probiotic bacteria, residing in your microbiome. This exposes you to all sorts of adversity from poor digestion and malabsorption.

Heavy metals and toxins are another monkey wrench in neurotransmitter production, because they can interfere with production directly. Mercury, for example, destroys nerve cells. Whereas toxins such as bisphenol-A (BPA), can attach themselves to cells' receptor sites and mimic the substance for which the receptors are intended. Toxins then block a process from happening altogether. Or they can trick the cell into using the toxin as a building block in protein production. Glyphosate, for instance, is structurally similar to glycine, so proteins get made with defective materials. When mistaken identity of this sort happens, the defective neurotransmitter, hormone, or DNA causes the body to work overtime preventing or repairing any damage that may result.

Hormones. In the case of BPA, the body mistakes it for estrogen, which causes problems in young women, such as increased risk for breast cancer and early puberty (100 years ago, many women went through puberty, age 16–20).

Medications. Pharmaceuticals force the body to do something it doesn't want to. Good examples: drugs such as steroids, statins, birth control pills, and blood pressure meds steal nutrients from cell repair, digestion, and extinguishing inflammation.

Stress consumes extra nutrients and co-factors needed to make cortisol, dopamine, and adrenaline for perceived emergencies.

Lack of building blocks needed to make neurotransmitters. GAPS individuals tend to eat limited diets because (1) pathogens in the gut increase cravings for sugars and carbs. And, (2) being persistently low on pleasure chemicals, GAPS people tend to fall into addiction, which junk food satisfies like a drug. When you eat foods that deplete minerals, and your diet is not very nourishing, you lack building blocks to make the neurotransmitters by which brain centers communicate.

Imbalanced microbiome. Probiotic bacteria manufacture vitamin A, vitamin K$_2$, essential fatty acids, and most of the B vitamin group. Probiotics also help the digestion and bioavailability of nutrients such as: copper, calcium, magnesium, iron, manganese, potassium, zinc, proteins, fats, carbohydrates, sugars, milk, phytonutrients and cholesterol.

The importance of diet and nutrition should not be underestimated when healing not only ADD/ADHD symptoms (behaviors), but also underlying mechanisms (biology). Fixing hyperactivity is good. But restoring full functionality of the brain, body, and immune system is even better when you fix root causes such as nutrient deficiencies.

Conversely, what happens when you target *symptoms* with drugs, instead of *causes* with nutrition? You generally get results ranging from tolerable to pretty good, but rarely ideal. To illustrate the influence of underlying mechanisms: Nutrient deficiencies are thought to be a big reason that drugs such as Ritalin and Adderall can lose effectiveness over time: you deplete minerals required to make neurotransmitters, thereby settling for temporary half-measures, instead of more complete fixes.

The neurotransmitter production process

When your digestive system is healthy, probiotics break down foods into vitamins, minerals and amino acids. This starts the chain of digestion, absorption, biochemical production, utilization and recycling. For example, proteins make L-tryptophan. L-tryptophan makes 5-HTP. 5-HTP makes serotonin. And serotonin turns into melatonin. These processes require zinc, vitamins B_1, B_3 and B_6, stomach acid, folate, iron, calcium, magnesium and vitamin C. Beneficial bacteria themselves also make aromatic amino acids like tyrosine and phenylalanine, which are used as precursors in the production of all-important neurotransmitters dopamine, epinephrine and norepinephrine.

But, when the gut is corrupted, deficiencies in minerals, vitamins, amino acids, and enzymes impair neurotransmitter production in systems such as the liver, adrenals, and gut wall itself. Toxic substances circulating in the body from a leaky gut don't help either. All this is crucial to brain function, because 90% of serotonin is made by cells of the gut lining in communication with bacteria; more than half of your dopamine is made in the gut; and about 30% is made in the kidneys. So, oddly enough, the brain is responsible for making only about 10–20% of neurotransmitters that it uses.

Achieving perfect brain function with drugs is darn near impossible

Over 120,000 SPECT scans confirm the brain's ability to wake up in some areas, calm down in others, and work normally after correcting neurotransmitter imbalances with pharmaceuticals. However, finding the right combination of drugs to replicate the body's own neurotransmitter balance is easier said than done.

Decades of clinical experience has proven that pharmaceuticals can work wonders treating the symptoms of ADD. But finding the perfect combination that gets your brain working exceptionally well, with no adverse effects or tolerances – not just the absence of hyperactivity – can be extremely difficult. Which is to say that *improving* brain function with drugs is easy. But getting it to work flawlessly, without side effects, is a tall task.

Perfection can be a moving target, because the innate intelligence of the body's own internal pharmacy is difficult to approximate, let alone duplicate. It can take several months to quarters of adjusting drug types, dosages, brands, timing, combinations, diet and lifestyle choices to get to 'okay' or 'better.' But if you're looking for 'excellent' and 'sustainable,' you may be looking for a needle in a haystack. We'll talk more about tailoring a drug regiment in Chapter 19: Managing the Symptoms of ADD.

The steps from a corrupted gut to noticeable symptoms

When you follow the chain of events in either direction – from environmental exposures to observable effects, or from problems back to their source – all roads lead to a corrupted gut as the core component of most cases of attention deficit disorder. How the steps link together:

- Antibiotics, glyphosate, heavy metals, chlorine/chloramine in water, sugars and carbs, prescription drugs and fluoride cause
- probiotic demise and pathogen overgrowth, which is responsible for
- a corrupted gut, which creates
  - o nutrient deficiencies
  - o immune system hyperactivation (exacerbated by vaccines)
  - o tight junction damage and leaky membranes (the gut, blood–brain barrier, blood vessels, and kidney tubules), producing
- increased toxin flow from your GI tract, which
- upsets your biochemistry, triggering
  - o degeneration of brain cells
  - o neurotransmitter imbalances, materializing as an
- underactive prefrontal cortex and other brain centers, leading to
- poor control over brain function (e.g., executive function and attention deficit), resulting in
- learning, behavior and social problems.

Either way you trace the pathway of disease, you arrive at gut dysbiosis and leaky membranes as the source of ADD and GAPS. The intertwined comorbidities break down your body's defenses, leaving you exposed to intrusion and injury from environmental threats. By chain of events, the body then loses its ability to control nutrient absorption, neurotransmitter production, detox capacity, brain function and attention span.

Simply put, ADD (whether hyperactive or not) originates in the gut. Psychological and social factors, such as learned behaviors and parenting style, surely influence how the "ADD cake" looks, once it's baked. But ADD is essentially a digestive disorder, caused by a dysfunctional gastrointestinal tract, which is itself caused by too few probiotic microorganisms protecting and nourishing you, and too many pathogens wreaking havoc on the body in potent, yet sometimes sneaky, ways.

ADD cause #2: Toxicity damage (chronic)
A trigger event of autism and ADD: disintegration of the blood-brain barrier lets toxins into the brain

The human body is filled with protective barriers that act as dynamic, living filters. They're designed to let beneficial things through, while keeping unauthorized substances out. The most important of these barriers are in the gastrointestinal tract, brain, kidney tubules and blood vessels. As we discuss in other chapters, these barriers are held together by the body's dynamic protective mechanisms, called *tight junctions*, which act like Velcro.

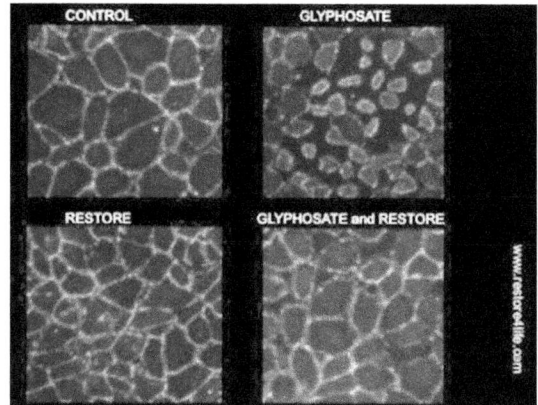

Image used courtesy of Dr. Zach Bush

To illustrate, when they're healthy, tight junctions keep cells of the endothelium (interior surface of blood vessels) firmly attached to each other. But, when they sense tissue damage or a microbial infection on the other side, they unzip themselves to let white blood cells through to defend and repair wounded cells. Cells then close up the hole like it was never there.

But over the past fifty years, Big Ag has been hybridizing and selectively breeding wheat to increase yield. Along the way, its gluten content has just about tripled, as has gliadin, a break down product of gluten. The problem is, gliadin powerfully stimulates zonulin production. When there's too much zonulin around, tight junctions not only open erroneously, they stay open too long. Cells then separate from their neighbors as if their Velcro had melted, holes develop in the membrane, and undigested food, chemicals and microbes leak into the bloodstream, GALT and brain. This explains how toxins crossing membranes trigger autism in people.

Alcoholic fermentation

What if I told you that the process by which alcohol is made in beer, wine and vodka is identical to a digestive process happening inside the tummy of those with a corrupted gut? What if I told you that scenario causes hundreds of poisonous substances to intoxicate the brain and body of ADD and GAPS individuals – more or less all the time? Well, this is exactly what happens every time a person with a corrupted gut eats sugars and carbs: the pathogenic yeast and bacteria in your gut consume the refined carbs you eat, turning them into hundreds of toxic metabolic waste products, which slowly, continuously enter the bloodstream and poison you with a never-ending flow of alcoholic beverages.

It's like having an I.V. pump slowing dripping vodka into your bloodstream as you try to concentrate while, at the same time, your liver does its best to remove those toxins. And pure grain alcohol (ethanol) is just the beginning. When pathogens predominate in your inner ecosystem, they setup nano-breweries inside your tummy. To brew their spirits, they need refined carbs, which they order from you by giving you food cravings.

They run their breweries at low volume when not being fed. But, when you give them lots of refined carbs, they ramp up production and kick the party into high gear. Pathogens serve pure grain alcohol to all the cells of your body that they can access, along with a dizzying array of other toxic brews – depending on which species of pathogen live in your gut. They have themselves a ball, and leave you with the bill (medical bills), the mess (sickness), and the hangover (literally).

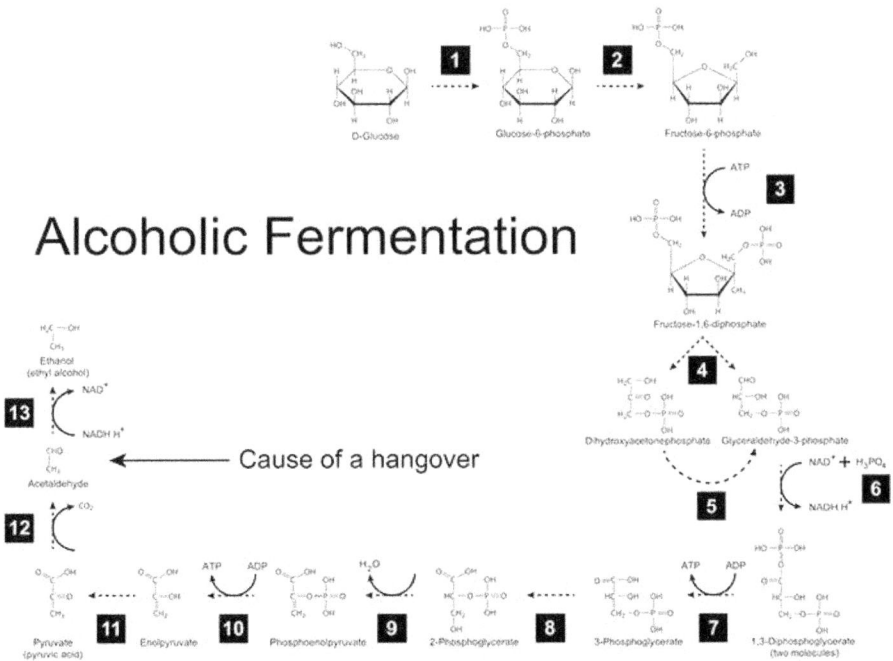

Alcoholic Fermentation

Cause of a hangover

Candida hijacks glucose metabolism and makes pure grain alcohol
In healthy people, normal metabolism converts glucose into lactic acid, water, and ATP through glycolysis. But, in people with yeast overgrowth, candida hijacks the glucose and digests it their own special way, called alcoholic fermentation. Through this mischievous process, candida and other yeasts convert glucose into alcohol. The liver then converts some of that alcohol into acetaldehyde, a highly toxic metabolite responsible for giving heavy drinkers a hangover. Acetaldehyde also dissolves tight junctions that hold the cells of the gut wall together. This is one of the mechanisms causing leaky gut, as well as leaky blood-brain barrier, placental barrier, blood vessel lining, and other barriers of the body.

Drunk without drinking a drop

This process of endogenous alcoholic fermentation was first described in adults who appeared to be drunk without consuming any alcohol. Employers, clinicians and law enforcement officers – even friends and family – assumed they were lying. Everyone thought these people were alcoholics who had a secret stash from which they were sneaking themselves a drink when no one was watching. But, after thorough examination and isolation, it was found that these people had yeast overgrowth in their gut, causing them to be permanently drunk – particularly after eating a big meal of carbs.

And this is exactly what's happening to many GAPS people: Their brains and bodies are continuously exposed to hundreds of different poisons that disturb mental function, coordination, digestion, detoxification, immunity and physical well-being. Adding to that, alcohol and its sister byproducts are small molecules, which make it easier for them to cross membranes, intact or not, and cause problems. This is why pregnant women are advised not to drink alcohol.

Common effects of alcohol, acetaldehyde, and their byproducts

- liver damage and clogging of detoxification pathways (impaired ability for the liver to dispose of worn-out neurotransmitters, hormones, and metabolic waste products is another way that cognitive deficits take place)
- damage to gut lining, mal-absorption, nutritional deficiencies
- brain damage, nerve damage, muscle damage
- immune system injury
- amplified toxic effects of drugs, chemicals and toxins
- decreased pancreatic enzymes that digest food
- reduced stomach acid
- altered metabolism of proteins, carbohydrates and lipids
- deficiencies of nutrients, such as vitamin B_6, by occupying receptor sites on proteins. You could get plenty of B_6 in your diet, but it can't do its job and ends up being useless.

How to make rats hyperactive and autistic for 30 minutes at a time

Dr. Derrick MacFabe and others at The Kilee Patchell-Evans Autism Research Group and University of Western Ontario have shown that **propionic acid (a pathogen's metabolic waste product) causes autism and hyperactive behaviors in rats.** In his group's research, Dr. MacFabe periodically shot propionic acid directly into the cerebrospinal fluid of rats, bypassing the gut entirely.

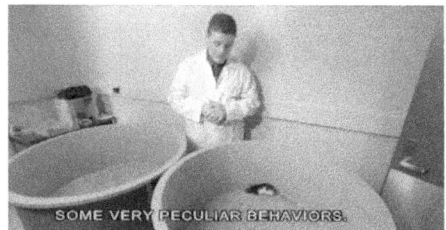

SOME VERY PECULIAR BEHAVIORS.

Dr. Derrick MacFabe pictured above.

This caused psycho/social problems such as

- hyperactivity
- repetitive movements
- fixation on objects
- sensory sensitivity
- impaired socialization.

After the propionic acid leaves the system via metabolism, the rats return to normal behavior. The entire cycle takes thirty minutes and is repeatable. This is the smoking gun, proving that toxin exposure alters behavior, sensory perception, learning and socialization in rats – and undoubtedly in humans too.

Propionic acid 101: The pathogens clostridium difficile (C. diff) and propionibacteria (causes acne) produce propionic acid is a waste product of their metabolism. These microbes like to feed on gluten and casein. So they make autistics and GAPS people crave wheat and dairy. Proprionic acid and its chemical cousins, called propionates (PPA), are also commonly used as a preservative in wheat and dairy products as an anti-fungal agent. That's another way you get PPA.

Toxin exposure caused behavior changes that look exactly like autism and ADD

Rats are normally social, calm, inquisitive creatures. But, when they're given small doses of propionic acid, they become hyperactive and antisocial.

- They display disordered movement, such as walking backward for no reason, limb flapping, back arching, and stretching their legs.
- They develop tics and anxiety.
- They stop socializing, preferring inanimate objects over other rats, which is unusual for them.
- They acquire obsessive/compulsive ritual behaviors, like taking three steps to the corner of their cage, pausing, taking another three steps, and repeating.
- They turn in place incessantly.
- They learn mazes as well as normal rats, but cannot forget them when put in new mazes.
- They suffer seizures of spacey-ness.

But the clincher is that these behaviors begin immediately after being given propionic acid. And they subside thirty minutes after it is metabolized out of the system. The rats then return to behaving normally. Furthermore, these effects get stronger each time the experiment is repeated, in what Dr. MacFabe calls a "kindling response." It's as if the brain gets sensitized – remembering and increasing these effects with each successive exposure. And, for extra proof, his tests were placebo controlled, scientifically scored, and measured electronically.

Now, while we can't assume that humans will respond to toxins the same way that rats do, that's exactly what researchers have found. The mechanisms of brain and behavior dysfunction observed in rats is in perfect alignment with what scientists have found studying humans: Human biology responds the same way to these toxins that rats do.

And, germane to autism and ADD, the effects of propionic acid increase in duration and severity relative to vitamin B_{12} and biotin deficiencies, as well as the presence of ethanol (common in GAPS conditions). What's more, the GAPS population is slower to metabolize propionic acid than others. Being both fat and water soluble, PPA not only enters the brain more easily than fat- or water-based substances alone, but it stays in the system longer and is more disturbing.

Propionic acid also

- affects the basal ganglia (motor movement and procedural learning);
- increases inflammation and oxidative stress, but doesn't kill brain cells;
- impairs glutathione metabolism, making your brain more sensitive to environmental toxins and mitochondrial dysfunction;
- releases auto-antibodies and changes immune system function;
- messes with fat metabolism by depleting carnitine (carnitine transports fat into cells so mitochondria can burn it as fuel);
- turns genes on or off.

Dr. MacFabe and colleagues believe that exposure to propionic acid early in development can cause effects later in life by controlling the genetic switches regulating brain development, aggression, anxiety, craving, addiction and movement. And, central to this discussion, they say PPA seems to exert long-term epigenetic control over dopamine and adrenaline production, thus inhibiting neurotransmitter production on a genetic level.

Basically, **scientists have found a way to create autism/GAPS, on purpose, in the lab.** The effects begin immediately. They look exactly like autism and ADD. They wear off in thirty minutes, they are repeatable and cumulative. This gives us extremely convincing evidence that exposure to certain toxins alters brain function, sensory perception, motor function, behavior, learning, and socialization identical to autism and ADD.

So, from now on, there can be no question that the presence of particular pathogens in the body, and/or eating foods containing certain chemicals, undeniably causes psychological and social disorders ranging from peculiar to severe. The net being, these pathogen populations and preservatives cause/contribute to the behaviors and symptoms we call ADD or autism (along with other factors). It's a fact.

Other toxins and effects

As if those effects weren't enough, pathogens also elevate ammonia, formaldehyde, malondialdehyde, histamine, and morphine in the blood. Common in the autism spectrum, parasites in the intestinal tract produce morphine as a waste product. Morphine shuts down rhythmic contractions of the intestine that mix and move contents through the gut (called peristalsis). In addition, new research is showing cell phone signals, and some vaccines such as the MMR, open the blood–brain barrier to intrusion.

Hyperactivity

The prefrontal cortex is supposed to control the direction of attention

Normally, your prefrontal cortex is able to focus your attention on sensory information that's relevant to you, like a friend calling your name. At the same time, the PFC lets you ignore *un*important sensory input, like clothing tags or nearby conversations in a crowd. But, in ADD individuals, this filtering mechanism is only partially effective. An underactive PFC simply doesn't have the processing power to determine what's important to you and what isn't, so it lets sensory information slip pass your screening mechanism that should be blocked.

When your "awareness filter" is leaky, your conscious perception gets bombarded with more noise than it can handle. It then can't filter important information from the unimportant, and you get unsettled by noise, light, clothing, people, or commotion that wouldn't bother a high-functioning PFC. That's why many ADD individuals find busy environments like a nightclub both stimulating and fatiguing: the conscious mind is being forced to do a job that it's ill-equipped to do. That job was intended to be done by a much more robust, yet less discerning, functionality of the brain called the "reticular activating system."

Toxin exposure assaults the prefrontal cortex

When the brain's executive function is able to suppress reactions to toxins – as it does when the PFC is working – you might experience mild to moderate symptoms. For example, after a "normal" person eats a big meal of questionable food, they might say they feel sleepy, icky, or mentally unsharp – but nothing clinically significant.

On the other hand, when the brain's executive center is partly disabled from neurotransmitters shortages, the brain then can't subdue the feelings of unrest from intoxication/poisoning/food allergies. When toxic reactions go uncontained, impulses turn into hyperactivity, altered brain function, and poor behavior control. Through this mechanism, many ADD symptoms come from toxic reactions going unchecked by brain centers that suppress anomalous sensations, before they're expressed.

The toxic response, and lack of internal supervision from the PFC, combine to create bad behavior. That's the biological basis of what causes classic ADD symptoms: an underpowered PFC that can't block toxic reactions before they get externalized into behavior problems, learning difficulties and hyperactivity.

Food additives trigger hyperactivity when PFC function is weak

As Dr. Ben Feingold and others have shown in some ADD individuals, hyperactivity can be caused by adverse reactions to ingested substances

- refined sugars and carbohydrates
- artificial food colorings (particularly colors followed by a number, such as red no. 40 and yellow no. 5)
- artificial flavors, fragrances and sweeteners (particularly sugar substitutes like aspartame)
- preservatives (including BHA, BHT, TBHQ)
- chemicals/toxins (including aspirin and salicylates)
- partially digested foods.

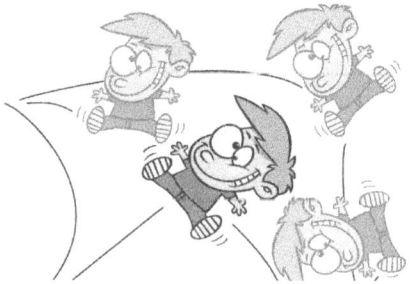

Refined sugars/carbs. Refined carbohydrates produce the infamous blood-sugar roller coaster. First comes a manic state in which elevated blood-sugar makes excessive energy available to the brain, muscles and nervous system. This is followed by a crash in which low blood sugar and high insulin produce an anxious and jittery feeling, which is quieted by muscle activity and release of dopamine and adrenaline. The commonality between *mania* and *crash* is *physical activity*. *Movement* is a primary outlet to dissipate the feeling of unrest that occurs when the PFC can't focus the mind. This is a biologic basis for hyperactivity.

Artificial colors, flavors, preservatives, ingredients and fragrances in food. After World War II, the petrochemical industry didn't know what to do with all the extra oil that American companies were producing. So their scientists set out to find new uses for petroleum to keep the rigs, refineries, and companies in operation. They came up with countless uses, including many intended for internal consumption. The problem is, these chemical additives are so foreign to the human body that our biology doesn't accept them as food, is not equipped to process them, and so we have a hard time getting rid of them.

In addition to overburdening detox pathways, these petroleum-based food additives can cause reactions that look like allergies or intolerances. They can disrupt a wide variety biochemical processes. And they can contribute to chronic, systemic inflammation that stays in "destruction mode" by hyperactivating the immune system. Simply put, ADD individuals have got a lot of imbalances, deficiencies, and vulnerabilities going on, causing chemicals that would merely irritate others to act as neurotoxins and allergens to the ADD brain, gut and nervous system.

Petroleum-based food additives literally poison you on an on-going, low-grade basis, rather than a catastrophic occurrence. These toxins expose you to vulnerabilities, until they can be cleared through the person's already overloaded detox pathways. Meanwhile, a person's underactive PFC isn't policing brain activity like it should. That's a simplified account of how hyperactivity happens.

Nutrient deficiencies. Mineral and vitamin shortages cause/contribute to hyperactivity in two ways: inability to relax due to magnesium deficiency, and trouble calming the mind and body due to lack of neurotransmitter building blocks.

Calcium activates nerves and muscles. Magnesium calms and relaxes

Magnesium and calcium are sister minerals that work as a team. Calcium contracts nerves and muscles. Magnesium helps them relax so you can sit still, focus, learn and behave. They are the "yin and yang" of tension-relaxation cycling. So you need an equal supply of each. However, the average person has plenty of calcium and a deficient of magnesium. In fact, 80% of the general population is magnesium deficient – perhaps more in GAPS people due to sugar cravings and resulting mineral deficiencies.

Magnesium deficiency is more common than calcium deficiency, even though magnesium is more important to watch because it's used in a wider variety of sensitive processes. For instance, magnesium is involved in nerve, muscle and mood signaling. It's used in over 300 enzyme reactions. It reduces inflammation. And it's critical for energy production and glucose absorption. When you're magnesium deficient you might be tight, irritable, crampy and moody. You might be constipated or fatigued. You might have heart palpitations or angina. Or you might be anxious, depressed, or have trouble falling asleep. Most people aren't getting enough magnesium in their diet. And they're doing things to deplete their stores faster.

TOP TEN MAGNESIUM FOODS

1 SPINACH 157 MG. (40 DV) 1 CUP
2 CHARD 154 MG. (38 DV) 1 CUP
3 PUMPKIN SEEDS 92 MG. (23 DV) 1/8 CUP
4 YOGURT 50 MG. (13 DV) 1 CUP

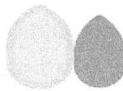

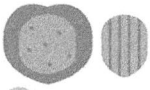

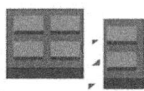

5 ALMOND 80 MG. (20 DV) 1 CUP
6 BLACK BEANS 60 MG. (15 DV) 1/2 CUP
7 AVOCADO 58 MG. (15 DV) 1 MED

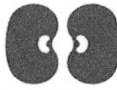

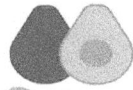

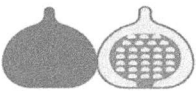

8 FIGS 50 MG. (13 DV) 1/2 CUP
9 DARK CHOCOLATE 95 MG. (24 DV) 1 SQU.
10 BANANA 32 MG. (8 DV) 1 MED

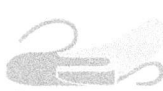

8 signs of magnesium deficiency

1. leg cramps
2. insomnia
3. muscle pain
4. anxiety
5. high blood pressure
6. type 2 diabetes
7. fatigue
8. migraine.

Magnesium deficiency systemically winds people up, and keeps them that way, until physical activity gives them an outlet for release. It's usually caused by poor diet, stress and diuretics. Poor diet, particularly refined sugars and carbs, depletes magnesium, as we have talked about. Stress consumes magnesium in the body's effort to combat tension. And diuretics such as coffee, alcohol and blood pressure medication reduce magnesium by increasing elimination in the urine. The body also excretes magnesium after use. It doesn't recycle it the way that it does with calcium. These are reasons why most people are magnesium deficient.

Here are a few ways to elevate your magnesium levels: cut refined sugar/carbs, caffeine, alcohol, diuretic drugs like blood pressure meds (check with your doctor first), and reduce your stress level. Eat more raw spinach, kale, sesame seeds, brazil nuts, almonds, cashews, molasses, quinoa, buckwheat, hazelnuts, millet, pecans and avocados. And make sure to get plenty of vitamins D_3, B_1, E, B_6 and selenium to help your body use magnesium.

Mercury displaces magnesium

One of the many troubling effects of a corrupted gut is that you lose much of your protection against heavy metals. Studies have shown that probiotic bacteria chelate 99% of the mercury they encounter in the digestive system. Your friendly critters attach themselves to mercury molecules and escort them out of the body so they don't harm you. Without these friendly microbes patrolling the gut, around 90% of the mercury you eat in fish, for example, gets into the bloodstream because pathogens don't protect you nearly as well. Mercury then bonds to receptors sites normally occupied by magnesium. It displaces magnesium and prevents it from relaxing the body, which exacerbates hyperactivity.

Summary on hyperactivity

People who have attention deficit with hyperactivity have got two situations combining to form ADHD: they've got an underactive prefrontal cortex, which controls behavior, impulses and attention. With less impulse control to keep manic behavior in check, their surplus energy and adverse reactions build up like a pressure cooker, until an outlet for release is found in physical activity (sometimes taking the form of heel tapping, rocking, or pacing). Therefore: *manic energy seeking an outlet + inability to relax + lack of behavior control = kids bouncing off the walls.* Key point: If your child displays clinical hyperactivity in childhood, it's likely they have attention deficit too, and will continue to have it into adulthood – even if they find a way to control the hyperactivity.

ADD cause #3: Cellular degeneration and atrophy

In gut-based ADD, the total amount of cell death that has occurred determines how much healing can ultimately be achieved through treatment *vs.* how much of your symptoms will remain after treatment. Residual damage that can't be fixed is what this section is all about.

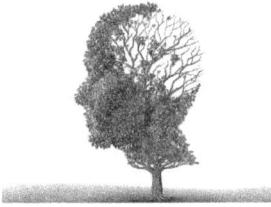

Cellular degeneration caused by the *waste products* of pathogens

When protective barriers fail, toxins, partially digested food, pathogens, and their waste products enjoy unhindered access to the body's sensitive equipment. Degeneration starts from this. Giving toxins the keys to go anywhere, brain structures get damaged and atrophy. Chemicals and toxins land on receptor sites, disrupting hormone production and reception, as well as cell reproduction. Biochemical pathways get blocked, causing a variety of physical damage around the body.

The longer this goes on, the more extensive the cellular degeneration. The longer a person has a corrupted gut, the harder it is to reverse damage to the brain by healing the gut. So, after many years, a fair amount of damage becomes irreversible. However, do not be discouraged from endeavoring to heal your gut – whatever your age or state of health. Cells are constantly renewing themselves, and improvements are always possible, no matter how much damage has been done. It's never too late to enhance brain function.

Cellular degeneration due to *atrophy*

The brain is like any muscle: it atrophies when idle for too long. Atrophy is a gradual weakening and loss of function from lack of use. It's one of the deficits that's most challenging to reverse when healing ADD, because atrophy is as much a result of structural decay as it is a neurochemical and behavioral/developmental malady.

Over a course of years, a brain that's severely underutilized will atrophy and degenerate. Whether that's because (1) areas of the brain go to sleep, (2) the body's built-in pruning mechanism decides some neurons are no longer needed, or (3) some dysfunction prevents brain cells from reactivating, the human brain does shrink from years of abuse or neglect. When any part of the brain sits idle for long periods, the body, having lots of competing priorities, will reallocate resources to areas of greater need. Cell degeneration will take place, and the brain loses performance.

Consequently, if you start healing a child of a corrupted gut prior to the age of six, there's much greater chance of reversing the causes of injury and bringing their brain completely back "on line." They can start challenging their brain, or at least exercising it, and they might be able to catch up developmentally with others in their age group.

On the other hand, the same treatment on a person in their twenties or beyond will almost certainly have lasting effects because of all the damage done over decades of exposure. And they'll be far behind developmentally and socially. Most of the difference between good outcomes and ideal ones is the amount of atrophy that's taken place – physically and psychologically. This determines how much improvement is possible.

Atrophy can also be caused in long-term medication users by way of the "lazy internal pharmacy effect" (not a real medical term). This is when the body gets used to making and recycling biochemicals in the presence of pharmaceuticals. However, when you stop taking these drugs, the body can forget how to make adrenaline, dopamine, and other neurotransmitters on its own (and you're screwed until it remembers).

Mental health professionals see this frequently when a person comes off psychoactive drugs. It can take weeks or months for the body to get back up to speed making brain chemicals on its own. The good news is, when you eat right, production capacity often returns to normal before the gut is healed. Rarely will a lazy internal pharmacy prove to be permanent.

What you can do to reverse atrophy

The best ways to improve brain function after suffering any of these woes is the four basics of healing most ADD conditions: (1) Heal your inner ecosystem, (2) nourish the body thoroughly, (3) detoxify deeply, and (4) put your brain to work. Challenge yourself mentally. You may not be able to recover 100% of your brain's ultimate potential. But every little bit you do to improve brain function can improve your quality of life.

Cellular degeneration due to lack of *restorative sleep*

Irregular sleep cycles can play a significant role in cellular degeneration. Medical experts say that the body does most of its building and repair while you're sleeping – particularly in REM sleep. Unfortunately, much of the population does not get enough restorative sleep – some due to stimulant use, some due to life circumstances, and a fair amount as a result of health conditions such as sleep apnea or GAPS.

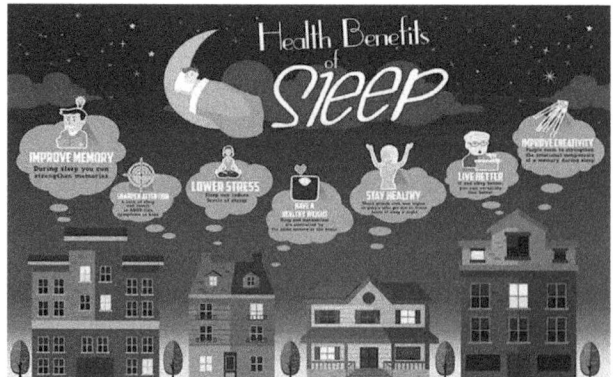

Maintenance and repair. New thinking in the field suggests sleeping difficulties rob the body of time to perform vital maintenance and repair. Neglecting maintenance can weaken organs and biochemical systems when sleep deficiency becomes chronic. This can have an indirect effect on a person's ADD symptoms by causing a long list of problems such as headaches, fatigue, weight gain, high blood pressure, diabetes, stroke, heart failure and depression. It's all connected. Doctors see these problems a lot in sleep apnea patients.

The importance of paralysis. The body does most of its muscle and tissue restoration while you're paralyzed in REM sleep. While you dream in REM sleep, your body performs a variety of chores such as cell repair and replacement. Of course, you can't be using muscles and repairing them at the same time, so your "maintenance crew" completely immobilizes muscles to do its repair. You also don't want to be talking or acting out your dreams while you're asleep, so muscles need to be disabled.

Therefore, sleep circuits deactivate skeletal muscles only while you're in the short, cyclical phases of REM sleep. A complex symphony of chemicals and structures in the brain keep some muscles turned on such as heart, lungs and swallowing muscles, while paralyzing others not needed during sleep, including muscles of the back of the tongue, tonsils and throat.

The problem is, millions of people aren't getting enough good sleep, which instigates a cascade of problems, because REM sleep is the first to suffer when you're not sleeping right. When this happens, the body postpones maintenance on everything it can possibly defer, such as replenishing hormones and neurotransmitters, detoxifying, fighting infection and completing digestion.

Obstructive sleep apnea. Each apneic event causes a multitude of health-eroding effects to build up over time. By definition, sleep apnea is when you stop breathing in your sleep for ten seconds or more. This can happen 5–20 times per hour, depending on acuity. When you stop breathing, oxygen saturation in the blood plummets to harmful levels. Blood pressure rises quickly to dangerous levels, and drops just as fast when you resume breathing. Blood glucose levels stay high all the time. Carbon dioxide builds up in the tissues and brain, and can cause headaches when you wake.

With each apnea event, the brain, sensing a need for oxygen, elevates you out of REM sleep into a lighter stage. It reactivates the muscles of the tongue and throat that were blocking the airway. You may fidget, thrash, snore, wheeze, gasp, or even wake up completely with each apneic event. This can happen repeatedly all night long – as if someone was choking you for ten seconds to two minutes at a time.

Whether disturbing or potentially deadly, you don't get the restorative REM sleep to reset neurotransmitters, hormones, brain, muscle and organ function back to normal. This leads to a chronically tired brain, weaknesses and imbalances all over the body, and inability to quiet the body's inner angst. Most important to understand, daytime sleepiness and diminished executive function of the prefrontal cortex go hand-in-hand. That means the PFC is like employees of a department store on Black Friday: they're short-staffed, overwhelmed, and sometimes trampled by demand.

As you've undoubtedly experienced yourself, of all the areas of the brain impacted by a sleep shortage, the PFC is probably the one most affected by a lack of REM sleep. Creative ability, complex thinking, planning, and foresight are the first to go when you're tired, followed by emotions and habits when deeply deprived, followed by hunger and autonomic nervous system function when you're critically deprived.

You need sun. Some experts blame sleep problems on a lack of sun and vitamin D (the sunshine vitamin) – especially during fall and winter. This would make sense, because we're designed to get less sun, and sleep more, during short winter days. Yet, we stay up almost as long in winter as we do in summer, thereby exhausting our supply of vitamin D and causing neurotransmitter imbalances, sleep problems, chronic disease and mental disorders. Indeed, vitamin D is involved in so many vital functions, some call it a hormone, instead of a vitamin.

This would explain a constellation of symptoms, effects, and problems now epidemic throughout society. Lack of sun causes low vitamin D, which affects serotonin, melatonin and dopamine production. Melatonin and serotonin help us sleep properly, while dopamine and serotonin help our brains perform at a high level. Vitamin D deficiency not only contributes directly to sleep difficulties and neurotransmitter imbalances, it can also cause a long list of degenerative conditions. Substance abuse, psychological problems, and physiological problems aren't helping people's sleep cycles either. These lead to longer waking times and increased vitamin D consumption. It's a vicious cycle that most people know nothing about.

Sleep problems rising. It's estimated that half of Americans suffer from sleep difficulties. Whether from lack of sun, nutrient deficiency, or excesses of modern living such as smoking, smartphones and energy drinks, we're not getting enough sleep. And these sleep disorders are causing a wide variety of mental and physical problems in people from all walks of life. Whatever the source may be, we can say that sleep disorders have risen dramatically in the past few decades in lock-step with chronic, degenerative diseases. We can say many northerners don't get enough sun. We, as a society, are mineral deficient. And our technology-ladened lifestyles are stressing our minds and bodies to the point of disease.

Heavy metals from chemtrails
(aka: geo-engineering, stratospheric aerosol injections, solar radiation management or climate engineering)
Geo-engineering has to be mentioned when discussing mental health problems, because the toxins raining down on all of us are a big component of ADD and GAPS. Along with glyphosate, they are contributing to health problems more than you'd ever suspect. This means the best healing, nutrition, and lifestyle changes won't get you to optimal wellness when you've got nano-particles of heavy metals and radioactivity assaulting your brain and endocrine organs continually.

I just did a challenge-rechallenge test with my Magnetico Sleep Pad to confirm my beliefs. After sleeping many months on 30-gauss, earth-type magnetism, I tried sleeping without it. Result: I woke up repeatedly through the night for no reason (unusual for me). I'm now positive that the Magnetico, as claimed, is one of the very best modalities you can use to improve your sleep quality, recovery, and biochemistry. See Recommended Resources section at the back for contact info.

The devastation it's already done is horrific. And it's accelerating

The damage to vegetation is obvious to everyone paying attention. Just look at plant life in your area. You'll see severely distressed vegetation – from drooping limbs to crooked tree tops to patches of missing foliage to branches with a scorched look to bark burned off the south-southwest side of trees exposed to late afternoon and evening sun. You'll see many trees are already dead, for no apparent reason.

As this is being written (~2017), maybe 40% of trees and bushes in Portland, Oregon (where I live) look seriously distressed, and about 5–10% look to be in critical condition. These are mature trees in their natural environment that haven't been sprayed at ground level. What's more, the damage being done to plant life mirrors the damage happening inside all of us. But you can see loss of health in trees. You can't see loss of health and healing capacity in people, until it's almost gone.

Update 2022: Where I live, most trees now look like they're struggling. After a rain or snow storm, roads are shut down everywhere from fallen trees and branches so brittle, they look shattered by an explosion. Maintenance crews are so overwhelmed by downed power lines that they don't even bother to clean up all the branches along busy streets anymore. They leave big ones right up next to white border lines.

Plant life is being damaged by
- **Glyphosate.**
- **Nano-sized heavy metal particles.**
- **Radiation.**
- **High surface temperatures** from geo-engineering schemes chronically stress plants (enzymes that run photosynthesis slow down above 68°F, and shut down above 104°F).

Clearly, the burning of petroleum products is not helping. But it's just the scapegoat in this narrative. Blaming climate catastrophes on carbon emissions takes the attention off of atrocities being done by the elite.

New World Order types are spraying millions of tons of heavy metals particles into the atmosphere

This is recorded in government and military documents, over 300 patents, international treaties, and forums such as the UN. The technology has been proven in practice beyond any doubt. And you can see footage all over the Internet of plane nozzles cycling on and off with their aerosol sprays. This proves to anyone with eyes and critical thinking ability that chemtrails are done with intent and not incidental contrails.

Furthermore, climate scientists in the system not only admit that geo-engineering is being done at the present time, they're publicly campaigning for more. They're openly calling for more geo-engineering in public conferences, articles and think tanks. Major countries such as China even admit to using weather modification technologies before the 2008 Olympics in Beijing. And, to top it off, you can see pictures of at least one US president touring a plane equipped with geo-engineering equipment.

Governments around the world can control the weather

World powers now have excellent to near complete control over when and where it rains. They have the ability to keep it from raining in an area almost indefinitely, or cause a hurricane on-demand. Some parties can make earthquakes happen using HAARP technology. And they have very good control over steering weather patterns to control temperature as well.

Most atmospheric aerosols are a hazy, wispy white, or rainbow hued. Due to different densities of material, sections of them form streaks across the sky as they descend and disperse in wind currents. To put it simply, they're weird-looking formations that don't look or act like normal clouds. On the other hand, real clouds are usually puffy white, flat on the bottom, and don't disperse or descend. Their top sides change shape as they move across the sky, seemingly stuck to a set altitude.

The Powers That Be have been doing geo-engineering so long that normies still believe chemtrails are normal clouds. These psychopaths brainwash the people into believing that aerial abominations are regular clouds – going so far as to invent names for atmospheric formations that didn't exist before, like "cirrocumulus," "altocumulus" and "virga."

What's in stratospheric aerosol injections?

The nano particles exactly match those named in geo-engineering patents, whose purpose is to deflect sunlight. Composed primarily of aluminum, barium, cadmium and strontium (and things far more grotesque), these heavy metals accumulate in our fatty tissues such as the brain and heart. They're now being found in Northern California ground and air samples at 50,000% higher than normal concentration.

Some effects that geoengineering has on the body

First, the particulates in aerosols disturb the lungs, causing asthma and allergies. Next, the toxins upset the GI tract with accumulations from the ground. As they circulate in the blood, they settle mostly in the brain and nervous system, fatty tissue and vital organs. To our detriment, heavy metals cause neurologic dysfunctions such as Alzheimer's, dementia, loss of motor skills, and dumbing down. They contribute substantially to most modern diseases by interfering with biochemical, enzymatic, hormonal, nutritional and detoxification process.

I, myself, have recently noticed I've been having trouble finding and articulating words, loss of physical coordination, less mental clarity, and respiratory weakness – all unusual for me, but exactly what you'd expect from increased intake of heavy metals. Aluminum, in particular, is known to damage neural pathways (e.g., Alzheimer's), contribute to neuro-muscular disorders (e.g., Parkinson's), interfere with detoxification and immunity, make people complacent, and cause memory problems. Aluminum is also a fire accelerant, which is causing forest fires around the globe to burn much hotter and faster than they ever have.

ADD cause #4: Structural brain damage (event-based)

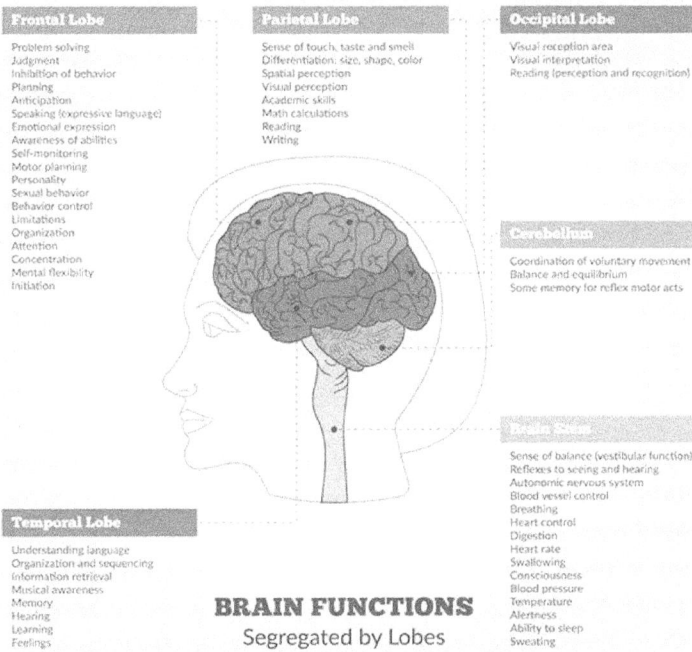

Frontal Lobe

Problem solving
Judgment
Inhibition of behavior
Planning
Anticipation
Speaking (expressive language)
Emotional expression
Awareness of abilities
Self-monitoring
Motor planning
Personality
Sexual behavior
Behavior control
Limitations
Organization
Attention
Concentration
Mental flexibility
Initiation

Parietal Lobe

Sense of touch, taste and smell
Differentiation: size, shape, color
Spatial perception
Visual perception
Academic skills
Math calculations
Reading
Writing

Occipital Lobe

Visual reception area
Visual interpretation
Reading (perception and recognition)

Cerebellum

Coordination of voluntary movement
Balance and equilibrium
Some memory for reflex motor acts

Sense of balance (vestibular function)
Reflexes to seeing and hearing
Autonomic nervous system
Blood vessel control
Breathing
Heart control
Digestion
Heart rate
Swallowing
Consciousness
Blood pressure
Temperature
Alertness
Ability to sleep
Sweating

Temporal Lobe

Understanding language
Organization and sequencing
Information retrieval
Musical awareness
Memory
Hearing
Learning
Feelings

BRAIN FUNCTIONS
Segregated by Lobes

A small minority of ADD cases are caused by traumatic head injury, birth defect, or acute infection. These injuries are relatively permanent.

Toxin exposure in the womb damages brain cells and neuronal wiring

Many babies are exposed to toxins in the womb that cause the brain to develop abnormally, resulting in a GAPS conditions. Sharing in the blame, the barriers of the body break down when the gut's a mess, including the placental barrier. And, even when it is intact, far more substances can cross the placenta than previously thought. You see, gluten and glyphosate in the mother's diet create leaky barriers, which opens baby up to toxin exposure such as mercury from dental fillings, chemicals sprayed on crops, toxins in personal care products, legal and illegal drugs, and industrial chemicals such as bisphenol-A, flame retardants, and non-stick cookware.

What happens next is a sad, but necessary, survival mechanism built into our biology. In an effort to give the mother and her future children the best chance at survival, the mother's body treats the developing fetus as a toxic waste dump for heavy metals and toxins.

Whether by design or biologic accident, the mother's body sees the developing fetus as a new place to get rid of toxins, so it concentrates them in umbilical cord blood at a higher level than that of her bloodstream. That is why so many mothers miscarry one or more times before they can carry a baby to term. It's toxicity damage. And it's the reason first-born children are far more likely to have a GAPS condition than their later-born siblings, as Dr. Natasha has seen in her practice.

Head trauma

Flagrant damage to the brain has been studied for hundreds of years (like a railroad spike through the skull). But you may be surprised to learn how little it takes to damage the brain from a blow to the head. Even an ordinary concussion can cause permanent brain damage and, along with it, personality and behavior changes. You don't even have to lose consciousness to suffer a permanent damage.

That's because the skull is very hard and filled with sharp, bony edges inside. While the brain is very soft, like warm butter, and can tear more easily than you think. So doing "headers" in soccer, using forceps in birth, or falling off your bike and landing on your head – even with a helmet on – can damage small blood vessels and connective tissues of the brain. This can halt blood flow to a region, and disrupt communication between brain centers.

In fact, Dr. Amen has seen ADD due to head trauma so much in his practice that his standard intake procedure includes asking new patients five times if they ever got hit in the head hard enough to lose consciousness. But, oddly enough, people often don't remember they were knocked unconscious one or more times, until they're prompted multiple times to recall. Amen does this to find out if there's a physical reason for dysfunction that he's seeing on a SPECT scan. And so he knows how to treat the condition better.

The neo-cortex

The brain's higher functions are controlled by its "newer" components (evolutionarily speaking), which are located toward the outer surface and toward the front of the head. The "neo-cortex," as this region is called, is known for its rational, abstract thinking and decision-making. The prefrontal cortex is that portion of the neo-cortex infamous for causing ADD symptoms when it malfunctions.

Essential to understanding ADD, the neo-cortex is a precision instrument that needs many components to run properly for the whole to work well. That is, the architecture needs to have developed properly and be undamaged. The supply of brain chemicals needs to be balanced. And communication between brain centers needs to flow freely and precisely, in order for the neo-cortex to function optimally. For these reasons, the neo-cortex is far more vulnerable to injury from head trauma, as well as insults from toxins, than the older "reptilian" brain.

The hind brain

In contrast, the brain's more primitive functions, like regulating heart rate and body temperature, are controlled by the lower parts in and around the brain stem and cerebellum, often called the "hind" brain. They're housed deep in the center of the head, as far away from injury as possible so they can survive severe head trauma and continue operating.

Is the mind separate from the brain?

Although we can't prove it, the way the brain operates appears to agree with spiritual scholars who believe that our high-level human thinking is actually done non-locally. This explains why high-level thought is far more susceptible to transmission, reception and decoding errors: Rational thinking requires two-way communication with external sources. On the other hand, lower brain functions are done locally in the brain stem. Autonomic functions are handled internally and require no transmitting or receiving.

To put it differently, many believe the thinking portion of our brain is a two-way radio of sorts that transmits and receives signals from a non-physical place where your spirit resides. Communication between mediums happens instantly and is not location-dependent. So when the brain is physically damaged, or impaired for reasons that we're discussing, it can't send or receive signals properly and dysfunction happens. Like a cell phone with bad reception, you get dropped signals, miscommunication and static between your brain (the grey matter in your head) and your mind (non-local). At the same time, autonomic functions like heart rate and breathing are protected at all costs by virtue of the hind-brain being a fault-tolerant, entirely self-contained unit.

In summary, by its very nature of being a super high-tech piece of equipment, the brain only works perfectly when it's running in a flawless state of tune. When something goes wrong, it still works, but in a compromised way. These slight deviations from the norm, such as low dopamine and serotonin, cause symptomatic effects that we call ADD.

ADD cause #5: Emotional trauma

It's well established that severe emotional trauma and abuse can cause lasting psychological damage. Here are some of the more unusual effects:

Trauma and heavy metal retention

Areas of the brain that store memories of abuse and trauma have been known to hold on to mercury so that it resists chelation efforts. On the other hand, when a person successfully deals with traumatic memories, the brain will suddenly release its mercury, scrubbing both your psychology and physiology. On the other side of this mechanism, if a person does an aggressive detox, and they get the mercury out, it's as if their emotional baggage is suddenly easier to process and remove of its negative charge. Could it be that positively-charged heavy metals stick to negative emotions like a magnet? Food for thought.

Two ways that severe emotional distress can cause ADD symptoms

1. **Psychological distress can create a pattern of physiological imbalance.** Emotions can cause neurotransmitter imbalances through "habit." A perfect example: depression lowers serotonin level, *or* low serotonin can make you feel depressed. Low serotonin depresses mood, alters thinking, affects sleep, suppresses appetite, and makes you obsess over negative thoughts. At the same time, it's not uncommon for depression to alter dopamine, adrenaline, and GABA, which can upset brain function and cause ADD symptoms. When that happens chronically and/or acutely, residual effects can linger out of habit – even after you remove the source of distress. That's because neuro-inflammation of the glial cells (immune cells of the brain) gets stuck in the 'on' position, thus interrupting cellular communication, healing and brain function.

To illustrate, have you ever known someone that always seemed to be stuck in a rut? They just couldn't stop thinking or behaving in unproductive, anti-social ways, no matter how much they wanted to change? That's what "behavioral-biochemical habit" (I made that up) does to a person chronically. And, let's not forget, even when your conscious mind is able to block out traumatic memories from your conscious mind, your subconscious still replays it and has to deal with it. As a result, trauma can be like a record skipping in the back of your mind.

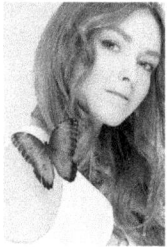

2. **Emotional trauma can trigger the brain's ultimate defense mechanisms.** The mind has built-in fail-safe mechanisms that protect the individual from catastrophic collapse, should they experience situations too ghastly to deal with conventionally. When a person is confronted with real-life trauma too gruesome to take, it stores those experiences in a virtual partition of the mind that some mental health professionals call an "alter." This special container will split off from the rest of the mind so as to avoid contaminating the person's consciousness with horrific experiences. They then won't be able to recall the bad memories, unless prompted to by a therapeutic intervention or accidental "leak" in this protective filter.

Trauma effectively rewires certain aspects of the brain in order to preserve the person's sanity. It's a deeply-rooted survival mechanism that's built into the way we're wired. And it can sometimes overlap with ADD symptoms. Specifically, people that experience ritual abuse, torture, rape, armed combat, or bad car accidents can have their mind messed up in ways that mimic ADD.

To recap, **severe emotional trauma like torture or sexual abuse can create ADD symptoms in a small percent of atypical cases.** I think of trauma-based ADD and gut-based ADD as coming from two separate places, yet arriving at a common destination: neurochemical imbalances and a biochemical rut. We won't focus much on trauma-based ADD here because it's truly an occult science. And the field of psychiatry hardly knows what to do with trauma-based psychological disorders because they don't want to acknowledge it. But there are enough people in therapy that look like classic ADD, but damaged much deeper than gut dysbiosis, that we ought to acknowledge it.

Other causes/comorbidities of symptoms
Sticky symptoms can be the result of bad habits

Procrastination, impulsiveness, and poor coping skill are three symptoms that can stick around after root causes are removed, due to behavior patterns that are hard to break. This is one of the few instances a good psycho-therapist or coach can help as much as fixing your microbiome.

Medical conditions often mistaken for ADD/ADHD

- food sensitivities
- blood-sugar swings
- lead/mercury poisoning
- autism spectrum
- hyperthyroidism/hypothyroidism
- nutrient deficiencies such as B_{12} deficiency, iron anemia
- sensory processing difficulties
- bipolar
- sleep disorders
- drugs such as anticonvulsants, antihistamines or psycho-depressants.

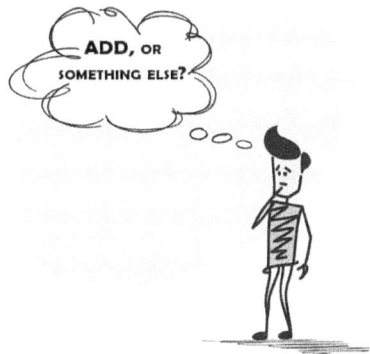

Unpacking one disorder and understanding it top-to-bottom is confusing enough without arguing about where one disease ends and the other begins. But what we can say is that the causes of disorder are complex. Comorbidities (co-existing conditions) are common. And there's a lot of overlap in symptoms. So let's get to fixing underlying problems, and not worry so much about labels.

Diagnosing by symptom clusters, as psychiatry has done for decades, is such an old-fashioned way to define mental disorders, it's of limited value in our healing efforts. Besides, how much use is a doctor's diagnosis in getting a prescription regimen right on the first try? Not much. In case you're not aware, doctors typically prescribe drugs based on educated guesses and experimentation – not facts and data. Through many trials and adjustments, doctor and patient usually settle for moderate improvement of symptoms, with tolerable side effects.

Instead, let's transition our analysis and efforts to root causes, mechanisms of action, and solutions without compromise. These do require a more thoughtful approach and determined effort, but the outcomes can get you to a better place overall. Our knowledge of biochemistry is at a point where we should be examining origins and outcomes moving forward, instead of diagnostic labels and FDA-approved treatments. The unknowns that Western medicine faced in the '80s and '90s are being replaced with legitimate answers, so why not?

ADD wrap up

When our understanding of ADD was in its infancy, diagnostic manuals defined a cluster of behavioral and cognitive issues as attention deficit disorder. When hyperactivity was present, people called it ADHD. But with the advent of routine SPECT scan imaging to correlate symptoms and behaviors with visible brain activity, we've outgrown that definition.

Although everyone is not quite onboard yet, the fields of psychiatry and developmental sciences are moving in the direction of defining ADD as executive dysfunction, chiefly in the prefrontal cortex. We now know that learning, behavior, and social difficulties come from a PFC "gone wild." And so there's no sense in defining ADD by symptoms anymore when we can trace them back to physical deficits and events upstream. Until you do that, you don't truly understand what caused ADD in an individual, what those defects are doing to them now, and how to fix problems so they stay fixed. You're only guessing. You're treating symptoms, not causes. And you're rarely getting the best outcomes.

Granted, ADD is not simple, any way you look at it. It's one of the more complex disorders to understand and treat. And, more often than not, multiple chains of causality coalesce to create symptoms that we can see. That's why attention deficit disorder has remained such a mystery up to this point, and why it takes a multi-modality approach to get a good handle on it. It really takes a holistic way of thinking to uncover the truth about ADD and discuss it in detail the way we are now.

But it's now possible to at least create the beta version. We have the technology. The consolidation of ideas you have in your hands is just that: part user guide-part repair manual for attention deficit disorder, in one. It's sure to gain clarity and refinement as our understanding of the science and mysteries of ADD matures in the years ahead.

14

THE VEIL OF CONSCIOUSNESS

**When your brain works well, you perceive your
thinking to be done entirely by your conscious mind**
But, far from it, the mind actually communicates with a variety of non-physical sources and weaves their information into your stream of consciousness, as if they were your own. Therefore, your thoughts are a mixture of communication from five sources:

1. Your conscious, waking mind
2. your subconscious or soul (sometimes called the "super-conscious")
3. your Higher Self or the collective consciousness
4. other people in your vicinity
5. spiritual entities from other realms (e.g., God and demonic forces).

Some people call messages from unexplained sources "the other side." Some are considered otherworldly. Point being, they are not you, but you can mistake them for being you. And that becomes problematic when entities are intent on butting into your stream of consciousness and causing you trouble. You see, under normal circumstances, this combination of communications is so dominated by your conscious mind that you interpret other channels of information to be intuition or inspiration, rather than sentient beings trying to communicate with you. Feeds from other sources normally come across so fuzzy and faint that their messages feel more like a guardian angel nudging you, instead of intelligent, structured communications with a purpose.

Now, most of the time, the mind isn't aware that it's incorporating external sources into your thoughts and feelings. What happens is, the mind senses when messages are coming from external sources. It interprets and edits their meaning. And it mixes them into your thought stream so that your conscious awareness can't tell the difference between your thoughts and those from elsewhere. To keep you from going crazy, your brain listens to all sources, runs them through some filters, and translates the collection into a form such that your conscious mind believes it's operating independently. This is how it's supposed to work when all areas of the brain are working properly: other sources can't intrude into your stream of consciousness and taint what's being said – or hijack your thoughts altogether. Simply put, your conscious mind is supposed to maintain primary authorship of your thoughts and feelings.

This non-physical filtering function of the mind has been called "The Veil of Consciousness"

The Veil of Consciousness is a semi-permeable screen separating your conscious mind from all other sources that can communicate with your conscious mind, influence, or commandeer it – including your own sub-conscious. It's one of the characteristic features of the human mind that's said to be unique to this planet. The Veil basically turns the volume down on communications from the other side and obscures their "resolution" so they're unintelligible to undetectable, under normal circumstances.

The Veil is designed to give you a strong sense of sense. It helps us maintain our sanity, as opposed to hearing voices. So it keeps you from going crazy, were you to hear all the crosstalk coming at you from several sources. Through its efforts, you're able to maintain the illusion that you are your own person, separate and distinct from everyone and everything around you. So anything you then hear, see, feel, or sense through The Veil is deemed to be coming from a mysterious compartment of the mind that's inaccessible to your conscious awareness.

7 phenomena can cause The Veil to break down and let non-native information bleed into your stream of consciousness

1. **Mental illness.** #1 is considered a mental disorder.
2. **Drugs and alcohol.** #2 is chemically-induced.
3. **Sleep disturbances.** #3 is caused by compromising circumstances.
4. **Trauma and extended hyper-vigilance.** #4 has been used to transfer control of the mind to others.
5. **Hypnosis/trance.** #5 has been the subject of great mystery and speculation throughout the ages.
6. **Invitation/invocation.** #6 can be a can of worms you regret opening.
7. **Prayer.** #7 is done with faith and hope in mind.

1. Schizophrenia, psychosis and paranoia

One of the more extreme manifestations of mental illness occurs when The Veil of Consciousness breaks down in schizophrenics, psychotics, and the clinically paranoid, causing them to receive inappropriate messages from otherworldly sources. These people basically hear voices that no one else can hear or explain. This makes observers think the affected individual is crazy, and in need of treatment. This is an unsatisfactory explanation, at best. Here's a more accurate interpretation:

Structural defects and/or disturbed brain chemistry cause the filtering effect of the Veil of Consciousness to malfunction, thus allowing unauthor-ized access to your thought stream. Demonic forces sense when a mind is too weak to protect itself against intrusion. Trickster entities then establish a connection with an individual and inject messages into their consciousness.

Common in psychotherapy, impositions such as this are presumed to be voices coming from pathological aspects of a person's own consciousness that they can't control. However, a more accurate description is that demonic forces enjoy messing with people just for fun, stealing their energy, and giving them demented energy for them to deal with.

So, what can a person do to protect themselves? Talk therapy can strengthen a person's control over their thoughts – like exercising the muscle that blocks evil entities from gaining unauthorized access to your mind. Medications such as lithium can dull all sources/voices across the board, to the point where demonic forces are easier to ignore, or can't be heard at all. A third option is to heal your corrupted gut, and correct your brain biochemistry, to improve your brain's executive function. This strengthens your control over the sources forming your thoughts.

Whichever method you try, start with just saying 'no'. Oddly enough, this universe is built upon the principle of free will. So entities with evil intentions are prohibited from violating yours. They're only allowed to do what you invite them to – or passively agree to by not objecting. In other words, they'll do what they want, unless/until you terminate their permission to meddle in your affairs. Believe it or not, some of the evilest, most-powerful entities must adhere to a code of conduct when dealing with others in commerce. This means they can't break the rule of *consent* overtly.

2. Drugs and alcohol

High doses of psychoactive drugs, particularly in combination, can breach The Veil, allowing malevolent entities to contaminate your thought stream. Overdosing on methylphenidate is one example. Artificially raising neurotransmitters such as dopamine to extraordinary levels can lower the barrier function of The Veil and make you hear voices that seem indistinguishable from your own internal dialogue. This can make you think extremely bizarre, paranoid thoughts – as if people, animals, or inanimate objects are talking about you and are out to get you.

It feels like your conscious mind has been hijacked, because you sense that your mind is saying things it normally would not say. Other entities are speaking through you, but you don't feel like a mouthpiece for some other source because it still feels like your mind is in control. You have to keep reminding yourself that it's not you doing the talking; it's some freaky force commandeering your self-talk like a puppet. It's probably the most haunting thing you can imagine.

Drug-induced lowering of The Veil is likely caused by suppression of those areas responsible for executive function and discernment, such as the prefrontal cortex, in combination with over-activation of those brain centers responsible for obsession and compulsion, such as the cingulate gyrus.

In this circumstance, excess dopamine causes confusion and inability to regulate the flow of information to and from the brain. It's as if prefrontal cortex function is accelerated and desynchronized with the rest of the brain. Neurotypical people will recognize this as the nervousness of public speaking, or being tongue-tied when approaching an attractive member of the opposite sex.

At the same time, as dopamine goes up, serotonin typically goes down. Serotonin calms the mind and helps it transition from one thought or movement to the next via the cingulate gyrus. So a serotonin deficit can entrap you in repetitive thought loops and compulsive behaviors. That's how intrusive entities create obsessional delusions in your head.

Habitually high doses of alcohol are known to cause similar effects. That is why alcoholic beverages are called "spirits": they're said to summon spirits who talk to you or through you. For example, absinthe, which was very popular among late-19th Century Parisian artists and writers, was notorious for conjuring spirits and causing mystical effects in its consumers. Made from the psycho-active herb wormwood, it was even banned in many countries, because it was said to have caused hallucinations and madness in people – supposedly from toxicity to its poisonous ingredients.

Only in recent decades have distillers brought absinthe back from obscurity with less-toxic versions of old recipes. They removed the substances thought to be most poisonous, which were also the substances that caused the most mind-bending trips.

3. Sleep deprivation and dreaming

A third category that opens leaks in The Veil is when an otherwise normal person is critically sleep-deprived or dreaming. The Veil of Consciousness breaks down in most people after 48–72 hours without sleep, because the brain does housekeeping in REM sleep that it can't do while awake. Physically, REM sleep gives the brain time to rebalance its neurotransmitter levels. Metaphysically, mystics and shamans say dreaming gives the conscious mind downtime to convert and upload daily memories into long-term memory, which is stored non-locally. So sleep deprivation prevents your short-term memory buffer from flushing its data at the end of the day.

To speculate further, dreaming also allows spiritual forces that have permission to communicate with you a channel in which to do so. This gives your Higher Self and other friendly entities a way to plant answers, inspirations, feelings, warnings, or suggestions into your mind, while your Veil is lowered. In effect, lowering The Veil during sleep allows information to be exchanged between "local, self-contained you" and higher powers that need to message you, while your conscious mind middleman is out of the way and bandwidth is unrestricted. Hence, messaging on this channel happens while you're asleep.

But when this process gets deferred too long, abnormal neurotransmitter levels cause you to dream while you're awake. And that can be weird. The brain can't wait any longer to do its housekeeping. So it directs your pineal gland to release a powerful psychedelic compound called dimethyltryptamine (DMT) to forcibly put you into a dream state in which your Veil of Consciousness lowers its shield. Through this coping mechanism, melatonin's role as the sleep activator is usurped.

Not coincidentally, DMT is the active ingredient in the psychedelic plant ayahuasca that Central and South American tribes use in religious ceremonies to induce a state of lucid dreaming. Whether dreaming in REM sleep, lucid dreaming, or under the influence of ayahuasca, DMT drops the Veil of Consciousness and allows the mind to communicate with spirits. Sometimes it's frightening. Other times it's fantastical. Many times it's awe-inspiring. But every time it's trippy.

4. Trauma and extended hyper-vigilance

Trauma can break down The Veil. When a person faces extreme danger, adrenaline is dumped into muscles to get them ready for action, should you choose to run, or stay and rumble. Just as important, dopamine and the fight or flight response speed up brain function to increase mental acuity and improve reaction time. The problem is, the flood of biochemicals released into the brain and muscles go unused. You're primed for battle, yet frozen in place. With no tiger to fight, or hungry beast to evade, the brain and body are put on high-alert mode, with no outlet to expend that energy. Imbalances of brain chemicals then cause the brain to behave badly.

As we just discussed, excess dopamine over-stimulates the PFC, causing synchronization problems and Veil permeability. When that happens, serotonin dips relative to dopamine. The 'too high, too low situation' upsets the brain's system of checks and balances. In this state, the brain is inundated with pro-excitatory brain chemicals that slam the aperture of your awareness wide open to take in as much information as possible to handle the situation. Yet, calming chemicals are not available to release that energy and concentration.

High dopamine and low serotonin can cause you to over-focus on thoughts and the fiends that sent them. Or, at the least, they give malevolent entities the opportunity to slip their messages into your stream of consciousness, while your discernment is porous. Perhaps our brain chemistry is meant to do this so we can pick up friendly messages from guiding angels in a crisis?

Whatever the case may be, if this is a survival mechanism, it comes with risks and side effects when the state of emergency doesn't end soon. Worst of all, extended trauma drops the Veil of Consciousness and opens the door for demonic forces to occupy the person's mind, possessing them. Or, in milder cases, trolls might only play tricks on you while the door is open.

Prolonged hyper-vigilance can be somewhat of a similar situation. Staying in crisis mode for many hours can exhaust the brain's supply of neurochemicals, temporarily puncturing The Veil. Two scenarios: if you were shot at for many hours in combat, or trapped overnight in a real haunted house, you might start to see and hear imaginary things. What happens is, when your brain is overloaded with dopamine, you are exposed to too much information, from too many sources, for too long.

Drinking from that firehose of information, your conscious mind gets fatigued separating appropriate information from the inappropriate. It starts leaking undesirable information into your consciousness. Aided by low serotonin, jokers from the spirit world can then message you against your will, because your obsessive/compulsive thought patterns resemble you 'listening' and giving them permission to keep talking.

5. Hypnosis/trance state
Another circumstance in which you can communicate with spirits is a trance state. Whether you're hypnotized, meditating, or using magik to alter your state of consciousness, a trance state can shut down that function of the brain responsible for separating "reality" from the supernatural. The clarity of communication in trance varies widely because, like cylinders of a lock, the alignment of multiple phenomena is required to open the gate and correspond with non-physical sources.

To give you some background, a state of trance quiets the conscious mind. The conscious mind acts as a gatekeeper to the rest of the mind, rather than the gate itself. Unbeknownst to you, the conscious mind catches unauthorized communications at the gate to the rest of the mind and ignores, or edits/re-authors, messages to obscure their source and meaning. The conscious mind actively tends this gate. Therefore, trance can circumvent this active filtering function and allow interlopers to bypass the conscious mind and put thoughts directly into your head.

But, even before that, the integrity of The Veil determines how clearly messages are received on your end. The Veil is the gate itself that protects the mind from unauthorized access. Once breeched, the conscious mind is the last line of defense against intrusive communications.

But, the thing is, hypnosis or meditation typically don't (1) lower The Veil *and* (2) "anesthetize" the conscious mind enough to let entities talk to you one-to-one. Both of these "shields" have to be down for communication to occur between realms. You typically have to give permission for hypnosis to lower The Veil. For this reason, hypnotherapists can only communicate clearly with your subconscious, Higher Self, or other spirits when you're in the deepest state of hypnosis, called the somnambulistic state. In this state, both The Veil and the conscious mind are disabled.

Further obscuring communications, your conscious mind casts its emotional shadow over your perceptions in light states of hypnosis – thereby projecting any fear, anger, doubt, or other emotions you may have onto people and events in hypnotic regression. Conversely, you have to completely shut down your conscious mind, with its emotional baggage, to talk directly to your subconscious and accurately recollect past events – usually for the purposes of learning about previous incarnations.

To illustrate, questioners of Edgar Casey were advised to tip-toe around the subject of religion when querying him about their health conditions, because Casey's religious beliefs were said to "color" what he said in trance. In doing so, his Higher Self was careful to avoid contradicting Casey's own (waking) religious beliefs.

6. By invitation (usually with dark forces)

Satanic forces "live" to corrupt and destroy. However, they can't carry out their indecent acts on earth by themselves. They need physical beings to do their dirty work. This means you need only ask demonic forces to communicate with, possess, and work through you, and they're only too happy to partner up. Of course, those who conjure evil spirits like to accessorize the invocation process with occult symbology, evil incantations, and the occasional blood sacrifice to liven up their late-night gatherings. Secret societies types and their overlords did invent the master-servant lifestyle and its trappings, after all.

Perhaps conjurers get their jollies from these sorts of tricks, having run out of carnal pleasures in which to get their fix. Maybe these are necessary evils to summon the biggest, baddest demons. Whatever the case, there's a reason occultist-types do these kinds of rituals. And they make no secret about paying homage to rulers of other realms.

Important to understand: Evil has to be directed at someone. That could mean just about anyone, at any time. But, usually, it means ill-will and wrong-doing are aimed at those who like to be of service to others and the greater good. To dark forces, the do-gooders of the world look like they've got signs on their backs that say: "I'll believe anything a government official, celebrity, or famous athlete tells me, so long as it makes me feel virtuous. Go ahead; use me and abuse me."

Which is to say, secretive fraternal organizations don't summon evil spirits and worship wickedness for mere entertainment. Rather, both conjurers, and the conjured, are intent on using everyone at every opportunity, to enrich themselves and satisfy their perversions. So don't think for a second that they don't take demonic possession seriously. Their very nature is to pervert all that is good in this world.

In summary, spirits are allowed through The Veil of Consciousness when they're invited – whether in ritual, or by contract known as a "bargain with the devil." My advice: Before entering into agreements you may regret, make sure you understand what you're getting yourself into. Be prepared to pay a hefty toll when the time comes to fulfill your end of the bargain. There are no takebacks.

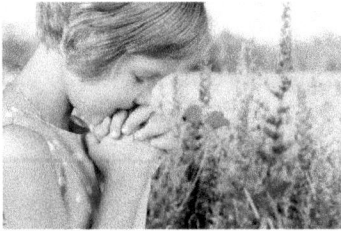

7. Prayer

A seventh way that people communicate with the other side is in prayer. Prayer is often defined as communion with benevolent beings. But it doesn't have to be. Whether you're religious, atheist, agnostic or satanic, prayer is a form of communication with spirits. Of course, the "reception" you get when talking with spirits is never as clear as a cell phone. But it can be improved with desire and dedication. They say faith can move mountains.

Veil of Consciousness summary

The Veil of Consciousness is a shield of protection that prevents unauthorized access to your thought stream when entities do not have permission to do so. This includes both benevolent and malevolent entities. Generally speaking, messages have some ability to influence your inner dialogue, no matter how secure an individual's Veil is. But the more permission and opportunity you grant an entity, the greater their ability to communicate with you, while your shields are up and fully operational.

Of the seven situations in which this can occur, the element that sets you up for unwelcome intrusions, more than any other, is having extremely abnormal brain chemistry, because biochemicals fuel executive function, discernment, and mental stability. In other words, contamination of your consciousness is caused by extremely imbalanced neurochemistry and/or serious physical dysfunction. They often go together.

One such collapse is having a faulty reticular activating system (RAS). The RAS is like a branch of The Veil that filters sensory information from your surroundings (as opposed to higher dimensions) so that your conscious awareness does not get overwhelmed with information. When the RAS is lowered for any reason, the conscious mind is unable to fully process stimulus from around you. **Overwhelmed with sensory input from the material world, the conscious mind then has diminished capacity to control unwanted intrusions from spiritual sources.**

Unfortunately, this happens more in ADD individuals than the general population. And when it lines up with one or more of the seven "veil-breakers," that's when you hear voices, are influenced or controlled by the other side, or can even become a vessel for demonic forces who'd love the use of a human body. Bottom line: when you're sleepy, drugged or extremely fatigued, you're vulnerable to influence from unfriendly forces. But, when you're well-rested, well-nourished and in-balance, your conscious mind is at its most protective against intrusion from evil entities.

The Veil serves as a reality check

The Veil actively monitors all transmissions to and from the mind in order to separate fact from fiction. It's the primary defense mechanism that separates a stable mind from one that we'd call delusion or psychotic. But that's not to say a leaky Veil automatically makes you crazy. As mentioned, the voices people hear are not imaginary. They're just coming from sources and places that science and psychology cannot explain.

Instead, it's an individual's response to voices, and ability to manage Veil permeability, that determine their level of sanity. And that's done mostly by the conscious mind, led by the PFC. Executive function is your mind's "bouncer" that actively controls your ability to reject unfriendly forces that want to corrupt your thought stream… Or, if you're fortunate, invite positive presences into association with you.

For instance, many of history's greatest inventors, authors, painters, and scientists admit to getting their best ideas from the other side. Geniuses and prophets such as Nicola Tesla, Albert Einstein, Vincent Van Gogh, and Edgar Cayce openly credited their best work to inspirations planted in their mind when in an altered state of consciousness. Their minds effectively molded background chatter from higher powers into remarkable works of science and art. However, you need a strong, yet receptive, conscious mind to do that without "losing it" over time.

It's for this reason that there's a fine line between genius and insanity, because if your Veil is leaky, and your conscious mind isn't sturdy enough to control the tapping process, you're at the mercy of mischievous forces that would like nothing more than to drive you insane, just for the hell of it.

A potential superpower of ADD: Enhanced creativity

When communication flows freely through The Veil, you have greater potential to be creative, because disconnecting the mind from rational thinking and concrete reality frees the mind to receive far-out ideas that could be valuable. Indeed, that's where creativity comes from: thinking outside the boundaries of conventional thought. Whereas, regular people – people that spend most of their time thinking *inside the box* – can't access creativity as easily or abundantly. Thus, creativity is a talent in which many ADD folks have an advantage over ordinary people – provided you can control the crosstalk in your head and put it to good use, instead of it controlling you.

PART 4

Solutions to Gut-Brain Problems

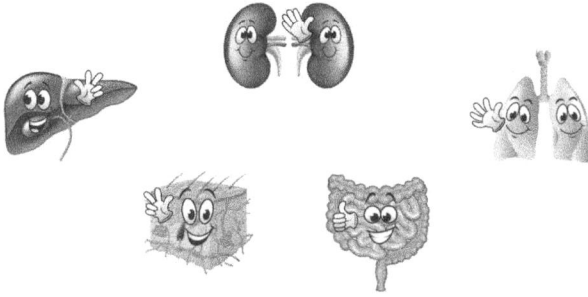

DETOXIFICATION AND
ELIMINATION

**Every day, your body is fighting desperately
to get rid of toxins faster than you're taking them in**

Detoxification is a never-ending battle between wellness and disorder. For most of us, that means the rate of toxins entering the body is high, and the speed with which they leave is somewhere between barely scraping by to not nearly enough. Both contribute to a high toxin load. However, it can take decades to notice slow detoxification, because symptoms tend to show up only after storage sites are full and your coping mechanisms are empty.

No one is unaffected. But, almost everyone on the ADD/GAPS spectrum is living with an elimination system that's in some state of dysfunction. Total body burden is important to watch because toxin exposure is a core component of psychological disorders, modern diseases and autoimmune conditions. It's a big reason that many healing efforts fall short of their goals. Most people will never know how important detoxification and elimination are to their wellness. But you can certainly feel it when toxicity causes adversities such as brain fog, hormone/endocrine dysregulation, or autoimmune skin problems.

Here, we'll examine how the detoxification system works, what causes it to break down, and steps you can take to increase the rate at which you detoxify. This chapter is all about turning your innards into a pristine environment where imbalance and disorder can't reside for long because mental and physical dysfunction are totally out of place in a system that's clean, in good working order, and has resiliency to spare.

Common types of toxin
- **Industrial and consumer chemicals,** such as plasticizers, household cleaners, flame retardants, industrial solvents, manufacturing chemicals
- **crop amendments,** such as herbicides, pesticides, fungicides, GMOs
- **heavy metals** in dental amalgams, big fish and air pollution
- **unhealthy food ingredients,** such as preservatives, artificial flavoring, food coloring, fillers and binders, artificial ingredients
- **personal care products,** such as makeup, hair care products, sunscreen, soap, lotion, nail polish, antiperspirant, toothpaste
- **antibiotics** for people and livestock

- **pollutants** such as car exhaust, smoke stacks
- **medications** now found in our drinking water
- **pathogens,** including bacteria, mold, fungi, yeast and parasites
- **non-native electromagnetic frequencies and nuclear radiation.**

Our bodies are processing and elimination machines

The majority of the body's organs and activities play some role in nutrition or elimination. From the mouth to the anus, and most organs in between, our anatomy is built to break down, distribute and absorb nutrients from food, then get rid of the material we can't use. Meanwhile, our elimination organs collect and expel

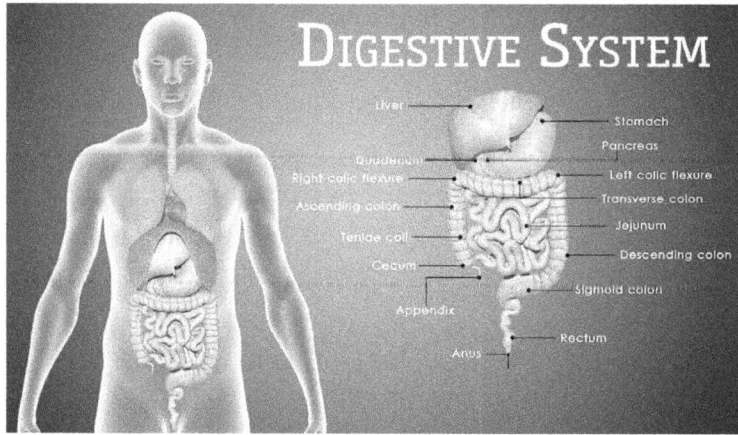

substances out of that nutrient stream that can harm us.

Not surprisingly, unless there's a reason to do otherwise, we only notice things that we ingest/absorb intentionally, such as food, air, water, and personal care products. We tend to not think about the environmental toxins hidden in personal care products, heavy metals in fish, chemicals used to disinfect water, and herbicides sprayed on plant matter. When, in reality, everything beneficial in what we eat, breathe and absorb needs to be separated from that which is harmful.

So there are a lot of steps that can go wrong in digestion, absorption, metabolism or excretion. Fortunately, the body takes care of all of it, without any thought or effort on your part. It's only when some-thing goes wrong that we learn to appreciate what a magnificent job our elimination and detox organs do for us day after day, year after year.

Four factors of toxin injury

1. rate of intake/exposure
2. rate of excretion
3. total volume of accumulated toxins (aka "total body burden")
4. your body's reaction to toxins.

Think of *exposure* (1) as filling your "toxin bucket." *Total body burden* (3) is how full that bucket is currently. And *detoxification capacity* (2) is the rate at which you're draining it. If your detox system is unable to keep up with demand, it stores toxins that it can't excrete in fatty tissues such as the brain, heart, nerves and endocrine organs. On the other hand, when your rate of excretion is outpacing your rate of intake, your system is getting cleaner and you are getting healthier, which is the goal of any detox treatment.

1. Rate of intake

Exposure level is how much of a toxin that you swallow, inhale, absorb through your skin, inject, or otherwise get into your system. Rate of intake is the quantity of toxin that you ingest over a certain timeframe.

Not much needs to be added to the topic of toxin intake at this time, other than to remind you that a corrupted microbiome lets 90% of mercury into the bloodstream through a leaky gut. While an intact gut lining blocks 99% of the mercury that you swallow in food. To put that in simpler terms, a leaky gut can let ten times the amount of toxins into the bloodstream than an intact gut wall.

2. Rate of excretion (detoxification capacity)

Detoxification capacity is the rate at which your detox system excretes toxins. Like a pump's capacity to transfer water, the rate at which your liver, kidneys, skin and lymph system are able to capture and remove toxins from the body is half of the equation in toxin injury. Improving the throughput of your detox organs is one of the two main focuses of modern detox treatments, cutting exposure being the other. Nothing new with either aim here. It's the new mechanisms we have to increase excretion rate that are changing the game.

Three things you can do to increase your detoxification rate: (1) Get plenty of trace minerals. Natural sea salt and certain kinds of ocean water are excellent sources. (2) Increase your intake of fat-soluble vitamins A, D, E and K. Without these vitamins, heavy metals are inaccessible to detox processes. (3) Get plenty of sleep. Detoxification is one of the last things the body focuses on during a night's sleep, so if you consistently short yourself of sleep, your detox organs must work harder during the day.

Finally, we need to get Roundup and glyphosate out of our food supply. They interrupt cytochrome P450 enzyme activity (a family of 50 enzymes, crucial to the liver's detoxification efforts). That means the liver can't break down toxins as well as it should. And that makes all the toxins it is trying to remove that much harder to mobilize, and a lot more toxic.

3. Total body burden

The sum total of toxins stored in your body affects your ability to remove newly-ingested toxins. Along the same lines, "toxic load" is a general term that means the sum total of a toxin you have circulating and stored in your body. Often the term toxic load includes new exposure as well.

These variables are important to take into account. However, old-school practitioners typically look at indirect measurements to ascertain total toxin accumulation, often called "total body burden" because "that's the way it's always been done." To measure total body burden, traditionalists have used chemical chelators to coax accumulated toxins out of storage sites and into circulation. They then use the quantity of toxins they see in urine or blood to extrapolate how much of a toxin that the whole body has in storage, beyond direct measurement of these tests.

These "provocation" or "challenge" tests don't give you a perfect picture, because they may not accurately reflect your actual total body burden, what your body's response to those toxin will be, or what will happen with any new exposure. They don't tell you a lot of things that a practitioner would want to know, because there are more factors at play. However, they do give some useful information when used intelligently. Fortunately, the detox field has made huge progress in the last decade with more sensitive test equipment, better understandings of detoxification mechanisms, new detox agents, and advances in treatment protocols.

4. Your body's (individual) response to toxins

Why does one person suffer long-term kidney damage when they get their dental amalgams removed, a second feels under the weather for a few days and then feels fine, and a third doesn't have any adverse reaction to the same exposure as the other two? It's because toxicity is your body's *response* to a toxin, not just *amount of exposure* or *accumulated volume*. This can be described as *sensitivity* to a toxin. Everyone handles toxins differently depending on genetics, epigenetics and their immune reaction.

Genetics. Humans are genetically disposed to remove toxins at different rates. There are fast, medium, slow, and ultra-slow detoxifiers, much of which is based on how much glutathione your body makes (the body's master detoxifier). Genes have a lot to do with that.

What's interesting is, you can often tell who is, or is not, an efficient detoxifier just by looking at them. The people with the brightest eyes, clearest complexions, most youthful appearance, and radiant energy are often the best detoxifiers. On the other hand, some people are genetically susceptible to mitochondria dysfunction and/or poor methylation. Either condition can impair energy production which is needed for detoxification. As mentioned, detoxification is a lower-priority process in terms of energy used than activities such as circulation and digestion.

Epigenetics. Toxins change the way your genes are expressed – not just for you, but for your children and your children's children. Some toxins can bind to your DNA, concealing its original coding. The body sees the "unholy union" and replicates it that way. This alters the way your genes are expressed physically and biochemically, not just for you, but for future generations. For instance, exposure to certain toxins can derail glucose metabolism and contribute to type 2 diabetes, thereby slowing metabolism and causing weight gain.

Methylation is the transfer of one carbon atom and three hydrogens (CH_3) – called a "methyl group" – to another molecule. Methyl groups control detoxification through glutathione, immunity, inflammation, gene expression, repair of free radical damage, neuro-transmitter production for brain function, energy production, the stress response and more. Methylation defects are thought to contribute to autism and many other disorders.

What surprises a lot of people is that epigenetics may play a bigger role in which traits you exhibit than your own genes (particularly biochemical ones). Scientists now believe that your own DNA contributes less than 10% of the expression of certain traits, while epigenetics influences more than 90%. And prevailing wisdom says it can take one to three generations to return epigenetic alterations back to their original state.

Immune system reaction. Another level of toxin response is how the immune system attacks harmful substances. Through this mechanism, the immune system sees a foreign material that doesn't belong in circulation. It produces antibodies to fight the foreign material, and attacks the invasion with this TH_2 immune response. This creates another layer of sensitivity – another layer of toxicity. Glyphosate and GMO proteins are prime examples of substances that can set off an immune response.

Along those lines, sometimes the immune system can become so crippled that it can't even *begin* to mount an attack on a lingering infection. Detox specialists see this happening in cases where the body's immunological response to a disease (e.g., antibodies) is used to test for the presence of that disease, instead of measuring pathogens directly. Lyme's disease is one such condition. In cases like these, clinicians warn patients when starting an intensive detox regimen to prepare for fever and illness, if they may be harboring an infection that was not dealt with adequately before.

Immune system function is collapsed in these people. So, after immune function is restored with advanced detox protocols, the body is then healthy enough to go through the healing process. It's able to fight the infection and recover from it, rather than isolate it and adapt to side effects. This is a case where untrained observers might mistake fever for a bad thing when, the truth of the matter is, the body knows what it's doing. And, when it's strong enough, it will allow the immune system to activate fever and inflammation as healing mechanisms.

These actions and reactions determine your sensitivity to a toxin

Genetics, epigenetics, and immune system reactions are factors of toxin sensitivity that detox specialists are just beginning to get a good handle on. This is where the detoxification field is focused, moving forward: (1) finding the levers and switches that accelerate detoxification processes, (2) resolving immune system reactions by healing and sealing our corrupted guts, and (3) undoing damage to our epigenetic code by ending toxin exposures and addressing nutrient deficiencies.

Synergistic toxicity

Many (perhaps most) toxins react with other toxins, to amplify their combined effect. So instead of one level of toxicity plus another equaling two – we'll call this "additive" toxicity – two toxins combined might be 3, 10, 100 or 1,000 times as toxic. For example, lead and mercury

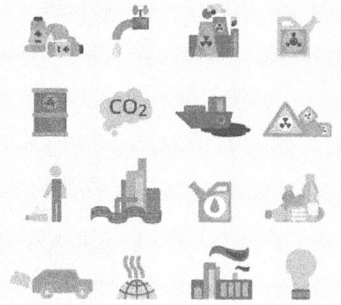

together are 100 times as toxic as either alone. But, the scary fact is, a tiny fraction of the 50,000+ chemicals introduced in the past hundred years have been tested for long-term toxicity by themselves. And far fewer have been tested for synergistic toxicity when combined with other toxins.

That's the elephant in the room that medical science, corporate heads, and public health officials shudder to think about, because the damage being done to the world's population is a train wreck crashing all around us, with potential solutions being few and far between. Indeed, synergistic toxicity is one of the biggest threats we face in our modern world. It's a major reason why most of us are either sick, suffer from chronic annoyances, or are one or two insults away from a health crisis. And it's not being talked about outside of the detox profession.

Trans-generational susceptibility

Accumulated exposure to toxins creates trans-generational susceptibility. That's when the offspring of an exposed parent are at multiplied risk of genetic mutation, injury, and death when exposed to the same amount of toxin as their parents. In other words, the amount of toxin that a person is exposed to at any point in their life, not necessarily their present toxic load, gets passed through epigenetic machinery to posterity so that they are affected "geometrically" more from the same amount. And this happens whether or not parent or child reduces their overall toxic load at some point in their lives.

For instance, scientists have found the first generation of frogs exposed to a given quantity of mercury display 'X' level of injury/mutation. But the damage done by that same amount doubles in the second generation, and doubles again in the third generation, until none of them survive. So, instead of gaining a tolerance, as is common with many biological processes, the frogs developed dramatically greater intolerance with each exposure, due to alterations in how toxins affect epigenetic expression.

They displayed increased sensitivity in future generations that makes them far weaker in resisting environmental threats, and correcting genetic defects. Most important in detoxification, this impairs biochemical processes such as detoxification capacity, DNA replication, and energy creation. In frogs, it increases each generation's risk of physical deformity, behavioral changes, and death – to the point that the entire third generation died.

Of course, skeptics may say that humans have stronger detoxification systems than frogs. And they would be right. But, then again, humans are exposed to more toxins, more often, in greater volumes, and over a much

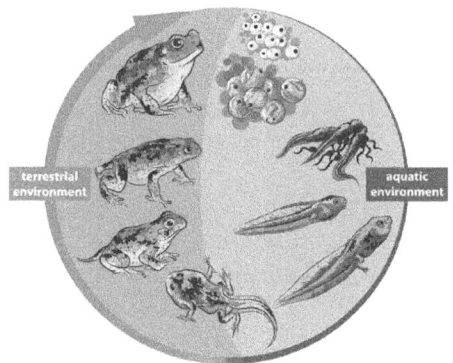

longer lifespan. Put into perspective, most of the Western world is about three generations into widespread use of mercury-based dental amalgams in much of the population. That's in combination with tens of thousands of other toxins developed since the 1950s.

Could it be that humans have developed an amplified reaction to mercury with each generation exposed, and are experiencing dramatically more health problems as a result, just like frogs do? Is it possible that each generation exposed to our hottest toxins increases psychological and physiological problems, which are now showing up in our public health statistics? Anecdotal evidence is saying it absolutely is.

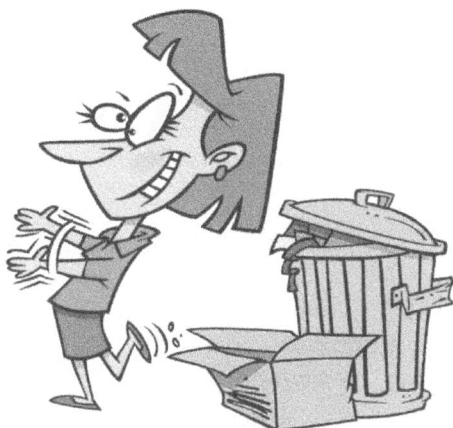

The 4 Phases of Detoxification

It's a common misconception that mercury, for example, stays in the body unless some external provocation forcibly extracts it. When, in reality, the body's own detoxification system is designed to never stop removing mercury. When each phase of the operation is doing its job, the body eliminates toxins roughly as fast as you take them in. And it stores the rest. This is the body's native detoxification system. Whereas, external detoxification products and programs are designed to assist the body with one or more of these phases, in doing what it does naturally.

Here are the most important steps in the body's innate detoxification system. Let's call them "The 4 Phases of Detoxification"

Phase I – Activation. Phase I prepares toxins for processing (mobilization) by making them more reactive. The reason for this is that many toxins are fairly non-reactive inside cells. Heavy metals are the exception. They're reactive by nature and don't need activation. Phase I basically turns a toxin into a free radical, making it more toxic.

Phase I is controlled by glutathione through its ability to catalyze reactions. Glutathione is the body's universal detox agent that's involved in removing hundreds of toxins from the body. It's instrumental in detoxification because it's used as a "substrate" (base material) for the production of many enzymes that catalyze reactions in later stages. Glutathione is also the body's most potent antioxidant.

Phase II – Mobilization. Phase II mobilizes toxins by prying them off of proteins or fats inside cells, and binding them to an enzyme called "glutathione S-transferase." This process is called "conjugation," and the new compound that's created is called a "conjugate." The conjugation process allows a toxin to leave a cell, makes it recognizable to the detox proteins in Phase III, and makes it water soluble so it can circulate freely.

Phase III – Transportation. In Phase III, active transport proteins – commonly called "multi-drug resistance proteins" – shuttle toxin conjugates out of the body in several stages. A different transport protein is used at each of these four stages: After being conjugated to glutathione, multi-drug resistance proteins carry the conjugate through cell membranes into the *bloodstream* (1), another transport protein pulls the conjugate from the blood into the *liver* (2), and still another protein moves it from the liver into the bile duct of the *intestinal tract* (3), so they can be passed *out of the body* (4). The same basic process applies to the kidneys as well. Key point: Substances don't readily cross cell membranes all by themselves. They need the help of transport proteins, the most important of which are made from glutathione.

Phase IV – Elimination. When the earlier phases are working well, toxins generally don't have a problem exiting the body. This phase is taken for granted in some people's minds. But the heavy demands we place on our detox systems today can add a fourth auxiliary category that must be met to complete the detox process. The Elimination phase consists of roads that the detox machinery uses to transport toxins out of the body... that is, unless a traffic jam clogs them up.

- **The skin.** Toxins can get stuck when exiting the skin, causing itchiness, irritation, rashes, eczema or psoriasis. Sweating and increasing circulation can help move toxins out faster. Avoid skin care products made from toxic ingredients. If you wouldn't eat a skin care product, use it on your skin sparingly/cautiously.
- **The lungs** eliminate a lot of toxins through breathing. You can help the body detoxify with more exercise, fresh air, and less pollutants.
- **The kidneys** collect much of the body's water-soluble waste from the blood and remove it through the urine. Increase your detoxing capacity by staying well-hydrated and eating less processed food.
- **The bowels.** The majority of the body's solid waste material leaves through the bowels. However, most people have some amount of impacted fecal matter in their bowels – particularly autistics and GAPS individuals. So you can facilitate the flow of toxins and prevent reabsorption by getting/taking plenty of <u>pre</u>biotic fiber to sweep the colon clean and feed your <u>pro</u>biotic bacteria. Enemas and colonics can produce stunning results. Of course, healing and sealing the gut with the GAPS protocol can help pretty much everything.

Together, *The 4 Keys to Detoxification* constitute most of your body's overall resistance to toxicity because they represent the speed and effectiveness with which your body removes toxins every day. When the productivity of any of these branches drops, your reaction to a given amount of toxin increases because more of it is sticking around and causing trouble.

What might not be obvious in *The 4 Keys* list is that detoxification involves biochemistry to make transport proteins, and physical equipment working together – including the liver, kidneys and bowels. So "detox pathways" are made up of a series of (1) *compounds* the body produces, such as glutathione, (2) *processes*, such as conjugation, and (3) *elimination organs* such as the kidneys that move material through and out of the body.

Transport proteins are the most important component, at least as far as detox therapy is concerned, because they're the scarce resource needed to increase your detoxification capacity. They're the actor that holds up the show when toxins aren't leaving as fast as you'd like – and the focal point of cutting-edge detox protocols.

The entire detox system depends on glutathione for its function and efficiency. That's because many compounds and process use glutathione as a raw material or catalyst to move things along. However, glutathione is somewhat powerless by itself. Rather, it's the most valuable player on a team of detox performers. Glutathione is the backbone, and most important element, of a system that depends on glutathione to keep toxins moving onward and outward.

Toxins need to be released from storage AND transported out
When you release toxins from their storage site, it's like you're stirring up sediment from the bottom of a lake. It then floats around and is free to go wherever it wants, and do whatever damage that it can do. So it behooves you to help your detox system get the toxins out more quickly with lifestyle choices such as exercise, therapies like lymphatic massage, organ support such as a liver cleanse, plant-based detoxifiers such as chlorella, or chelating agents like EDTA or DMSA. Otherwise, the toxins can get re-deposited elsewhere and cause new problems.

Important to know: when you do a detox therapy, toxins tend to get stored in batches, as certain toxins have an affinity for certain bodily tissues. For instance, heavy metals such as mercury, lead, aluminum, and arsenic are fat soluble. They tend to collect in high-fat tissues like the brain, nerve myelin, bone marrow, immune system and vital organs.

They then tend to come out sequentially in batches when you do a detox, as your detox system becomes competent enough to empty these caches one-by-one. This is one of the main reasons that detoxing can be such an unpredictable endeavor: you just never know exactly what is going to come out, when it will, and what kinds of problems are going show up in the process.

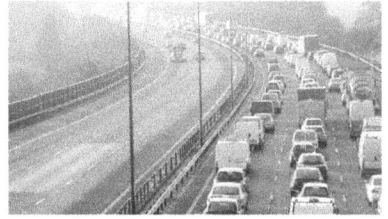

When the later stages of detoxification are blocked, earlier stages get turned down, and reabsorption occurs

When the flow of toxins exiting the body is restricted for any reason, those toxins can be reabsorbed and re-circulated through the detox system. Re-absorption (and reprocessing) is called "enterohepatic circulation." Specifically, when the body isn't producing enough end-stage transport proteins to keep up with demand, the entire system gets clogged with toxins waiting to get out, and the body cuts production of early-stage transport proteins. The entire system gets bottlenecked by this shortage, and detoxification slows to a crawl until more endogenous resources are available, or an intensive detox program restarts the system.

Minerals, vitamins, and other nutrients are needed to get the detox system out of its funk and revive its capacity. This often happens in quantum jumps. In some cases, mineral mega-dosing jumpstarts what was once a stagnant detox system.

Membranes should capture toxins on the way in, and mid-cycle

On the way into the body, the gut wall serves as an active filter that blocks unwanted things from getting into the blood, while letting nutrients through. Whereas, in the middle of a substance's journey through the body, other membranes do the same thing: The detox organs filter harmful things from the blood so they can be removed, while letting beneficial substances return to circulation to nourish cells.

However, when tight junctions are damaged by excess zonulin, harmful substances pass through breaks in the gut wall on the front end. And, not to be underestimated, leaky membranes in the kidneys, liver, colon, or blood vessels can't collect toxins from the blood. Toxins slip through filters and resume circulating. The intricate vasculature of the kidney tubules is the best example of a barrier/filter becoming holey from zonulin.

The takeaway from this topic: When your tight junctions come unglued, you've got more than one level of toxin leak: one that lets toxins enter the body like a sieve, and another that prevents detox organs from getting the darn stuff out. Increased toxin intake, coupled with decreased elimination, raises toxicity damage in GAPS individuals – the most severe of which can be found in autistic individuals.

Tight junctions help hydrate cells and remove toxins

Tight junctions enable electrical charge to build across cell membranes, which is the primary force that pulls water into cells and subsequently removes toxins. Hydration is essential to detoxification because water is the medium that transports toxins through cell membranes to the: bloodstream, detox organs and elimination pathways. Functional tight junctions keep hydration and detoxification going full-tilt.

INFLAMMATION

DETOXIFICATION

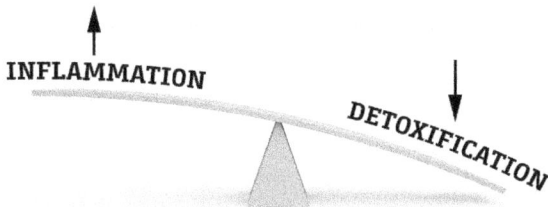

When inflammation goes up, detoxification goes down

Inflammation revolves around oxidation, because oxidation does the work of inflammation. Oxidation moves the process of inflammation forward, and reduction completes the job.

On the other hand, detoxification is mediated by antioxidant effect because the rate at which toxins move from one compartment to the next relies upon transport proteins. And the production of transport proteins is fundamentally a reductive activity. Specifically, the detox system conjugates toxins with glutathione S-transferase in order to create stable molecules for processing in *Phase II – Mobilization*.

The two are fundamentally-opposed processes: Inflammation loves to oxidize things (steal electrons), while detoxification reduces free radicals to make transport proteins. This is an antioxidative/reductive process.

This is important because when inflammation is running rampant, the detoxification system is unproductive. And most people in the Western world are living in a state of chronic inflammation all the time due to man–made vegetable oils, herbicides like glyphosate, processed foods, industrial chemicals, heavy metals and hormone mimics. Inflammation slows detoxification, so you and your health professionals should look closely at your level of chronic inflammation when you're trying to detox because it can undermine your efforts. And that makes you far more susceptible to health hazards that cause attention deficit disorder, GAPS, and many things that detract from your health and happiness.

When it can't expel toxins, the body has its favorite hiding places

When the liver, kidneys, and elimination organs can't get rid of toxins fast enough, the body stores them in out of the way places, and cleans them out later, as resources permit. It tries its best to store them according to how much damage will potentially be done in each location. First priority is to keep toxins away from vital organs. Next most important are the brain and nervous system. Then the bone and bone marrow. And then adipose tissue (fat).

So the body will store toxins in fat first. Then, when that's approaching capacity, it tends to store toxins in the bone and bone marrow. Then it deposits toxins in the insulation layer of the nerves, then the spinal cord, and the brain. Then, when those dumping grounds are full, it will store toxins in vital organs like the heart and lungs. There is always some equilibrating effect going on in the body. But, generally speaking, when you see toxins accumulating in locations critical to a person's survival, you know that person has a very high toxic load, because these are caches of last resort, only put there in cases of dire need.

Is fat made and retained for the express purpose of storing toxins?
Some have speculated that the body will purposely put on fat to create a place to put heavy metals or toxins that it has no other place to store safely. This could be one reason that a weight-loss diet or exercise program fails to work as well as expected: the body is protecting itself from toxicity damage. It could be why the first five pounds are far easier to lose than the last.

The body knows that losing fat would release huge amounts of toxins that its overwhelmed detox pathways are unprepared to handle. It knows if it were to burn off fat that contains well-insulated toxins, much of it will shift around and get re-deposited in another, more damaging place. So it resists weight loss until the detox pathways can handle more work.

Consequently, if you're thinking about starting a weight loss program, you might want to do a deep-cleansing detox first – both to catch up on removal of toxins waiting to leave, and to boost your detox capacity going forward. Healing and sealing your gut can help with that, as can a detox cleanse and daily support with EDTA, minerals, infrared sauna, etc.

Two reasons detox therapy fails: Starting too high or staying too low
Two common reasons that detox treatments fail to work as well as you'd like: One is starting out with an excessive dose and "burning" the person with a nasty Herxheimer reaction. And the other is never reaching a sufficient dose to elevate the detox system into overexpression.

When you start out with too high a dose of detox agents, you release too many toxins into the bloodstream, too quickly. With the detox system already working at full capacity in most people, and unable to handle more on short notice, the toxins circulate, cause side effects, and get re-deposited elsewhere. This makes the person feel cruddy or crippled (as in bad flu) for days to weeks, until the detox system can catch up. And this can sting people so badly that they never want to try it again.

The second mistake that practitioners make is never going high enough in dosage to jolt the detox system awake. You see, the detox system runs at its present rate, unless/until it sees a substantial increase in resources required for the job. When it sees it has production capacity it lacked before, it cranks up its efforts into overdrive. For example, you might need two or three times the minerals and vitamins as normal to upregulate detox pathways. In addition, getting plenty of sleep, exercising, and reducing stress chemicals tell the body that it's time for some spring cleaning.

The body then sees that extra "fuel and ammo" and encourages your detox system to go on the offensive in clearing out toxins. Instead of merely surviving, the body sees the surplus precursors and co-factors as an opportunity to kick start its waste removal efforts. It turns up oxidation activity. And that can be enough to suddenly, rapidly normalize problems that you've had for years. You do want to be careful, though, to increase dosages gradually to monitor the person's reaction, because detox pathways can be like an 'on-off' switch, rather than a dimmer. Turn it on, and it's on. Turn it off, and its stays off, until you turn it back on.

"Pulse" your dosing on and off to keep detoxing at the highest level

When you stay at a high level for more than about ten days at a time, the body habituates to that new level, and downregulates detox pathways to more typical levels. For example, if you take the same dose for thirty days, your detox rate may rise for fifteen days, and then fall back to where it started on the thirtieth day. So once you begin to approach what appear to be maximum dosing levels, start with five days on, two days off, and repeat. Slowly increase dosage levels. When you reach maximum dosage levels, go ten days on, four days off. That gives you the highest expression of your genetic detox capacity... and keeps it there.

Provocation testing: Savior, scam, or yesterday's news?

In the old days of detoxification (pre-2010), the test equipment that measured heavy metals in people was not very sensitive. The machines could measure mercury as low as one part per million. At that level, detox practitioners could not see mercury in the average person's urine without help. So clever scientists invented techniques to increase excretion rate to compare numbers – both in a single person 'before and after,' as well as between patients.

This method of testing is called "provocation" testing, or a "challenge" test. It involves injecting a person with a chelating agent such as DMPS or DMSA, and measuring what gets flushed out of the cells, into the bloodstream and kidneys, and then into the urine. The concentration of heavy metals in the urine using a provoking agent typically jumps 100 times, compared to non-provoked "ambient" level.

The problem at that time was, by artificially inflating the level by ten or a hundred times, virtually everyone looked like they were a toxic waste dump. So, in the eyes of skeptical regulators, these tests started to look like an excuse to treat everyone. In fact, one study found that 950 out of 1,000 people tested appeared to have dangerously high levels.

It didn't help that most people in the community were still comparing provoked numbers to ambient numbers (established years before). Regulators rightfully grew suspicious. They started cracking down on unsupported claims. And the detox profession earned its place on "quack watch" sites. Many laggards still use challenge tests and compare provoked numbers to ambient numbers.

Provocation tests can be misleading

Provocation testing also confused a lot of well-meaning professionals and patients in the past. For example, after eating fish such as tuna, the lower detection limit of most mercury testing equipment hovered around the three-day peak. By rising above the detection limit for three days, then falling below that level, it seemed like a typical person eliminates mercury in three days and it's gone. But that was completely flawed thinking.

They just couldn't see any mercury being excreted outside the three-day time window, so they assumed there was none. But, in truth, the equipment just wasn't sensitive enough to see that the true half-life of mercury is 40 days for fast detoxifiers, 60 for the average person, 100 for slow detoxifiers, and 120 days for ultra-slow detoxifiers.

Half-life: Time it takes to remove half the mercury from the system.

In other words, each time you eat some fish from the top of the food chain – for example, tuna, giant sea bass, shark or swordfish – it might take a little more than twice that amount of time before your system gets rid of 98% of the mercury from just that one exposure (equaling four months for the average person, over six months for slow detoxifiers!). It all depends on how well your detox system performs.

Christopher Shade to the rescue

Fast forward to today, thanks to Christopher Shade, PhD, and others in the detox community, testing equipment is now 100,000 times more sensitive than it was just a few years ago. Practitioners and patients can now see everything. Machines now measure mercury in the parts-per-trillion range. And almost no one falls below the detection limits. So we know what the true "time to eliminate" curve really looks like, and can say that most of the lingering 2% gets stored in fatty tissues such as the brain, nerves and heart. Moral of this story: Challenge tests have largely outgrown what little usefulness they once had, because they can give people the wrong impression, and we have far superior technology in use today.

Heavy metal detoxing

Endogenous detoxing. Detox regimens often target a particular toxin, like mercury, when symptoms seem to come from that metal. While there's nothing wrong with that approach, keep in mind that metals tend to leave in groups *through the body's natural detoxification mechanisms or a single organ detox* (as opposed to chelation treatments). That means the body's glutathione-transport protein system doesn't have a preference for one metal over another. When it has the resources available, it goes after one family of similar chemicals/toxins to eliminate. With some overlap, it then goes after another.

Detoxing by metal. The body redistributes caches of heavy metals such as mercury when there's a scarcity or abundance in any area. It does this faster than heavy metals are excreted through chelation treatment. So you can't target mercury and expect only mercury to come out when doing a liver cleanse, for example.

Detoxing by organ. That's why it doesn't do much good to target a specific area in the body to removal metals. You can't do a "mercury-brain cleanse" for clearer thinking, or a "lead-heart flush" to get rid of cardiovascular disease. The best you can do is support an individual organ for a cleanse, and see what comes out.

Systemic chelation. Chelators are better at targeting specific toxins than the body's own transport proteins or a single-organ cleanse. So you have to chelate the entire body via the bloodstream in order to reach an individual organ or metal. You have to let the body release heavy metals from wherever it will, and tissues will equilibrate by themselves. That's how to access otherwise hard-to-reach metals, and lower your total body burden systemically.

Mercury in dental amalgams inflames the gut and disrupts toxin flow through the body

If you've got mercury fillings, not only does a huge amount get stuck in cells of the mouth, but you also inhale it and swallow it constantly. When mercury reaches the gut, it causes inflammation that derails the transport protein "shuttles" that pass toxins from the blood into the liver, and from the liver into the gut. That backs up the flow of toxins making their way out of individual cells into detox channels.

Mercury also dysregulates the immune system. It inflames cells of the gut lining, which upsets the important work that enterocytes do involving digestion, absorption, barrier function and immunity. So you've got mercury blocking the doors out of the body for toxins. And you swallow it, directly damaging the gut wall and GALT. That's what makes mercury amalgam fillings double trouble for 75% of the US population.

How mercury poisoning is mistaken for other ailments

Mercury does so many unwelcome things in the body, that its toxic effects are often mistaken for other disorders. Mercury has such a strong ability to disrupt your biochemistry that it can lead to brain, nerve, and kidney dysfunction. It dysregulates so many processes that it can contribute to heart disease, nerve disorders, retention toxicity, and psycho/social problems,. And it acts synergistically with other toxins, particularly other heavy metals, to substantially increase the overall toxic effect on processes that the body uses to build, maintain and eliminate.

First and foremost, it does this is by blocking enzyme activity. The body relies on hundreds of different enzymes to catalyze reactions in digestion, cell repair, toxin transport, and virtually every aspect of our biochemistry. These enzymes are constructed around a good metal, such as zinc or magnesium, in the core of their molecules. Mercury and lead do their damage by infiltrating these enzymes and displacing the good metals, thus inactivating the enzyme. And that happens early on in many biochemical processes, which creates a cascade of negative effects.

The destruction of nerve insulation, for example, can manifest as any number of problems from multiple sclerosis to neuropathy to loss of fine motor skills. A collapse in mitochondrial function can lead to chronic fatigue, heart problems and autism spectrum disorder. A blockage in detoxification can show up as kidney failure, eczema or ADD.

In addition, mercury toxicity can be confusing to practitioners because it can lead you into polar opposite states. Neurologically, it can take you into depression. Or it can take you into anxiety. It can make you hyperactive. Or it can give you chronic fatigue. Its destructive ability is so widespread and deeply rooted, that its damage can be hard to figure out looking at causation, present symptoms or future consequences.

Consequential to all modern humans: Heavy metals like mercury, lead, aluminum, cadmium, and arsenic are incredibly toxic in minute quantities because they upset foundational processes of energy production, neurologic communication, digestion and absorption, cell replication, genetic expression, immune response and detoxification. That means mercury and company are capable of creating havoc with pretty much every microscopic and macroscopic element of your mind and body, depending on how your body responds to these exposures.

Mercury causes anxiety, obsession and compulsion

Mercury hyper-stimulates glutamate receptors in the brain, which amplifies bias toward a sympathetic tone. It promotes a state of fight or flight in a person, which makes you feel anxious and fixated. The longer you live in this state, the greater your feeling of fatigue and depression, as it burns you out from overstimulation.

For some perspective, GABA and glutamate are the two dominant neurotransmitters in the brain. They're polar opposites – another "teeter-tooter" pair of brain chemicals, in charge of controlling opposing tones in the brain and body. GABA is used to chill you out. It relaxes your mind and body so you can rest, digest and repair (parasympathetic). So it's your "zen" neurotransmitter.

On the flip side, glutamate is used to get you worked up. It puts you in an action-oriented, stressed state (sympathetic) so you can think and act fast. So it's one of your fight or flight brain chemicals. When mercury gets into glutamate receptors, it makes them over-fire. This puts your brain and body in a constant state of high alert. This can contribute to obsessive-compulsive disorder and Dr. Amen's ADD type 7: "Anxious" type.

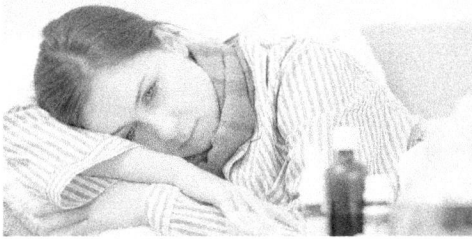

Herxheimer reaction

Killing pathogens too quickly – as can happen with antibiotics – releases their endotoxins (such as mercury) faster than your detox system can eliminate them from the bloodstream. This can produce flu-like symptoms such as headache, fever, joint and muscle pain, body aches, sore throat, general malaise, sweating, chills and nausea. This is known as a "Herxheimer reaction, die off reaction, or healing crisis." A healing reaction, as it's also called, floods you (the host) with 79-or-so pathogen waste products, as if you ingested a huge cocktail of poisons.

For obvious reasons, detoxing too rapidly through a cleansing effort can have the same effect – this called a "detox reaction." Detox reactions come from a rapid mobilization of toxins into the system, without a corresponding increase in the transportation and elimination steps of detoxification.

This creates congestion in the latter phases of detoxification when a person's detox system is already running at full speed, or is overwhelmed. The body can't produce enough transport proteins to get all the toxins out before they recirculate and cause irritation, inflammation, and immune system reactions. As a result, you feel terrible for a while, until your detox system can catch up and clear them out. When that happens, not only do you suffer any number of symptoms that make you feel sick. But those toxins may recirculate through the detox system, before they settle somewhere new (usually in fatty tissue).

But, as unfun as it may sound, when kept to a reasonable level, a Herxheimer reaction is nothing to worry about. It tells you that you're making progress and poisons are coming out – provided your symptoms are indeed from a Herxheimer reaction and not a new insult to the body. In fact, health practitioners have long used healing reactions to gauge detoxification speed. Take more and speed up the pace, if you don't have any reaction. Or reduce the dosage and slow down, if it's getting too unbearable. Meanwhile, support your detox system with additional products and protocols to increase detoxification capacity.

Genius tip from Dr. Shade: If you accidentally overdo it and find yourself in misery "herxing," a big dose of beneficial minerals stops a Herxheimer reaction almost immediately. A teaspoon of quality sea salt in a glass of water stops a bad reaction in minutes.

Rethinking Herxheimer

News from the cutting edge: The explanation of Herxheimer above is the way alternative healers have long thought about die-off reactions. But there's another possibility now gaining momentum among clinicians: Leading experts now doubt that there is any evidence to suggest that Herxheimer reactions are caused by a die-off of pathogens in the gut. Rather, it's an oxidative event.

Dr. Zach Bush explains that the normal process of cell death through apoptosis (programmed cell suicide) is a totally silent event with little chance of disturbing you the way practitioners once thought. It doesn't require the immune system. It does not escalate inflammation. Instead, he believes the so-called die-off reaction is due to a newly-introduced supplement (e.g., vitamin C or probiotic) or cleansing agent (e.g., antifungal, antibiotic, chelator or kidney cleanse) creating an immune system shift that releases a burst of reactive oxygen species that overwhelms your body's antioxidant reserves.

The immune system, after being provoked, floods the body with oxidative stress until the immune system can catch up and make more of the antioxidant glutathione, for example, to bring inflammation back to where it was. In other words, you're feeling the effects of the body's own threat annihilation system – inflammation – dealing with the change, not the pathogens dying, or the effects of the toxins alone. Time will tell which causality is correct.

Four primary organs of detoxification
The liver

The liver is one of the hardest working organs in the entire body. Over a hundred different functions have been identified thus far, with more still to discover. The jobs that it does are so essential to life that it's the only organ that is truly irreplaceable. You can survive on life-support machines doing the work of other organs, but not the liver. Its functions are too vast and vital to be replaced. It does so much for us that Nature even gave it the ability to regenerate. Injure or surgically remove up to a third of your liver, and it just grows back. Neat trick. But its most indispensable services involve detoxification.

Not only does the liver manufacture and coordinate the activity of transport proteins, but it collects and exports toxins down the detox mini-highway. Here's the short version of how the liver moves toxins: The first port of call for water soluble toxins to be gathered up for removal is the liver. The portal system routes blood through the GI tract to the liver. Some of the toxins in the liver enter blood flow going to the heart and then the lungs, where they are turned into a gas and are expelled.

The liver is also a recycling station for worn-out neurotransmitters, hormones, enzymes, and other biomolecules. But when the liver can't whip these important biochemicals back into shape, the partially broken-down molecules can't do their jobs effectively. As if falling behind on detoxification weren't bad enough, faulty dopamine and serotonin recycling then make GAPS conditions worse. They attach themselves to receptors sites and wreak havoc on brain and nervous system operation.

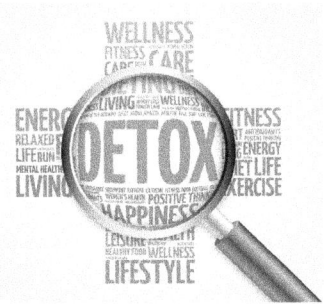

The lungs

The lungs are the second port of call for toxins. Toxins collected in the liver are transported to the lungs. When they reach the lungs, toxins that can be converted into a gas escape through the lungs in respiration. Toxins that can't be converted into a gas get consumed by immune cells called lymphocytes and macrophages inside the lungs.

Meanwhile, pathogens and toxins trying to enter the body through the lungs get treated to an escalator ride up and out of the body aboard the so-called "mucociliary escalator." First, these unwelcome guests get trapped in the layer of mucous lining the upper digestive tract. Then, microscopic hair-like structures called cilia push the encapsulated foreign material progressively higher and higher up the lungs and throat, where they can be coughed out as phlegm. Smokers and people who routinely inhale gross stuff know all about this detox mechanism.

The kidneys

The kidneys filter water-soluble toxins from the blood and excrete them out of the body through urine. But when the kidneys malfunction, you can't get rid of toxins, they recirculate, damage organs, and can threaten your life. What's to blame for this affliction of modern living? Pathogenic bacteria, leaky gut, and autoimmunity can contribute to kidney failure.

When your gut is corrupted, undigested food particles (particularly proteins), pathogens and their waste products, and other toxins get into the bloodstream. Some settle in the kidneys. Kidneys may get clogged with toxins. The bladder lining may breakdown. And the immune system may attack the kidneys with a TH_2 autoimmune reaction. When kidney function fails, you have major detoxification problems.

2022 update: The medical establishment thinks that kidney failure is caused by faulty blood flow/chemistry. They say it's due to poor circulation, diabetes, heart disease, blood pressure medications, or severe dehydration. These line up well with my explanation in *The Mitochondriac Manifesto* that kidney failure is a result of reduced electrical charge in the body, aka redox potential. Intimately involved with mitochondrial fitness and water structure… poor electrical charge in the blood/body manifests as low zeta potential; viscous, clumpy blood; deficient paramagnetic charge on the kidneys because the blood isn't charging them up; and endocrine organs that cannot attract hormones from the blood due to weak charge.

Zeta potential: Net negative charge around red blood cells that (electrostatically) keeps them from sticking to each other. This thins the blood and makes it easy-flowing. At the same time, the positive charge in the blood's fluid gives the blood cohesiveness.

The lymph system

Despite the fact that you have five times as much lymphatic fluid as blood, and the lymph system does much of the detox system's grunt work, most of the population still doesn't know a thing about it. Like stage hands working behind the scenes to put on a show, the lymph system supports the more celebrated cardiovascular system.

Composed of vessels, nodes, ducts and fluid, the lymphatic system sidesteps the liver and collects fat-soluble toxins. Using skeletal muscle contractions, it transports waste products through its slow-moving plumbing. The system then empties the mixture into a major vein for recovery of *wanted* material, and elimination of *unwanted* materials by other detox systems.

The lymphatic system also performs two specialized services that you can't live without: it transports disease-fighters such as white blood cells and lymphocytes where they need to go. And it absorbs excess fluid, metabolic waste products, pathogens and extracellular toxins.

The biggest problems affecting the lymph system are blockages and/or poor circulation. These are relatively common for people in poor health (whether by cause or effect) because the lymph system needs muscle contractions to drain properly. That is, the lymph system relies on physical activity of the individual to pump toxins through the lymph system, into detox organs, and ultimately out of the body. So if you aren't using your muscles much, lymph fluid stagnates and can become a cesspool for toxins that are both mobile and in an active form. Blockages due to swelling or infections also contribute to stagnation of lymph fluids.

Many practices through time – collectively called "drainage therapies" – have been used to drain the lymph system. From traditional Chinese medicine to European deep tissue massage to yoga, the ancient practice of toxin elimination is an established method to improve health and longevity. However, modern medicine seems to have missed that memo.

Avenues of excretion

When everything's working, toxins leave the body through one of four drainage routes for men, plus three addition routes (potentially) for women.

- breathing
- urine
- bowels
- skin/perspiration
- menstruation
- pregnancy
- breast milk.

Breathing

Breathing is the largest channel of detoxification. As the body's preferred path to get rid of substances that can be converted into a gas, 70% of detoxification takes place through exhalation. Not only does breathing expel metabolic waste products such as carbon dioxide and carbon monoxide, but more than 200 volatile compounds can be measured in expired air. This is why fresh air outdoors, and filtered air indoors, contribute to your "health bank account": fewer contaminants and irritants entering the lungs, and a cleaner medium to pull toxins out.

Urine

Urine works closely with its upstream partner, the kidneys, as one of the body's two best detoxification tandems. (The liver and bowels, the other.) The kidneys filter water, toxins, and other waste products from the blood to form urine. That solution then flows into the bladder for removal.

What's important to know about detoxification is that chemicals absorbed through the skin, and most metals that have been chelated, leave through the urine. These can damage the bladder. Some toxins can irritate the lining of the bladder, causing pain, infection, or inappropriate emptying of the bladder. However, generally speaking, once toxins accumulate in the urine, they have no trouble leaving. Urine doesn't get slowed down, or blocked up, as much as the liver, bile tract or bowels do. In this pathway, it's usually the kidneys that bottleneck the proceedings more often than the bladder.

Bowels (aka colon)

After the lymph system and liver have done their jobs, they pass their toxins through the gut wall, into the bowel. In the colon, these toxins are combined with food waste products, living and dead bacteria, and our own metabolic waste products to form fecal matter. Excess water is removed. And that's how stools are created.

That's the normal process. However, gut dysbiosis is notorious for upsetting the process, thereby producing diarrhea, constipation, or compacted fecal matter along the bowel walls. Key point: As fecal material is processed in your bowels, toxins can leech back into the bloodstream – particularly when the gut wall leaks. That's why diarrhea gives you get a tummy ache: reabsorption of toxins creates a sense of urgency.

Startling demonstration of this effect: Dr. Natasha has had autistic children speak their first words after cleaning out their bowels with an enema. Westerners may think it's weird. But that's how impressive enemas can be at dropping your toxic load. In fact, many traditional cultures have used enemas as a front-line treatment for sickness. As soon as a person started feeling ill, they were given an enema, because it's the fastest, most effective way to get toxins out, ease the workload on detoxification and elimination organs, while getting nutrition in.

Perspiration

We used to think skin was a barrier. And while it does block microorganisms from getting in, it's far more permeable than we ever thought. We now know the skin absorbs virtually everything else you put on it, including chemicals and medicines.

When you put makeup, lotion, sunscreen, or personal care products on your skin, they absorb in seconds and enter the bloodstream. For example, you can apply a garlic poultice on a baby's feet and smell it on their breath in minutes. In fact, the skin absorbs substances more readily than a healthy intestinal tract. Medical science is well-aware of this phenomenon, as transdermal medication patches have been used for decades when oral delivery is poorly absorbed or targeted.

What's more, when you absorb a substance through the skin, it doesn't go through the liver first, as it would when swallowed. Rather, anything you absorb through the skin goes directly into the bloodstream, and is filtered by the liver later. So personal care products – including makeup, soaps, and hair care products – expose you to substances day after day, without dilution or a toxicity check by the liver.

Fortunately, the skin also provides a path through which toxins leave the body. It's far more active than previously thought, and is actually the largest organ of excretion (by size, not volume or importance). It also does some filtering of its own, independent of major detox organs. How it works: Whenever perspiration leaves the body, whether visible as sweat or not, it takes toxins with it. Much of it settles on the skin surface, with some of it evaporating, and some getting reabsorbed, if it isn't washed off.

To illustrate how busy the skin is with these comings and goings, think about how salty that sweat is, or how a white shirt acquires ring-around-the-collar after a short while. Through these pathways, a variety of substances are leaving the body in perspiration. Acne, eczema, and psoriasis are three more examples of unfriendly substances causing skin problems as a result of toxicity – either when toxins linger too long and irritate the immune system, or when they feed pathogens that make more toxins.

You can use this effect to your advantage. If you spend a few hours a day sweating in a sauna, and then shower promptly afterward, you excrete so many toxins that you could actual live without kidneys. Intensive sweating is that effective at removing toxins. In fact, many potent chemical toxins, such as those from meth labs, can only be removed via therapeutic sweating. Conventional detox products/programs can't do it.

So, did Nature have detoxification in mind when it gave us a desire to shower after working out? I bet the urge to wash toxins off the skin before they're reabsorbed is built into our biology. And the blissful state after a shower just adds to the anchoring effect of bidding toxins goodbye.

Menstruation
Women have been clever enough evolutionarily to get rid of toxins and extra iron through their monthly cycle. That's one reason women tend to live longer than men: extra detox pathways that men don't have.

Poultice: A soft, moist mass of some substance, applied to the body for some medicinal purpose, and kept in place with a wrap of cloth or plastic.

However, some hormonal birth control pills decrease detoxification by delaying periods, or preventing them altogether.

Pregnancy

Nature designed pregnancy to be a "can't miss" opportunity to detoxify for the mother. It's one of the biggest opportunities to get rid of toxins that she'll ever have. But why does Nature do this? It wants to drop the mother's toxic load to protect her health, and that of her future offspring. It wants to give her <u>multiple</u> children the best chance at survival… not any one child in less than perfect health, raised by a mother who's compromised by toxicity herself. That's not sustainable for the human species.

In other words, one partially-healthy child doesn't bode well for survival of the species. You theoretically need at least two healthy babies from each couple to perpetuate humankind. So Nature designed the first pregnancy to clean out decade's worth of toxins in her body, when needed, to prepare for multiple future pregnancies. Rather than shielding the baby from toxins, as the placenta was once thought to do, the pregnancy process concentrates toxins in the umbilical cord and passes them onto baby. In fact, some toxin levels in cord blood have been measured at twice the level of mom's own blood.

This macabre detox method is the reason that first born children are significantly more likely to be affected by Gut and Psychology issues than younger siblings. That's why second or third-born children are rarely GAPS-affected, and not the first. And it's the reason many mothers miscarry one or more times before their body is clean enough to carry a pregnancy to term. It's because mother's body is using the 5–8 pounds of pristine cells as a quick and easy way to catch up on housecleaning it could not get to before. With pregnancy, it doesn't have to work so hard; mom's body just uses the pregnancy process as a serendipitous detox pathway.

From a "survival of the species" standpoint, it all makes sense: survival of the mother is Nature's first priority. Survival of some offspring (collectively) is the second. Survival of any one particular baby is Nature's third priority. Therefore, mother's body stores toxins (particularly fat-soluble toxins) that it can't get rid of in the least damaging place to her. Where else can the mother's body find that much fatty tissue to offload toxins into?

Knowing this, we need to teach our prospective mothers the importance of detoxing well before conception. And the best way to do that, while setting your children up for a lifetime of good health, is to normalize your gut flora and detox daily with quality foods and supplements.

Breastmilk

Lactating mothers excrete toxins through their breastmilk. Breastmilk is basically mother's whole blood with the red blood cells removed, and immune factors added. That means virtually everything in the mother's bloodstream gets passed to baby in her milk – including toxins, pathogens, stress hormones, and undigested food (e.g., gluten, cow's milk casein, and partially digested proteins).

Bloodletting

In the Middle Ages, medicine men (barbers, actually) used the curious practice of bloodletting to heal people. They opened up a person's veins and let them bleed for a while in order to heal them of all sorts of sicknesses both physical, mental and spiritual. While orthodox medicine has progressed in many ways since then (other ways, not so much), bloodletting does have the benefit of reducing the body's total body burden of iron and other substances that become toxic in excess.

Watch the Saturday Night Live skit about bloodletting, entitled "Medieval Barber Theodoric of York" for more information. https://youtu.be/ edIi6hYpUoQ

But you know what's crazy? Today's universal truths often turn into tomorrow's comedy routines, as history has a habit of invalidating beliefs we hold dear. As one saying goes, "Science is about most scientists being wrong about most things, most of the time." Who knows, maybe in a hundred years, we'll find out the bloodletters had it right all along and return to the practice? Case in point: Healers in some parts of the world have used leeches to restore circulation and remove waste products in cases of frostbite or poor circulation (like that from diabetes).

Others

The body also expels some toxins through saliva, phlegm, the tongue, tears, hair and mucosa – not enough to be meaningful routes of elimination, but useful for testing, as is the case with hair.

A story about toxin removal that will blow your mind: Kim Schuette (Certified Nutritionist and Certified GAPS Practitioner) saw a client that had hyperpigmentation around her jawline (a condition in women with weak adrenals during pregnancy). During an intense liver detox of heavy metals, she came into Schuette's office and exclaimed, "Look at my eyes!"

She used to have blond hair and brown eyes. Now they're completely green. In fact, she met her husband in high school, and he used to call her his "brown-eyed girl." The incident also reminder her that her eyes used to be hazel when she was a little girl. But, by her teens, they had turned brown. In her case, removing the toxins from her skin that caused hyperpigmentation appear to have removed superfluous pigmentation in her eyes, revealing their natural green color.

Situational detox events and cleansing show stoppers

When detoxification efforts fall behind in certain areas, the body can perform situational detox procedures as a form of emergency house cleaning. Dr. Natasha calls these cleansing procedures. You can think of them as urgent "detox events," rather than routine processes.

Just a temporary inconvenience in decades past, they came and went without serious incident or lasting effects. But widespread exposure and modern medicine have changed that. Now, after a child suffers a first-time asthma attack, for example, they're taken to a doctor to get a prescription to suppress symptoms. This can have devastating long-term effects, because it circumvents the body's natural cleansing mechanisms. Instead of removing toxins from an area, as a detox event is designed to do, the toxins accumulate. And when buildups turn into blockages, an asthma attack can become life-threatening.

Key point: Modern medicine has misunderstood the nature and purpose of these situational detox events. It's taught us for decades that detox events are harmful and need to be stopped. When, in reality, they exist to help. But when we interrupt Nature's restoration efforts for comfort and convenience in the moment, we risk amplified injury later.

Asthma attack

When toxins build up in a bronchial passageway to harmful levels, the immune system shuts down that motorway so its cleanup crew can remove all the garbage. This manifests as an asthma attack. At least that's the way it's supposed to work. But not anymore.

Historically, asthma was a benign condition – inconvenient and uncomfortable – but not life-threatening. Medical textbooks in the first half of the 20th Century instructed caretakers to have the individual stop what they're doing, rest, keep warm, maybe drink tea or lemon water, and the episode will pass in 10–20 minutes without harm. They could then go about their day as if nothing had happened.

Asthma attacks were no big deal; people recovered from them in minutes and no one died. But today, we use drugs to halt the bronchospasm. Without considering the ramifications, Western medicine prescribes an inhaler to stop an asthma attack when it happens. This shuts down the cleansing process that would normally close off that section of lung for 10–20 minutes while toxins are swept out by the immune system.

However, you can't repair a freeway when cars are still driving on it. So each time you interrupt the healing process, another section of lung is impaired. This damage accumulates each time the person uses their inhaler, because another bronchial tree gets shut down. Eventually, enough bronchial passageways are clogged that a life-threatening condition can occur, as the body tries to fix all of the accumulated damage in one go.

Epileptic seizure

When a dangerous level of toxins accumulates in the brain, the body tries to annihilate all of it with a series of powerful electric discharges, which neutralizes the tissue of pathogenic byproducts, heavy metals and chemicals. This is a cleansing procedure doctors calls an epileptic seizure.

Modern medicine sees the seizure as unproductive (at best) and prescribes powerful anti-seizure medication to stop the process. Unfortunately, anti-seizure medications can mess up a person's brain chemistry and turn a once-bright child into a zombie. What's more, the drugs are typically prescribed for many years. They're hard to come off of. And the effects often last for quite a long time. Once you start taking these drugs, your brain gets so addicted to its presence that detoxing can be quite dangerous. Brain chemistry often becomes so disturbed through the detox phase that a person experiences suicidal or homicidal thoughts.

But that doesn't mean seizures are a good thing. You just need to fix the real problem, toxins, so that the body's detox systems never need to trigger seizures. Fortunately, detox specialists have come a long way in the past decade at helping the body purge itself of toxins and restore balance.

Fever

Fever is a prime example of what happens when people perceive symptoms to be an enemy that they need to eradicate. When, really, fever is just like pain. It's a message to the self that all is not well inside of you. Most of the time, fever is a beneficial mechanism that the immune system uses to fight infection. It does this by kicking the immune system into high gear which, by design, generates heat. Fever is an ally in making you well, because pathogens can't stand the heat.

Fever is a natural healing process. However, fever normally accompanies a viral infection, bacterial infection, or some drastic insult to the immune system such as a vaccination. So alarmists among us blame a person's state of disease on the messenger: "Fever is threatening to kill poor Timmy. If we just give him something to bring the fever down, he'll be saved, and we can be happy again." Unfortunately, this is another circumstance in which Western medicine thinks it knows better than Nature.

We're taught that if a child is running a temperature, we're supposed to go see the doctor. The expectation being, the doctor will prescribe us medication that will fix the "problem." Of course, there are times when that's warranted. However, circumventing Nature's healing process can make matters worse for the person's long-term health and immune function. Typically, antibiotic/antiviral drugs are given to fight the infection, while anti-inflammatories such as aspirin or Tylenol are given to reduce the fever and make the person feel better as quickly as possible.

The problem is, each time you resort to medical interventions like this, the individual tends to pay for that comfort in the moment with a lifetime of problems related to a corrupted gut. You see, Nature intended for a person with this condition to feel bad for a while, she gets better, and her immune system becomes stronger after being beneficially stressed. But, as a result of man's high-and-mighty approach, these situations incrementally erode a person's long-term health, as their first- and second-line defenders (probiotic microbes and our innate immune system) become increasingly dysfunctional with each round of drugs that interrupt the healing process.

Sneezing

Sneezing is caused primarily by particulates such as pollen, dust, mold, or dander irritating mucous membranes in the nose and triggering this cleansing reflex. There are other ways to trigger it, but sneezing is usually an effort by the immune system to remove allergens from the nose and throat. Pathologically, sneezing can be indicative of leaky membranes letting allergens across nasal membranes to then over-activate the immune system, as is the case with seasonal allergies.

Diarrhea

Diarrhea is one of the most common cleansing procedures that you never knew it to be. It's the body's way of diluting disagreeable materials and getting rid of them fast, before they recirculate and cause harm. The instigator we all know about is food that your digestive system does not agree with, such as foods containing lactose, are spoiled, or are otherwise hard to digest such as beans. Heavy metals also leave through the bowels, as do many chemical toxins.

Whether toxins pass directly through the GI tract – never making it into circulation – or your detox system is releasing them through the bowels, after travelling around the body, both irritate the bowel when they stagnate. To speed things along, the body floods the colon with extra water and salt to dilute the toxin before flushing them out. But, until they are evacuated, the body provides extra motivation to get rid of them sooner rather than later by giving you a tummy ache. The idea is to get rid of the toxins before they get reabsorbed through the gut wall. That's the cleansing procedure we call diarrhea.

For the most part, modern medicine has left this cleansing procedure alone and not tried to convince us that our bodies are broken and need drugs to fix the occasional diarrhea.

Eczema and psoriasis

Eczema or psoriasis can be caused when toxins get stuck in the skin. Conditions like these are a result of the body objecting to toxins loitering in the skin where they don't belong. The immune system sees a buildup of toxins. It mobilizes its cleanup crew to neutralize them. And your own skin cells get damaged in the mêlée – sometimes presenting as white scale, other times as a red rash. Your skin cells, when mingled with toxins, take collateral damage from this "friendly fire" attack. Self-inflicted damage turns into autoimmune conditions that we call psoriasis or eczema, depending on presentation.

Of course, modern medicine prescribes steroids and medicinal ointments to suppress rashes and irritation. But these are yet more chemicals that the body needs to get rid of, rather than removing the source. Even more common, a lot of people get dry, itchy, flaky, sensitive skin in winter, as perspiration decreases and waste removal slows in winter. Similarly, dry wind itself and residual laundry detergent in clothing can cause dry, itchy skin. FYI: Moisturizers ease skin conditions mostly by diluting and mobilizing toxins (most are fat-soluble).

Tips to make your skin happy

- spend time sweating in a sauna
- exercise (sweating)
- improve circulation with natural supplements (e.g., EDTA, natto)
- hydrate with quality water
- earthing
- rid your spaces of nnEMFs.

Try not using soap all over your body when showering in the winter, if you don't need to. Many people find spot cleaning with soap, and rinsing with water, to be sufficient. That can go a long way in retaining your skin's natural oils.

In addition, low fat diets can deprive your skin of oils that help retain moisture. For this reason, many vegans/vegetarians suffer terribly dry skin – especially in winter. Pro tip: eat plenty of healthy oils in your diet such as saturated animal fats and fish oils. Try applying edible oils such as coconut oil directly to the skin. Many people find they work better than commercial moisturizers. At the same time, avoid seed oils. They're surprisingly bad for you.

Releasing emotional baggage
The mind and body are connected in ways than medical science refuses to acknowledge. So clearing past traumas of their energetic charge (their hold over you) can be just as productive in recovering your health as removing chemical poisons from the body. You literally need to detox emotional negativity from your mind in order for treatments and lifestyle changes to work as well as they're supposed to. This is an instrumental, often overlooked, element of detoxing. And there are solid reasons that this is true, to go along with metaphysical reasons.

Especially important for those who have trouble letting go, detoxing yourself of emotional baggage can be just as healing as any organ cleanse or chelation protocol. That's because emotional stress – whatever the source – affects the body the same as physical, mental, chemical or environmental stressors. You see, all forms of stress affect your endocrine/

hormone system (cortisol and adrenaline), digestion, detoxification, gut health, immunity and cell repair. Plus, emotional baggage contributes its own toxicity by keeping the adrenal system chronically activated.

Those are just the physical reasons past traumas are so important to confront with intention. Because until you move past them, the residual stress will consume your energy and contaminate your being. Same thing goes for self-limiting beliefs, being a worry wart, and negativity in general: they can blunt any healing efforts. So, what can you do about it? *Acknowledgement, acceptance, forgiveness, and gratitude* can do wonders to deplete bad memories and emotional wounds of their negative charge, leaving a positive frame of mind that attracts good things in their place.

Intermittent fasting/time-restricted eating

Intermittent fasting shifts metabolism from *living in the moment* to *making use of the past* (burning fat stores) and *preparing for the future* (regeneration and autophagy). Some physiological effects of intermittent fasting:

- lowers insulin levels
- enhances recovery and reduces inflammation
- boosts metabolism
- increases fat burning
- helps cell repair and replacement.

When you eat for fewer hours a day, you're probably eating less overall, which can help you lose weight. Intermittent fasting may help you

- increase fat burning
- lose weight and change body composition (i.e., leaner)
- lower blood-sugar level and insulin (possibly reverse type 2 diabetes)
- improve mental clarity and concentration
- increased energy level
- increased growth hormone (at least short term).

Hourly effects of fasting (time since last calorie intake)

4–8 hours
- blood-sugar falls
- stomach is emptied
- insulin production stops.

12 hours
- all the food you've eaten has been burned
- the digestive system goes to sleep
- the body starts healing processes
- human growth hormone increases
- glucagon decreases.

14 hours
- the body starts using fat stores for energy
- human growth hormone increases dramatically.

16 hours
- fat burning ramps up.

18 hours
- human growth hormone skyrockets.

24 hours
- autophagy begins
- glycogen stores are depleted
- ketones are released.

36 hours
- autophagy increases 300%.

48 hours
- autophagy increases 30% more
- immune system resets and regenerates
- inflammation response is turned down.

72 hours
- autophagy maxes out.

16   Intestinal Parasites

PARASITES
AND AUTISM

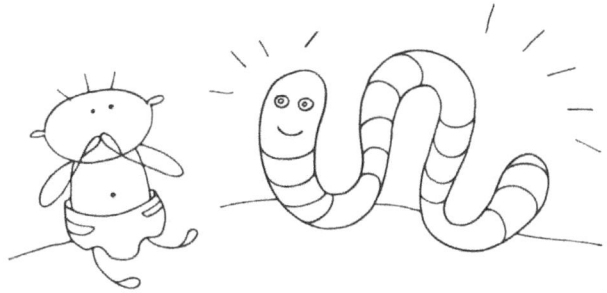

Parasites are a major source of toxins and hard to eradicate

They contribute to states of disease by stealing vitamins and minerals from their host, and dumping their toxic waste products into the digestive tract. So testing for their presence, and a parasite cleanse if indicated, should be considered in any GAPS or detoxification effort. Those on the autism spectrum should be considered highest risk.

Of course, getting rid of parasites is easier said than done, because they move around and multiply (many reproduce at each lunar cycle). And they have the ability to hide when threatened, like when they sense anti-parasitic drugs are being used. The most common varieties are rope worm, pinworm, ascaris lumbricoides, whipworm and flukes.

But as uncivilized as they sound to First Worlders, parasites have co-existed with humans since the beginning. So their presence is nothing unusual. Some figures say 90% of people world-wide carry parasites of some kind. And the World Health Organization says 25% of the world's population carries worms in particular. Yet most don't know they have parasites, since they don't exhibit any symptoms. It's only when they affect your health that a parasite cleanse seems important.

However, diagnosing the presence of parasites is far from customary practice. Conventional medicine pretty much ignores them entirely because they aren't good at testing or treating them. Their toxicology tests look for chemicals, heavy metals, waste products or microorganisms. While pathology labs look at blood tests or tissue samples to find signs of disease. Both are not setup to look for macroscopic parasites, so they just don't.

You pretty much need to send your samples to a parasite specialist that uses good old-fashioned microscopes to reliably detect parasites, count numbers, and identify species. Veterinarians and their labs still do this kind of testing with their patients. But not human healthcare providers.

How parasites wreck your health

The first reason that it's good to rid yourself of parasites is that they steal nutrients from you. They loot their host of B vitamins, minerals such as calcium and magnesium, as well as growth hormones. This can indirectly affect neurotransmitter levels. Even worse, parasites release ammonia, morphine, histamine, malondialdehyde, and formaldehyde into your digestive tract as waste products.

Parasites poison you with their toxic waste

- **Ammonia** can cause tremors, seizure, delayed growth, lethargy, and abnormal posturing, as well as loss of balance, coordination and muscle control.
- **Morphine** is dangerous long-term. Its presence slows movement of food through the digestive tract, causing fermentation, constipation and reabsorption of toxins. Its effects include euphoria, nervousness, drowsiness, restlessness, severe headache, irritability, loss of appetite, body aches, severe abdominal pain, nausea, vomiting, tremors, chills, goose bumps, muscle spasms, anxiety, insomnia, mood swings, amnesia, confusion and paranoia.
- **Histamine.** Excessive histamine can cause inflammation, immune dysfunction, and problems sleeping (neurons stay awake).
- **Malondialdehyde** is mutagenic. It alters the way genes are expressed into physical, biochemical, and neurologic traits. It changes the way you think, look, behave, and interact with others. Which is to say that it changes you mentally, physically and emotionally.
- **Formaldehyde.** Parasites involved in autism and GAPS constantly drip formaldehyde into the GI tract that detox organs do their best to remove. Widely used as an embalming fluid and tissue preservative, formaldehyde also goes into composite wood products and building materials, glue and surface coatings, as well as preserve vaccines, cosmetics, and household products.

Parasites are even suspected to consume growth hormone, stunting the growth of their host in their formative years and making the worms grow larger than expected. All of which contribute to corruption of the gut and neurological effects, such as sensory processing difficulties, cognitive dysfunction, developmental delay, and social impairment.

Parasites cause physical symptoms such as

- constipation, yellow stool or diarrhea
- bloating, abdominal pain or cramps
- cold extremities
- allergies
- anal, nose or skin itchiness
- leaky gut
- hemorrhoids
- fatigue;

Affect the central nervous system, causing emotional disturbances

- anxiety
- depression
- anger, irritability
- brain fog
- obsession;

Cause sleep disorders, including

- insomnia
- teeth grinding
- bedwetting
- multiple wakings
- drooling
- nightmares;

Cause developmental problems, for example

- stunted growth
- delayed intellectual development
- obsessive/compulsive cravings for sweets or particular foods
- stubborn weight gain or loss;

Cause muscle and joint problems like

- muscle spasms
- numbness in hands or feet
- pain in navel
- coronary arrhythmias
- cutaneous hypersensitivity
- auditory hypersensitivity.

So, as alluded to, parasites aren't just an autism problem. They affect many GAPS people, some ADD individuals, and a fair amount of the general population. So get checked out if you have a number of these symptoms.

Parasites are master manipulators, intent on their own survival

Like all life forms, parasites have a built-in survival instinct. To that end, leading parasite and autism researchers believe that the modus operandi of parasitic worms is to control your hormones, thereby controlling you. That means parasites don't care what you think. They care what you do. And the best way to do that is to control your cravings and behavior patterns through your hormone levels.

Somehow, someway, worms figured out that the best way to get what they want from you is to control your cravings and compulsions, rather than your thoughts (although they also do that as a secondary effect). And, unbeknownst to most people, they're darn good at it. Parasitic worms make you crave sugar and other carbs whose waste products get released into the body as endorphins. These endorphins give the nervous system a pleasure signal which turns the individual into an addict who's dependent on refined carbohydrates and processed foods to get their fix.

Causes of autism

Did you happen to notice that the symptoms of parasites matches up well with the symptoms of autism? If you didn't know any better, you'd think it *was* a list of autism symptoms. Coincidence? I think not. Let's put two and two together: The main driver of autism is pathogens residing in the digestive tract, including bacteria, viruses, candida, heavy metals and, most important, parasites.

These pathogens colonize the gut in a protective blanket called "biofilm," from which they continuously poison you with their waste products. This steady stream of toxins alters a person's biochemistry so profoundly that even seasoned clinicians assume that (1) autism is genetic, (2) it's been there since birth, and (3) there's nothing you can do about it: you're stuck with it for life.

I say, these people simply underestimate how upsetting a continuous flow of biotoxins is to the nervous system. They can't imagine how a non-stop assault of pathogenic waste products and heavy metals triggers neurological deficits, developmental delays and food sensitivities. And they've failed to realize how the poaching of nutrients messes up your health and resistance to disease, exposes you to genetic vulnerabilities, and interferes with your body's ability to correct problems that others can easily handle.

Biofilm

Biofilm is a slimy, tenacious layer of mucous-y membrane that houses and protects pathogens. Our area of interest is the gut, but biofilm can form anywhere. In nature, biofilm makes rocks slippery at the bottom of streams. In addition to microorganisms, biofilm is a composite material made up of extracellular DNA, proteins, sugars, and heavy metals encasing its population on the intestinal walls, largely out-of-reach from detection and correction by digestive enzymes or antibiotics.

Impressive to imagine: biofilm has its own nutrient intake and garbage removal system. Like a muncipal food delivery service, biofilm actually constructs mechanisms to pilfer nutrients such as calcium and magnesium from food products passing by. And it has utilities to move waste products out of the biofilm, into the digestive tract.

This more or less continuous stream of toxins from pathogens is what poisons the host's brain and body chronically and causes symptoms that we call autism. And it's this protective layer that can make pathogen removal so hard. Biofilm keeps its inhabitants safe inside, while keeping foreign invaders and therapeutic agents out. Some things can get inside with some difficulty. But biofilm, in general, is one of the reasons it can take many months of concerted effort to change your gut flora profile.

Chlorine dioxide helps reverse autism symptoms

A leading specialist in autism and parasite detoxing, Kerri Rivera, has developed protocols developed first by Jim Humble as a remedy for malaria, then by Dr. Andreas Kalcker and Miriam Carrasco specifically for parasites.

Rivera has taken their core parasite protocol and expanded it into a multi-modality therapy that's highly effective at reversing the symptoms of autism. Her protocol uses chlorine dioxide to break up the biofilm that harbors the pathogens causing autism symptoms. Dispersing biofilm is instrumental to driving pathogens out of their safe space, because it exposes them to "the elements" of relief – both internal and external.

Rivera's protocol can be described as a drip campaign that hits them mercilessly for weeks to months. At least eight times a day, you drink a solution that's a fraction of a drop of chlorine dioxide in several ounces of water (Rivera's book and website explain how to make it). Repeated dosing from morning till bedtime, for months at a time, is the only treatment strong enough on parasites, yet gentle enough on the host, to give you great results. Worms are just too resilient to get killed off by a pharmaceutical quick fix or surgical extraction.

Kerri Rivera's protocol to heal the symptoms known as autism

- diet (including gluten, casein-free)
- chlorine dioxide
- ocean water such as Quinton marine plasma
- diatomaceous earth
- lepidium latifolium extract or chanca piedra (stone breaker)
- pyrantel pamoate (brand name Combantrin®)
- mebendazole
- castor oil
- neem
- probiotic supplement (usually THERALAC®)
- chelation (sometimes)
- hyperbaric oxygen (sometimes)
- GcMAF (frequently).

Although other elements are important to the protocol's success, chlorine dioxide is the breakthrough that people in the autistic community had been waiting for. It was the missing piece that gave this protocol its potency, because chlorine dioxide is excellent at breaking up the biofilm that harbors pathogens. And it weakens parasites so other elements of the protocol can finish them off.

Neither chlorine dioxide, nor Rivera's protocol, should be considered a universal cure. But it's far more effective than any interventions offered to the autism community thus far. It's a lot of hard work for steady, consistent, improvement that takes anywhere from 3 months to 2+ years to achieve over 90% cessation of symptoms. And how well does it work? As of mid-2022, over 1,600 children have lost the diagnosis of autism, as measured by the Autism Treatment Evaluation Checklist (ATEC), with an ATEC score of 10 or below. The running total can be found on Kerri Rivera's site mentioned below. Compare that with the number of complete recoveries by conventional medicine: **ZERO.** No doubt, many more have achieved the same results, but were afraid to be counted for fear of reprisal by agencies such as Child Protective Services that intimidate families to keep quiet about effective treatments.

For more information on healing the symptoms of autism (may help ADD and GAPS as well), visit Kerri's websites: "kerririvera.com" and "cdautism.org." And get her book: Healing the Symptoms Known as Autism. It has pictures, descriptions, and the complete protocol.

Chlorine dioxide has been used for over 100 years disinfecting water outside the body. So why not in you?

Chlorine dioxide has been approved by public health agencies around the world as a commercial disinfectant in water treatment facilities, food processing, and mold treatment. And it has much lower toxicity and side effect profile than chlorine compounds such as chlorine bleach and chloramines. Chlorine dioxide has also been sold in camping stores for many decades to kill pathogens in wild stream water to make it drinkable.

In other words, chlorine dioxide is proven in a century of use to have no serious side effects, besides a die-off reaction if you ramp up treatment too fast. In fact, chlorine dioxide is inherently safe for humans at recommended doses because it produces no harmful byproducts as it *oxidizes* pathogens and their waste products. On the other hand, chlorine and chloramine disinfectants are widely known to hurt human health because they create highly toxic byproducts as they disinfect through *chlorination*.

How chlorine dioxide works its magic

On a molecular level, chlorine dioxide steals an electron from a pathogen, turning the chlorine dioxide molecule into sodium chlorite. Other chlorine dioxide molecules steal more electrons from that pathogen or its neighbors, until four electrons are added to the sodium chlorite molecule to form sodium chloride (table salt) and two oxygen atoms. Through this oxidation process, each chlorine dioxide molecule is able to oxidize five molecules in a pathogen's cell wall. That's the short explanation of chlorine dioxide's "oxidation capacity."

The missing electrons in the pathogen's membrane make it fall apart because electrons hold molecules together. This particular process leaves no unwanted electrons (free radicals), microbes, or molecules behind to hurt you. It's a "clean kill." Even better, it's impossible for pathogens to

Oxidant	Electrochemical Potential I (Volts)
Free Radical, (-OH)	2.8
Ozone atom (O)	2.42
Ozone, (O3)	2.07
Hydrogen Peroxide, (H2O2)	1.78
Potassium Permanganate, (KMnO4)	1.7
Chlorine Dioxide, (ClO2)	1.57
Chlorine gas, (Cl2)	1.36
Oxygen, (O2)	1.23
Bromine	1.09
Hypochlorous Acid, (HOCl)	0.95
Sodium Hypochlorite, (NaOCl)	0.94
Iodine	0.54

develop a resistance to this extermination technique because it happens at a molecular level, instead of a cell/nucleus/DNA level, which antibiotics use. Conversely, chlorine bleach and chloramines do leave toxic substances behind when they disinfect through chlorination. They exchange electrons in substances being oxidized, producing new substances – many of which are carcinogenic.

In short, the long-term safety and efficacy record of chlorine dioxide is beyond question. So if it is excellent at killing pathogens in water treated outside the body, and does not harm you, then why wouldn't it be good at doing the same inside the body, when taken medicinally? This is indeed the case: Whether disinfection happens outside the body or in it, chlorine dioxide is outstanding at killing pathogens and not harming you, or your gut microbes. That right there is the litmus test of a great medicine/therapy: deadly to pathogens, gentle on you and your tummy.

And how about real-world results? Jim Humble and the thousands he has trained have quickly and completely cured tens of thousands of people of malaria using only his chlorine dioxide protocol. It takes about four hours to improve a person's situation from being on death's door to being back on their feet, feeling great, joking around, and ready to go back to work the next day. Chlorine dioxide works that well and that quickly.

Chlorine dioxide's superpower is it only harms pathogens

Chlorine dioxide's special skill in detoxification is that it breaks down the cell walls of anaerobic microorganisms (non-oxygen breathing). Many pathogens are anaerobes that metabolize sugar for fuel, using no oxygen. A key feature of anaerobes is that they like acidic environments (low OH⁻).

The pH scale, which stands for "potential hydrogen," measures acidity-alkalinity via concentration of hydrogen molecules (H+) in solution. Acids (0–7 pH) are higher in H+, and bases (7–14 pH) are lower in potential hydrogens. The opposite way of measuring pH is by oxygen-hydrogen (OH⁻) groups, or pOH⁻. So, on either scale, as H+ goes up, OH⁻ goes down, and vice-versa.

Conversely, chlorine dioxide does not hurt aerobic microorganisms, because oxygen-breathers are higher life forms that like slightly alkaline environments (oxygen alkalizes). For aerobic cells, living in an oxygen-rich environment means that they have a natural ability to resist being stripped of electrons through oxidation more than do pathogens. Indeed, chlorine dioxide has just a little more oxidative pull on electrons than does oxygen. (See chart, above.) Consequently, the oxidation potential of chlorine dioxide is strong enough to steal electrons from pathogens, but not from probiotic microbes, or your own (healthy) cells. This makes it an ideal agent to kill parasites and other pathogens in your body, while leaving your own (healthy) cell unaffected.

In addition, chlorine dioxide oxidizes heavy metals that chelating agents can't reach. Since chlorine dioxide is negatively-charged, it's attracted to positively-charged heavy metals held deep within tissues. It bypasses your own negatively-charged cells, leaving them unaffected. In contrast,

"Chlorine dioxide is a universal antidote... able to destroy mold and fungus, as well as bacteria and viruses, with minimal harm to humans, animals or plants."
—NASA, 1988.

"Chlorine dioxide: the most powerful pathogen killer known to man."
—The American Society of Analytical Chemists, 1999.

chelation agents can only grab hold of heavy metals they can reach on the periphery of cells and then let the body redistribute repeatedly.

Another reason that chlorine dioxide is both potent and low in side effects is that it's only active for a few hours. A single dose attacks pathogens for about four hours. It then breaks down into a few grains of salt. Another key factor in chlorine dioxide's effectiveness is that it hits all the pathogens at once so they don't have time to hide, recover and repopulate the gut. Most important, it weakens parasites directly so other elements of the protocol can drive them out.

In summary, chlorine dioxide is uniquely qualified to affect a narrower range of cells than more potent oxidizers such as hydrogen peroxide. Thus, chlorine dioxide attacks only pathogens. But those affected are impacted more: It nabs about 2½ times as many electrons as ozone. And, being good at neutralizing toxins, chlorine dioxide is good at cleaning up the waste products that spill out when you blow up a pathogen (causing Herxheimer).

Chlorine dioxide also treats Lyme's disease

Lyme's disease is a serious, chronic problem brought about by strains of bacteria such as borrelia burgdorferi and borrelia mayonii, acquired from infected ticks. It can cause flu-like symptoms, including joint and muscle pain, swelling and stiffness, chronic fatigue, fever, malaise, brain swelling, and neurological problems. In fact, it's one of the more common ailments known to undermine a person's health for many years unless/until you diagnose and treat it. Good thing for millions of suffers aware of its presence, chlorine dioxide is very effective at conquering Lyme disease for the same reasons that it wipes out parasites.

Summary of parasites

Parasites were the more demanding element of autism to deal with, because they actively pollute the gut with their toxic waste products. They're hard to drive out due to their defensive biofilm. They continue to reproduce until they're stopped somehow. And they steal nutrients from their host – making you weaker, and them stronger. But thanks to Jim Humble, Kerri Rivera, Dr. Andreas Kalcker and others, we now have protocols that consistently work well at reducing parasite populations in the gut and, with it, the symptoms of autism, Lyme's disease and also ADD.

In addition, Ken Rohla recommends GHC's *Oxy Powder Intestinal Cleanser* to amp up oxidation of parasites. It floods the GI tract with oxygen to weaken and kill anaerobic parasites. He also recommends "The Terminator Zapper" from worldwithoutparasites.com. It emits weak, negatively-charged square-wave electrical pulses that (positively-charged) parasites and pathogens can't stand.

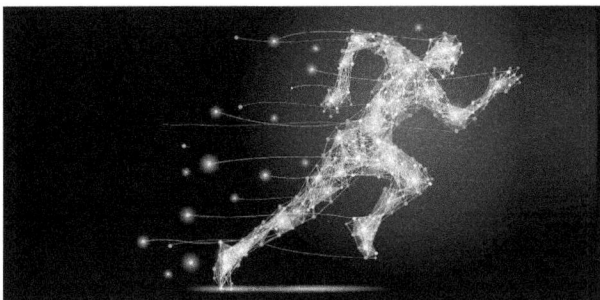

17

ADRENAL ENERGY AND THE STRESS RESPONSE

Everything that the body and mind do requires energy:
digesting food, using your brain, removing toxins, suppressing inflammation, fighting infection, making hormones, replenishing neurotransmitters, repairing cells, combating aging, and especially handling stressful situations. You can't name a bodily process that does not consume energy. Yet we tend to take our energy level for granted until we're unable to count on it being there when we need it. Like all innate aspects of being human, we don't appreciate what energy does for us until it's gone.

We have core energy needs such as respiration that are active full-time. And we have flexible needs, such as managing stress and removing toxins, which consume additional energy, on top of that used to keep you among the living. So, if you're like 99% of people, you need more energy. We all do. You can never have too much energy, because the body uses it for so many functions that we never think about. By this, I mean we all need more naturally-derived energy – not stress hormones squeezed from the adrenals.

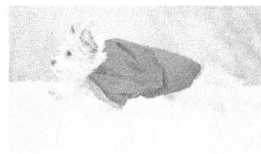

As we all should know by now, emergency energy is taxing on the body and in limited supply. Whereas real energy is healthy, empowering, and never needs to be repaid. To help Average Joes understand the difference between wholesome, native energy and "adrenal energy," we'll examine how the adrenals and thyroid raise our stress level and alertness to meet daily demands.

The stress response

The adrenals are designed to help you get through two types of situations that make the body and mind work harder: routine, daily demands, as well as acute and threatening emergencies. Your adrenals pick you up at times in the day when *routine daily tasks* require a higher systemic stress level. And your adrenals summon extra energy and alertness from your backup supply in order to cope with *emergency situations*.

Normal, daily stresses: Your adrenals help regulate normal, everyday activities, including waking and getting going, staying alert when blood-sugar drops after a meal, standing after squatting, and even shifting to a more intense task. In a normal day, the adrenals are designed to help you overcome significant, but temporary, *physical* stressors. Everyday activities like these normally don't put you into an energy debt.

Classic, acute stress: The classic example of acute stress is when a caveman had to fight a saber-toothed tiger in a kill-or-be-killed situation. When that happened, the incident occurred and it was over in minutes. So recovery time from stressful *events* like these were trivial.

Mental/emotional stress: Much harder on the body are our modern forms of acute and prolonged stress that tend to be more mental/emotional in nature, happen more often, last longer, and lack a physical outlet for expression. Examples would be repeatedly facing gunfire on the battlefield, working in a high-pressure sales job, moving to a new town, finding a new job, going through a breakup, or the death of a loved one.

Important in understanding the body's stress response, most situations from man's ancient past requiring adrenal intervention were employed to produce both a physical and mental response. That is, situations of-old were often both physical and mental challenges. For that reason, the adrenal system does not differentiate between physical, mental, or any other type of challenge. It treats all threats the same by releasing the same biochemicals – including stressors that fit into two newer categories: chemical and environmental stresses.

(Modern) Chemical and environmental stressors: Exposure to stressors such as bisphenol-A, artificial light, irregular sleep patterns, temperature extremes, and even high levels of fructose, create a persistent stress response from the adrenals, just like traditional kinds of stress.

Past (and future) stressors: Traumatic events such as early childhood trauma, rape, or war-related stress can permanently hyper-sensitize your stress response, unless/until you successfully process them psychologically. Obsessively worrying about future events, by itself, can chronically raise your baseline stress level.

So whether threats are physical, mental, emotional, chemical or environmental… whether they're in the past, present or future… whether they're real or imagined… your adrenals are constantly being tasked with the job of keeping you on top of all the challenges that your body and mind face on a daily and minute-by-minute basis. And the adrenals respond to these extra, sometimes extraordinary, demands on the body and mind by releasing more of the same stress-management chemicals that routine mental and physical challenges employ in order to activate certain mechanisms in the body, while deactivating others.

Key point: All these stressors have a cumulative effect on the adrenals and body. All these stressors "stack up," one on top of another, to form your total stress load. The sum total of all stresses in your life(style) turn into chemical wear and tear on your body. When any stressor occurs too frequently or too intensely, the persistent presence of stress chemicals disturbs the body's biochemical balance, which can lead to physical damage to cells, organs, and systems from the increased energy consumption (ATP) and decreased recovery (e.g., sleep).

Emergency energy consumption also tends to borrow energy and alertness from the future, which encourages you to keep borrowing from future reserves in the form of more stimulants to get you through each day, and each situation… or else suffer through an energy shortage we call a crash. Simply put, the use of your adrenals to survive emergency situations like these is increasingly stressful to sustain the longer it continues. And there's a variety of prices to pay for unrelenting stress in its many forms.

The adrenals activate the stress response through hormones

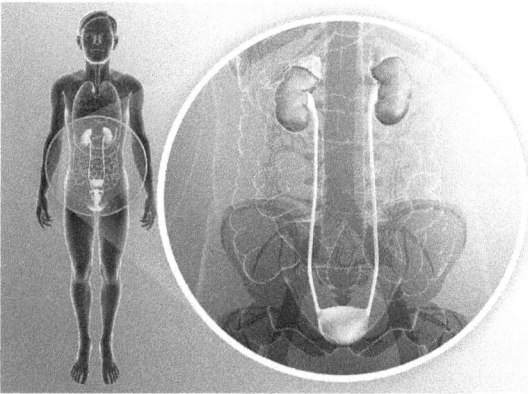

The adrenal glands are tiny, triangle-shaped organs sitting atop the kidneys. They are the body's pharmacy, making over fifty hormones that control virtually every endocrine-related function including the stress response, digestion, metabolism, immune system and sexual function. Specifically, the adrenal system makes hormones that help control blood sugar, blood pressure, stomach acid, electrolytes, blood pH, biorhythms such as sleep cycles, inflammation and sexual response.

Stress hormones turn on the body's "survival mode"

The adrenal system is responsible for releasing the stress hormones cortisol and adrenaline (also a neurotransmitter). Both help you cope with stressful situations by diverting resources away from bodily functions that can be postponed, toward organs and functions crucial to your immediate survival. To help you rise to an occasion, cortisol is designed to work in tandem with adrenaline to activate crisis programs. For example

- High cortisol shuts down production of **stomach acid,** because digesting food is less important than running or fighting for your life.
- Cortisol floods the body with **glucose** and inhibits **insulin production** to prevent that glucose from being stashed away in muscles.
- Cortisol directs **blood flow** away from visceral organs (e.g., stomach, intestines), toward muscles in the extremities so you can fight or flee.
- Cortisol shuts down the **immune system,** because fighting infection is a longer-range priority than fighting an adversary in front of you.
- Adrenaline raises **blood pressure.**
- Adrenaline raises **alertness and mental acuity.**

Together, cortisol and adrenaline prepare the body and mind for survival situations by calling upon every coping mechanism that the body can muster. As you might expect, this causes a number of adverse effects that grow from minor to major the longer they go on. The most important of which is that heightened adrenal activation turns off ordinary operating processes that burn food and make energy. And it turns on "survival mode" processes that store food for later use.

Key point: When you're in survival mode, the food you eat is not being converted into conventional energy to power everyday processes. Instead, it's being converted into fat – particularly belly fat – as a way to shortcut digestion. That lack of everyday energy tends to make you feel physically drained, emotionally spent, and mentally cloudy because the body shifts fuel consumption away from regular sources such as ATP, onto cortisol and adrenaline, thereby increasing wear and tear. Cortisol and adrenaline are the biochemicals released by the adrenals that flip the internal switch to either burn food or store it.

Especially important in GAPS conditions, about half the adrenaline released goes straight into the gut, stimulating pathogen growth such as E. coli by some 10,000 times. As a result, adrenal activation and stress hormones contribute to corruption of the gut. Cortisol is also the body's strongest anti-inflammatory, so elevated cortisol suppresses healing. And, as you're probably aware, over-activation of the adrenal system contributes to heart disease, sleep problems, physical exhaustion and mental burn-out. Yet, this is all when the adrenals are working properly.

Adrenal dysfunction
Mainstream medicine is just learning how to diagnose and treat adrenal dysfunction

Western medicine sometimes calls the inability to make stress hormones "Addison's disease." "Adrenal insufficiency," as it's also called, is autoimmunity of the adrenals. Other causes and conditions tend to be discounted. Western medicine pretty much dismisses adrenal fatigue as a figment of people's imagination because (1) doctors don't have a way to *test* for adrenal function, (2) they don't have a drug to *treat* it, (3) they don't have a surgery to *correct* it, and (4) the adrenal glands themselves rarely suffer from disease and dysfunction. Consequently, doctors tend to ignore that which they cannot diagnose or treat.

On the other hand, many alternative healers think the condition they call adrenal fatigue or adrenal exhaustion is just a mild case of Addison's. Disagreement is common about causes, conditions and names because the body's stress management systems are still a relatively new science. Medical science has yet to fully understand exactly which imbalances, processes and dysfunctions, coming from which organs and biochemicals, cause which symptoms and diseases. It's just within the last 15–20 years that leaders in the field have figured out what the body does when it's working properly, or is trying to do when it can't make enough energy.

Adrenals malfunction in three different ways. Think of them as

1. **Arrhythmia.** Here, nothing is wrong with the adrenals themselves, but they appear to be malfunctioning because their timing is off, causing surpluses or deficits at inappropriate times in the day.
2. **Overuse.** They're working properly, but not doing what you want. This is relatively quick and easy to fix (often completely) because there's nothing physically wrong with the thyroid and adrenals.
3. **Collapse.** They fail to make stress hormones because the thyroid itself is broken. 95% of the time, this is due to an autoimmune attack on the thyroid gland, producing Hashimoto's Disease.

The three categories of dysfunction have three different causes, and three distinct ways of treating them. So there is no blanket treatment to fix all adrenal or thyroid issues. You can't just take a thyroid support supplement and hope it will fix your energy issues. You might do exactly the wrong thing for your situation and make it worse.

1. Adrenal *arrhythmia*

Adrenal arrhythmia occurs when your daily rhythms are out of sync with your local light cycles. It's caused by a lack of natural sunlight on your eyes and skin, combined with excessive exposure to an altered light spectrum through most glass, glasses, sunglasses or contact lenses – as well as light from screens and artificial light sources. These sources modify or make light that is then unnatural.

When exposed to an altered light spectrum, your biorhythms fall out of sync with your environment due to too much blue light at night, and not enough ultraviolet and infrared exposure during the day. This dysregulates your circadian rhythms by releasing excessive hormones and neurotransmitters at the wrong times of day, thus depleting your stores. At the same time, your system isn't making biochemicals at full capacity due to lack of natural light. Full spectrum sunlight on the eyes makes biochemicals.

Conclusion: Adrenal arrhythmia is mostly a timing issue of your biochemistry that can be reversed by changing your daily routines.

- Correct your daily cycles of sleep, light, diet, stress level and stimulant intake. Read this book's sequel, *The Mitochondriac Manifesto,* for more information about light and seasonal eating.
- Watch the sunrise by looking in the general direction of the sun without glass, glasses or contacts for 30–45 min/day if you're unwell, 3–4 min/day done regularly. And watch the sunset, if possible. This sets your hormonal and neurotransmitter rhythms for the day.

- Avoid blue-spectrum light emitted by smartphones, computer screens, and LED lights after sundown. They expose you to colors unnatural for that time of day, which de-synchronize your circadian rhythms. The body releases dopamine, cortisol, and adrenaline in response.
- Get apps for your gadgets that shift color balance from blue to red.
- Button shirts to the top or wear a turtleneck to block blue light from hitting your throat area (blue light penetrates the skin 5–8cm, dysregulating the thyroid, which sits just below the surface).

Note: when wellness coaches say "blue light" we mean bright white light with a bluish tint.

To make it simple, follow Nature's rules, do what Nature does, and avoid man-made technologies.

2. Adrenal *overuse*

The adrenal system is designed to help you survive the occasional intense situation that doesn't last very long. However, if you're like many modern humans, you can't help but exhaust your adrenals day after day by (1) living in a perpetual state of stress – emotionally, mentally, physically and chemically; (2) not replacing nutrients after your adrenal system uses them up; (3) not getting enough quality sleep with which to renew; and (4) obsessing over social media, drama, smoking, risky behaviors, or worse to make up the deficit. To complicate matters, many people raise their alertness with chemical stimulants such as Ritalin, Adderall or caffeine.

Unfortunately, you have to repay some portion of tomorrow's energy that you expend today. There's a price to pay for energy debts and deferred maintenance, because even when stress hormones are being made and used properly, *adrenal overuse* creates problems such as nutrient depletion, sleep disturbances, weight gain, immune deficiency, and poor regeneration of cells and mitochondria.

"Adrenal fatigue" is a misnomer. For perspective, a leading expert in thyroid and adrenal health, Dr. Alan Christianson, believes "adrenal fatigue" is mis-labeled, or at least misleading because the adrenals are seldom exhausted to the point of incompetence, as the term "adrenal fatigue" suggests. Meaning, the literal description of adrenal fatigue is inaccurate. The adrenals are not fatigued in most cases, just you. The adrenals are still responding the way they should, in most people.

Thus, he and other experts now think the body is designed to debilitate you with cortisol and energy shortages to force you to slow down, recuperate and repair. The body does this by sending (or failing to send) hormonal signals along the "hypothalamic-pituitary-adrenal axis" (HPA axis) that tell the adrenals to cut cortisol production on purpose.

This condition, sometimes described as "HPA axis dysregulation or dysfunction," is a huge deal because it now affects a majority of people in the Western world to some extent, causing tiredness, "the blahs," and brain fog. HPA dysfunction is a more accurate term to describe what most people call adrenal fatigue. I'm calling it *adrenal overuse*.

Recovering from adrenal overuse

Most adrenal dysfunction is caused by poor signaling between the hypothalamus, pituitary, thyroid and adrenal glands. In most cases, the adrenals still respond to instructions from the hypothalamus and thyroid. They're just not getting the right messages to the right organ at the right times because of hormonal disturbances resulting from chronic inflammation, nutrient deficiencies and toxins – on top of complications with sleep cycles, light exposure and circadian rhythm.

Unfortunately for those hooked on modern medicine, there's no pill or powder you can take to reset your adrenals. Treatment usually involves lifestyle changes such as reducing your stress level at home and work, getting out into nature, sleeping better, reducing your dependence on coffee and stimulants, exercising regularly, and eating better to replenish nutrients that the adrenals need, such as vitamins C, B_5, B6 and B_{12}. You need to stop doing the things that exhaust your adrenals, and start doing the things that support them.

Glycogen. Glycogen is the body's most efficient form of energy. However, it takes 8–14 hours to make it – mostly from carbs. Therefore, you want to concentrate your protein consumption to earlier in the day to minimize blood-sugar spikes. And you want to concentrate your carbohydrate consumption to later in the day to make glycogen while you sleep. This means when you don't sleep enough, you don't make as much glycogen, and your body has to run on stress hormones, instead of regular fuels. You can also eat more fiber and green, leafy (alkalizing) vegetables throughout the day to moderate blood-sugar level.

The good news is, adrenal overuse problems are relatively straightforward to solve, considering how debilitating the symptoms can be. Most cases are fixed in under three months using standard treatment protocols. However, be aware of speedbumps such as…

Visceral fat increases cortisol. Belly fat (created by adrenal activation) increases cortisol. Visceral fat, as it's called, stores cortisone (a weaker version of cortisol). Every day, some of this cortisone is converted into cortisol, and back again, so that extra stress is built into each daily cycle. To put that another way, belly fat adds a certain amount of stress hormone (and timing) to your intrinsic circadian rhythm.

Visceral fat increases stress hormone in circulation, which promotes fat storage. Therefore, fat does more than just store calories. It's actually a pseudo-endocrine organ that influences hormone levels – just like the thyroid, adrenals and pancreas. The end result being, belly fat itself creates a stress response, in addition to more belly fat.

Talk to your holistic health professional for help in restoring adrenal function (mainstream doctors generally aren't good at fixing adrenal issues).

3. Adrenal *collapse* (aka "adrenal exhaustion" or "adrenal insufficiency," which is true dysfunction)

An even bigger problem than the first two conditions is when your adrenal system is completely unable to respond to daily ebbs and flows, no matter how much coffee you drink. In this situation, the adrenals truly don't work anymore. When this happens, the adrenals can't make enough cortisol (and sometimes aldosterone) to control essential body functions such as blood pressure, blood sugar and wakefulness. Lack of stress hormones is a far more serious problem to have than adrenal overuse, because a severe shortage of stress hormones causes systemic problems such as chronic fatigue or blood pressure so low that you can blackout just from standing up.

At the heart of this serious condition, the adrenals make most of the hormones that run the body. But when cortisol is not being made, for example, your adrenals also can't make the other cholesterol-based hormones, including estrogen, progesterone, aldosterone and testosterone. Lack of sex hormones testosterone or estrogen can make it hard for you to feel a sense of vitality.

Equally troubling, one of cortisol's most important functions is that it shuttles a wide variety of hormones into cells. So if you're deficient in cortisol, your system may be producing enough hormones, but they can't get where they need to go, which can impair endocrine-hormone function all over the body. In more serious cases of adrenal collapse, you can't even respond to daily demands like getting out of bed in the morning or showering. That's when adrenal collapse can cause physical and mental effects ranging from debilitating to life-threatening.

Adrenal collapse is caused most often by an autoimmune attack on the physiology of the adrenal glands. So it's treated with autoimmune protocols, such as a healing and sealing the gut lining, gluten and casein elimination diets, and anti-inflammatory efforts.

So adrenal fatigue is not just one thing

It's usually caused by some combination of mis-timing, overuse and true dysfunction. Therefore, successfully treating adrenal dysfunction may take a bit more understanding and effort to untangle the three forms of impairment that produce similar symptoms. It all starts with knowing what's really happening in the body when you're given the blanket diagnosis of "adrenal fatigue."

Thyroid

Dr. Christianson jokes that alternative healers tend to think everything's a thyroid issue, while mainstream doctors think nothing is caused by the thyroid. As a result, alternative healers tend to over-treat, while mainstream doctors tend to under-treat. The question then becomes 'is your tiredness due to rare dysfunction of stress organs? Or is the body simply telling you to slow down; you're overdoing it?'

Thyroid dysfunction can make your engine run slow or fast

The thyroid – which works in partnership with the adrenals – can also play a huge role in energy deficits, because it acts as the body's idle speed regulator and thermostat. When it's underactive, your systems related to energy production and consumption slow down and you feel sluggish all the time. **Hypothyroidism,** as depressed thyroid function is called, can cause symptoms such as

- extreme fatigue
- weight gain
- weakness
- cold hands, feet and body
- hair loss
- brittle nails
- dry skin
- constipation
- poor memory
- depression.

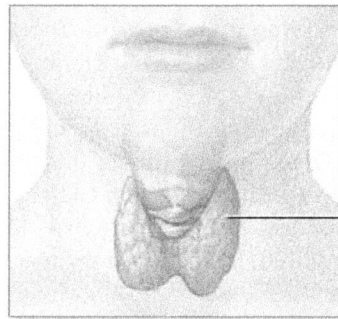

Thyroid gland

On the other hand, when the thyroid is overactive, you feel wired and often overstimulated, as if your internal engine is idling too fast. **Hyperthyroidism,** as it's called, can cause symptoms including

- unexplained weight loss
- tiredness and weakness
- difficulty sleeping
- heart palpitations
- increased sweating
- shortness of breath
- trembling in hands and fingers
- vision changes
- nervousness, irritability, and mood swings.

Important in GAPS conditions, thyroid problems can cause or worsen symptoms, similar to other sources of ADD. Underactive thyroid can decrease the activity of certain brain centers, leading to

problems with alertness, attention, memory or depression. On the other
hand, overactive thyroid can increase the activity of certain brain centers,
leading to a persistent anxiousness, irritability and moodiness.

Hypothyroidism and hyperthyroidism often cause hormonal and
neurotransmitter imbalances that can mimic other sources of attention
deficit, or overlap with them, which then complicate treatment. So these
are things you should look at when diagnosing and treating ADD,
especially when physical symptoms are present. Thyroid problems,
particularly hypothyroidism, are also known to cause infertility in women,
which conventional medicine is not good at diagnosing or treating.

The root of thyroid problems

Thyroid problems are quickly emerging as a major source of problems
(often going undiagnosed) in high-tech societies. A major cause: The
thyroid needs iodine so badly that it sucks up every bit of it that it can get
from the bloodstream and concentrates it. The problem is, it mistakes many
toxic substances for iodine – notably fluoride and chlorine – and actively
hoards these potent toxins. This includes radioactive isotopes of iodine and
other metals, resulting in radiation damage to the thyroid and whole body.

Further contaminating the thyroid are gluten, soy, perchlorates, PCBs,
dioxins, flame retardants, pesticides, plasticizers, antibacterial agents and
heavy metals. The immune system then attacks the toxins and accidentally
damages thyroid cells with friendly fire. The result being, either an
underactive condition called Hashimoto's thyroiditis, or an overactive
condition called Grave's disease – both autoimmune-related.

Hashimoto sufferers are often found to be deficient in selenium, vitamin
D, vitamin B_{12} and thiamin – which can then help reverse symptoms
when supplemented therapeutically. Seek a qualified thyroid and adrenal
specialist if your symptoms appear to indicate either condition, as both
Hashimoto's and Grave's forewarn of other autoimmune conditions.

A third less-serious thyroid problem is an enlarged thyroid, called a
"goiter," that may not bother the person at all. Goiter can be caused by
iodine deficiency or hormone imbalances, not primarily autoimmunity.
See the Recommended Resources page at the back for products to detox
radioactive substances from the body.

18

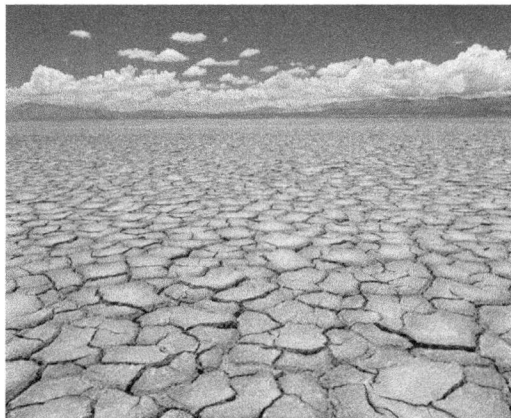

HYDRATION AND DEHYDRATION

We're all dehydrated inside cells... where it counts

We've all heard that it's important to stay well hydrated. But do you really know why? Do you really know how? What does water actually do inside the body when it's plentiful? And what happens when you don't have enough? There's a huge gap between what people think they know about hydration, and the real story of the vital role that water plays inside us. The surprising facts involve how water actually gets into cells, and what it does while it's there.

This is some of the most influential material in the *Gut-Brain Secrets* saga. And its influences are felt in nutrient delivery, energy usage, detoxification, disease resistance and anti–aging efforts. Hydration plays a crucial role in all aspects of human physiology. Whatever your state of health or dysfunction, water, properly utilized, is one of the best medicines you can take to optimize the performance of *your body of water* that you live with.

How do we get so dehydrated?

First, we drink too many diuretic (dehydrating) beverages like coffee, soft drinks, energy drinks, fruit juices and alcohol. Second, we don't drink enough pure water – many times due to a loss in sensation of thirst. Third, we've moved away from eating foods that are naturally abundant in water – toward processed foods that are relatively dry (e.g., breads and meat). Fourth, the water we drink doesn't get into cells for the reasons we'll discuss in a bit. And fifth, environmental threats like glyphosate, gluten, and pharmaceuticals interfere with the movement and usage of water throughout the body, which we'll also be discussing.

Daily water loss

Each day, we lose about

- 1.5 liters in urination through the **kidneys.**
- 0.5 liters in perspiration through the **skin.**
- 0.3 liters in bowel movements through the **colon.**
- 0.2 liters in breathing through the **lungs.**

Total water loss for an average person is 2.5 liters per day. Unfortunately, drinking more water is not necessarily the answer to raise hydration level, because we gradually lose the ability to get water into the interior of cells as we age. At the same time, many people perpetuate a state of dehydration by purposely avoiding water because it makes them visit the bathroom more than they'd like, or because their feet swell.

To give you a sense for how dehydration progresses in a lifetime: when we're born, the total volume of water inside our cells compared to outside is 1.1 to 1. By the time we're 80 years of age, this ratio drops to 0.8 to 1. That may not sound like a lot percentage-wise. But that 27% drop represents not just a reduction in cell volume. It represents a great deal of the aging process, because the body loses efficiencies in the absence of water, and must employ coping mechanisms when it doesn't have enough.

Misconceptions we have about water

False belief #1: Drink plenty of water and you must be hydrated. For babies in perfect health, and less affected by toxins, hydration is easy. However, as we age, we lose the ability to get water from the bloodstream and extracellular space into cells, where it can do its job. To rephrase, if you drink more water, and it doesn't get into cells, you're just going to pee it out without accomplishing the more important things that water is supposed to do for us. Think of it this way: From birth to death, our ability to get water into cells drops steadily from 100% to let's say 35%. That number, as we'll discuss in a minute, determines the rate at which we age biologically. Bottom line: The ability to get water into the cell, and the ability to clean toxins out, is a majority of the aging process.

False belief #2: Clear urine means you're well hydrated. We've all been told to drink enough water so that your pee is lighter in color. That means you're well-hydrated, right? Well, not exactly. Clear urine simply means that water entered and left your body with no cellular waste products to darken its color. On rare occasions, it means you drank enough water to dilute a healthy flow of waste products to a clear state. But in the majority of cases, especially in advanced age, it might mean that water never saw the interior of a cell. It got into the bloodstream, circulated around, and did little more than bulk up your blood volume. This is not the same as true hydration. So, whether you drink copious amounts of water, or you receive many liters intravenously in a hospital setting, having lots of water in the bloodstream does not necessarily mean it's getting to where it really needs to go: inside the cell.

False belief #3: Thirst indicates dehydration. Instrumental to the aging process, we lose the perception of thirst as we get older. It's like dryness becomes the body's new normal as time goes by, and so we don't even realize when our cells are starving for water. Consequently, we don't drink as much as we should. Thus nutrients don't get in. Toxins don't get out. Inflammation persists. And aging accelerates.

That's why this information is so crucial to the wellness and longevity of us all: It's a subtle, secret driver of the entire aging and decrepitude process. On the flip side, replacing your declining sensation of thirst with an active hydration program can work wonders in outsmarting the aging process and staying young on a cell level.

False belief #4: If it's fluid, it can hydrate like water. The truth is, nothing hydrates the body as well as pure water. Milk, for example, is basically food in a liquid form. Although milk does contain plenty of water, it carries baggage that restricts its ability to hydrate the body. It takes a lot more work for the digestive system to separate water from milk's other constituents. Same thing goes for vegetable juices, soups and smoothies. They do have high water content. But it's nowhere near as plentiful or accessible as pure water, because they contain other substances that complicate the process.

False belief #5: Dry mouth is a reliable sign of dehydration. Some people say that the presence of dry mouth indicates dehydration. But, really, it's not the greatest way to diagnose dehydration, because a variety of situations can make you misread your state of hydration. First, the body places a high priority on chewing, swallowing and digestion. So it puts salivation high in its pecking order of water allocation – even when the rest of the body is dehydrated. Plus, the mere thought of eating can make a person salivate in anticipation. On the other hand, nervousness is notorious for shutting down salivation and causing "cotton mouth" – even when the body is fully hydrated. Bottom line: A dry mouth is one of the more severe signs of dehydration. So you can't rely on it to tell you when you need more water.

False belief #6: Solutes (particulate solids) do all the work in the body. Medical science has long thought that the stuff dissolved and transported around in water does all the work. The assumption was, the therapeutic agents and nutrients dissolved in water performed all the biological functions that science cared to examine, and that water has no direct metabolic role in these processes. They believed water was merely a taxi cab in biology. But researchers in recent decades have come to understand that water plays as many essential roles in human physiology, if not more, than the substances it solubilizes and shuttles around. It's much more of an active participant than a means of transportation.

False belief #7: The body's water regulation mechanisms don't change during a person's lifetime. As we age, we gradually lose the ability to get water in and use it to full effect. This is the crux of the aging process (unless we take steps to tame it).

What happens when you're dehydrated?
(Water-rationing programs, crisis calls, and disease complications)

Dehydration disrupts a wide range of processes we count on every day for our bodies to run properly. Here are some hidden consequences of water scarcity in the body:

This list is from the book Your Body's Many Cries for Water, *by Dr. Fereydoon Batmanghelidj.*

1. **Back pain.** 75% of our upper body weight is supported by fluid in the discs of the spine. 25% is supported by fibers around the discs. So prolonged sitting, standing, or exertion basically squeezes water out of the discs and fibers, thereby compressing the supportive structures of the back, leaving no cushioning to relieve the stress. Using simple hydration strategies, many people are shocked to find that their back pain goes away simply by drinking more water instead of soft drinks, fruit juices and coffee.

2. **Stomach ulcers.** The stomach's protective layer of mucosal lining is made mostly of water. So it's one of the first areas to be impaired by dehydration. The remedy: You can support the stomach's natural barrier to acidity by drinking a glass of water thirty minutes before eating. This thickens the mucosal wall, thereby protecting the walls of the stomach from its hydrochloric acid, and preventing ulcers from forming. Avoid drinking too much as you eat though, because fluids dilute stomach acid and can impair digestion.

3. **General pain.** Nerve endings interpret a high acidity level in tissue as pain. So locally-produced pain (as opposed to pain produced by the central nervous system) can be caused by a shortage of water to wash acidic compounds out of tissues.

4. **Asthma.** The body uses the neurotransmitter histamine to regulate water use, and to manage drought. What happens in cases of asthma is, histamine constricts the bronchial tubes in an effort to minimize water lost through respiration of the lungs.

5. **Allergies.** Excess histamine in drought conditions hyperactivates the immune system in the nasal sinuses (i.e., inflammation), leading to an allergic-type reaction to pollen, dust and dander. Consequently, many people are amazed to learn they can reduce or eliminate allergies just by drinking more water. This is shown to calm down inflammation and allergies – even if someone has had allergies since childhood.

6. **High blood pressure.** In dehydration, little capillary networks shut down to conserve full blood volume in other vessels. With more resistance to flow, and less vasculature to distribute the load, pressure has to be increased to keep the blood pumping.

7. **Edema.** The body so desperately needs water when chronically dehydrated that it sometimes stores water as edema, and tries to force the water into cells by increasing blood pressure and retaining salt.

8. **Headache.** Brain cells shrink from lack of water, causing headache.

9. **Hormones and insulin issues.** Drought messes with hormones, and can contribute to metabolic problems. In dehydration, prostaglandin E (a drought regulator subordinate to histamine) lowers insulin production as a coping mechanism to keep sugar, potassium, amino acids, and water out of cells. Water can then be used for more critical needs such as digestion and the brain (that doesn't use insulin). All that contributes to insulin dysfunction and metabolic issues.

10. **Hard, dry stools and constipation.** The colon removes water from fecal material to form stools. So, in an effort to conserve water, the colon is ordered to save every last drop that it can, which can make stools overly firm, dry, and possibly hard to move.

11. **Weaker oxygenation.** The smallest air sacs of the lungs, called alveoli, use moisture to exchange CO_2 with O_2. So when you're dehydrated, the lungs can't completely get rid of all the CO_2 wanting to leave the bloodstream, and you lose oxygen–exchange capacity.

12. **Joint pain/rheumatoid arthritis.** Cartilage lubricates joint movement. To do that, it needs to hold water in its structure. So in a well-hydrated state, the friction and normal wearing away of cartilage is minimal. But when water is withheld, cartilage shrinks and becomes abrasive. It then wears away faster than it can be replaced.

13. **Digestive problems.** In the mouth, saliva solubilizes and lubricates the food we chew and swallow. In the stomach, the very act of breaking down food requires gastric juices in order to turn solid material into a nutrient soup. After the stomach, the pancreas needs water and salt to make the sodium bicarbonate solution that neutralizes the acidity of material leaving the stomach. All these depend on water to make them go. And digestion is a high-priority activity. So, in mild dehydration, the body takes water away from other processes to make sure digestion proceeds as planned.

14. **High cholesterol.** In a well-hydrated state, water gets into cells through gaps in their membranes. But in a drought, the body plugs up those holes with cholesterol to retain water. So rehydrating alone is shown to reduce cholesterol levels.

15. **Disturbed brain function.** The brain is a hydroelectric system. It contains the highest percentage of water of any body tissue. But in prolonged dehydration, brain cells shrink, blood flow diminishes (particularly in capillaries), minerals aren't broken down properly, and amino acid levels (the precursors to neurotransmitters) suffer. Water is also supposed to deliver neurotransmitters to nerve endings. So no hydro, no brain function. As a result, dehydration can cause or contribute to depression, negative thought patterns, multiple sclerosis, ALS and Alzheimer's.

All of this goes to show that a plethora of problems is caused, or worsened, by poor hydration in the cells: Water can't get in. Minerals and glucose can't get in. And detoxification slows. The geometry of proteins changes so they don't work properly. And aging accelerates. Are you beginning to see how water deprivation is making us sick and tired, without us having the slightest clue why it's happening, or how to fix it?

Dr. Fereydoon Batmanghelidj (author, *Your Body's Many Cries for Water*)
"We are beginning to understand dehydration manifests itself in as many ways as we in medicine have invented disease conditions. We in medicine, not knowing that dehydration becomes symptom-producing, and lack of water in the body is pathology-producing – we have labeled states of dehydration, and complications of dehydration, as disease conditions… and most often diseases of unknown origin. When the body has been calling for water, it has become [standard practice in medicine] to give it toxic chemicals."

Minerals/electrolytes
The body needs minerals in its water
As you know, sweat, tears, blood, and most bodily fluids taste salty. The reason is, once water enters the body, it is not normally present as pure water. Instead, the body needs water to be in a solution of minerals (electrolytes). Water must contain minerals because pretty much all biochemical reactions take place in a bath of water and minerals. That's what makes body fluids taste salty: it's the minerals.

Therefore, problems can arise when bodily fluids have too much water, and not enough minerals. For example, people have died from drinking too much water in water drinking contests. Likewise, people can die when they sweat profusely for many hours and replenish with mineral-free water. The point is, the body needs minerals to perform critical tasks such as sending nerve conduction signals that run the heart, brain and nervous system. So when the concentration of minerals in water drops too low (or too high), delicate processes all over the body can malfunction and cause medical emergencies

Natural water bodies are full of electrolytes
Lakes and streams have mineral compounds of sodium, potassium, chloride, calcium, magnesium, and phosphate that make water electrically conductive. It's these electrolytes, and resulting electrical conductivity, that pulls water into cells. But, to our detriment, civilization separates us from the high-electrolyte water that our ancestors used to drink and bathe in which offered them full hydration.

Today, to reduce contamination and disease, sanitation methods such as reverse osmosis, distillation, and carbon filtration remove the beneficial minerals that move water across cell membranes. This means the water we drink today has been substantially disempowered of its hydration ability, for the sake of mass consumption. As a result, our efforts to drink more water give us some fraction of the nutritional, energetic, detoxification, anti-inflammatory, and anti-aging benefit that pristine water sources once did. When water is devoid of electrolytes, it loses ability to get inside cells. And when water can't get inside of cells

- Minerals, vitamins, and therapeutic agents pass through the bloodstream, without giving you their full benefit.
- The body has a harder time cleaning out oxidative compounds (inflammatory waste products) from inside and outside of cells. This perpetuates inflammation.
- Detoxification in general is compromised because, like a slower moving stream, there's less water to rinse away waste material.

Salt does many things for you

Water and salt work as a team in hydrating the body. Too much of one, and not enough of the other, can cause unexpected problems that can be difficult to diagnose. So make sure to include sea salt in your hydration hacks, or else you may cause imbalances like the following:

- Nerve impulses are electro-chemical in nature. And salt is one of the main ingredients needed to **conduct nerve signals** between cells.
- **Muscle cramps** are often caused by salt depletion from prolonged sweating and dehydration.
- Salt is a strong **antihistamine,** so it can be used in conjunction with water to relieve asthma and allergies.
- Salt deficiency derails digestion because **stomach acid** is made from salt and water. So when you're low on salt, minerals don't get broken down properly, causing deficiencies of zinc, magnesium, manganese, selenium, copper, chromium and molybdenum.
- Salt helps **break down mucus plugs and sticky phlegm** in the lungs, thereby unblocking congestion and stuffiness.
- Salt is vital for **bladder control.** Low salt, plus high water intake, can cause muscle weakness and leaky bladder.
- The sodium portion of salt carries glucose across the brush border of the gut lining. Without sodium, **glucose absorption** is stymied in the gut. That's one reason people feel lackadaisical on a salt-free diet.
- The brain needs salt to **maintain alkalinity.** Cells have pumps that let one molecule of salt in for every (acidic) hydrogen ion released. This flushes acidity out of the brain.
- Salt helps you **sleep** – naturally.

- Salt inhibits excess **saliva production** when you sleep.
- Physicians tells us that salt is a primary cause of **high blood pressure.**
  This is inaccurate thinking. When the body retains salt, what it's
  really trying to do is hold on to water to maintain full blood volume.
  So the solution is not to increase urination with diuretics to excrete
  salt. It's to increase water intake. This reduces blood pressure, and
  the need to retain salt.

As a general rule, every two liters of water that you drink each day should
contain three grams (½ tsp.) of quality salt somewhere in your diet.

Magnesium moves insulin, thus raising hydration capacity and ATP

We know that insulin drives glucose into cells. But far fewer have heard
that the movement of insulin from the liver into the bloodstream, then
the bloodstream into the cells, uses magnesium. You can't move insulin
and glucose around without magnesium. Therefore, when you increase
your magnesium intake – whether in food or by supplementation – you
expand your insulin availability, which carries glucose into cells better.
More glucose feeds mitochondria better, which increases energy
production and hydration ability.

Float tanks give you mega doses of magnesium

Magnesium is one of the best electrolytes to increase water's electrical
charge. It's also among the most desperately needed to calm the mind and
relax the body. Yet, most of us are substantially mag deficient because we
no longer get it from natural water sources like we used to. That makes
float tanks a superb shortcut to get magnesium into your system quickly
and safely, without inconveniences such as loose stool. In fact, floating for
just an hour or so in a 25% solution of magnesium salt lets your skin
absorb the equivalent of several months' of dietary intake. Many people
even report transcendental experiences, similar to states of deep meditation.

Water's role in toxicity and aging

The hydration cycle in biology

Hydration in humans begins with water being extracted from food in the
intestines. That water is transited across the gut lining, into the
bloodstream. From the bloodstream, it gets into the extracellular matrix
(between cells) so it's available to the cell. At that point, electrons (and
their electrical charge) originating from the electron transport chain can
pull water inside the cell. On the way out, the kidneys filter toxins out of
the blood, and the colon forms stools by removing water.

Fouling up these processes, toxins like glyphosate, gluten, and alcohol
break down the tight junctions that hold cells together into cohesive
barriers. These living, intelligent barriers are supposed to actively

modulate the movement of water and materials across the gut, brain, kidneys and vasculature. However, when tight junction damage breeches the gut barrier, electrical charge can't be maintained across the gut membrane. Water then can't get into the bloodstream and extracellular space. The kidneys also don't filter toxins properly on the way out. And the colon loses control over the amount of water it leaves in stools.

Hydrological mayhem makes it more difficult to get water into cells. So the first step of improving your hydration ability is to support tight junction integrity, and the barriers they form, so that the body can direct water through the bloodstream, tissues, cells, kidneys and colon.

Nothing scrubs toxins, acidity, and inflammation out of the cell better than water

Water is the ultimate cleanser. Water dissolves, dilutes, and carries away toxins, as well as oxidative compounds and metabolic waste products. However, the average person drinks only a liter of water per day – despite the fact that the kidneys filter over 200 liters of fluid a day. So, if you only put back a liter of fluid to the volume with which the body can do its work, you handicap its ability to separate the "wheat from the chaff" and rinse the waste away.

As an adaptation mechanism, the body then borrows essential amino acids such as tryptophan, tyrosine, methionine, cysteine, and histidine to de-acidify those waste products, where they are stored. The body basically can't wash the toxins out of the cells. So it does the next best thing to minimize the damage: it takes neurotransmitter precursors out of circulation and uses them as antioxidants to make the intracellular garbage less toxic where it is.

This further depletes the body's neurotransmitter availability – regardless of how the shortage affects brain and nervous system function. In consequence, oxidative compounds accumulate in cells, and inflammation lingers. Without reacting chemically, water also reduces acidity throughout the body simply by making more urine and washing away acidic substances that salt helped to draw out.

"Phase angle" can measure hydration potential and biologic age

Phase angle is one of the best measurements of biologic age. It is read by: (1) sticking electrodes on the wrist, finger, ankle and toe; (2) laying the person flat; (3) keeping respiration at a resting rate; and (4) measuring electrical resistance between the electrodes. The electrical resistance (and reactance) shown in your phase angle tells you **the capacity of single cell membranes to hold an electrical charge,** which indicates the cell's ability to draw in water, **due to voltage differentials inside *vs.* out.**

Phase angle ranges from 3.5–10, or higher.

- A phase angle of 10 or higher, indicates ideal health and youthfulness. When you have a phase angle of 10–12, the electrical charge held across a single cell membrane (just a few microns thick) is estimated to be greater than 10,000 volts!
- Those in good health (i.e., most people) register between 6 and 8.
- Cancer tends to happen below a phase angle of 4.5.
- And death happens below a phase angle of 3.5.

One point in phase angle represents about 10–15 years of biologic aging. If you were to go up a point, your risk for getting a chronic disease plummets because you've turned your biologic clock back a decade or more in the factors that cause aging. For example, when you improve your phase angle, you increase your hydration ability substantially **without drinking more water.** On the other hand, if you drink more water with a low phase angle, you're likely to pee out most of it before reaching the interior of a cell.

Phase angle is a foundational, long-term indicator that changes very slowly over time. So you don't lose whole points off of your phase angle just by eating crappy on vacation, missing a few days of sleep, or stressing out making a deadline. Conversely, you can't eat right and drink lots of fluid for a few days to make your phase angle go up significantly. Instead, it might take 6–12 months of consistent effort to improve your phase angle by a single point. Why so slowly? It's measuring your body's ability to produce electrical charge, hydrate, detox, heal, and resist aging via mitochondrial productivity – all core drivers of health or sickness.

In years of measuring phase angle in his patients, Dr. Bush has never seen a person come into his clinic complaining of sickness, having a phase angle above 7. That's because when you've got a high phase angle, it's very difficult to get a life-threatening cancer, as an example. On the other hand, it's very difficult to beat cancer if your phase angle is low. You see, cancer isn't a disease that pops up out of nowhere. Instead, it's a lack of water inside of cells that's causing an accumulation of toxins, oxidative damage, and DNA damage that virtually define the cancer process. Dr. Zach Bush: "If you look at human biology as either *water* or *not water*, cancer doesn't happen until you're so dry that you're nearly dead."

Dr. Zach Bush

"As we age, we lose the ability to get water from the vasculature, or the extracellular environment, [to the] inside of our cells. If we could stay perfectly hydrated in the intracellular environment, our aging would slow down, if not reverse. And the reason is: water is the ultimate scrubber [of toxins and cellular waste products]."

Dr. Zach Bush's hydration tips

1. Support tight junctions and barrier membranes. The first goal in hydrating the body is getting water absorbed from the digestive tract into the bloodstream. Leaky gut prevents water from entering the body's first interior compartment, due to the fact that tight junction damage inflames the gut wall and reduces electrical charge across it.

So the first order of business is to protect the tight junctions from injury by adding ION Gut Support to your regimen, and subtracting glyphosate, gluten, medications like NSAIDs and candida. This revives the gut lining's intelligence that was injured by excess zonulin. When the tight junctions are healed, electrical charge is reestablished. Water can then be pulled into the bloodstream and cells. And it can be moved out at the end of the hydration cycle, with toxins in-tow.

2. Reduce your nnEMF exposure. The EMF frequencies all around us are mostly microwaves. And what does everyone know about microwave ovens? They dehydrate. They bombard food with microwave radiation so strong that it shakes water molecules loose from their surroundings. That's why steam pours out of food heated in a microwave oven. And that's how cell phones, Wi-Fi, and IoT devices unquestionably dehydrate you in their presence. Microwave frequencies, in particular, disturb the efficiency with which mitochondria make ATP, thereby making less water (mitochondria make water). The solution? Stop using hand-held microwave devices, put more distance between you and the devices, drink more water, or all of the above. See also: *The Mitochondria Manifesto* for tips on how to reduce your nnEMF exposure.

3. Replace electrolytes. Water needs an electrical charge to get inside of cells the way that it's supposed to. This is the job of minerals/electrolytes. However, very few people have a drinkable stream or lake nearby. So you have to add electrolytes to replicate natural (unadulterated) water. Lots of powders and liquids have good formulations. Experiment to see which ones work best for you, and that you can tolerate. Liquids tend to be more concentrated. Go up in dosage until you start getting loose stools. Then back off, until find your bowel tolerance.

4. Hydrate and detoxify by alternating water types. Every thirty minutes, alternate between drinking four ounces of electrolyte–rich water, which gives minerals, to four ounces of distilled water, which pulls toxins out. This creates a pumping action at a cell level – basically pushing water and beneficial agents into the cell to start the cycle, and drawing waste products out to complete the cycle.

You see, distilled water is a "hungry" water. It's so devoid of minerals that it sucks them up like an empty sponge. In fact, distilled water is so eager to grab hold of charged particles, that even when it can't get inside of a cell, it still creates an osmotic gradient across the cell membrane that pulls toxins and waste products out. So when you don't have enough electrical potential to get water into the cell, no problem. Distilled water can still pull toxins out as it moseys by.

Through this method of pulsing your intake, you dramatically increase your ability to take nutrients and therapeutics in, and move toxins out. A good rule of thumb is to drink half your body weight in ounces each day. So a 160 lb. person should drink about 80 oz. of water a day. Pulse your water intake for most of the day, stopping a few hours before bedtime.

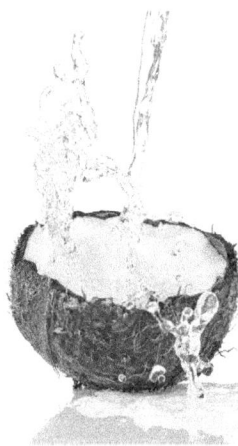

For more information, watch Dr. Joseph Mercola interview Dr. Zach Bush: https://youtu.be/FB Zfdmvn2aA, as well as "The Importance of Salt and Water", presented by Barbara O'Neill, ND: https://youtu.be/D m6fmiG4SAc.

Other hydration strategies

1. **Drink more water.** Duh. And purity matters. Make it easy on your detox systems by testing your water supply, filtering it, or buying water that helps your body remove toxins, not adding to your already high toxin load.

2. **Reduce beverages and foods that dehydrate.** Avoid diuretic beverages like coffee, soft drinks, and energy drinks because caffeine dehydrates. Stay away from fruit juices and sweetened beverages because sugar dehydrates as well. Their concentrated sweeteners are a burden on your system. Avoid alcohol for the same reasons. And cut down on salty foods when you can. They soak up water.

   Diuretic: Makes you pee out more than you drink.

3. **Barbara O'Neill's sea salt "hydration hack."** Dissolve a crystal of Celtic sea salt under the tongue as you drink some water, or before. It's absorbed quickly through the oral mucosa, and beats the water into the bloodstream. The salt then gets into cells first, which pulls water inside from the magnesium in the salt (it's hydrophilic). Just make sure not to put the salt directly in the water you drink. It will just absorb water before it enters the cell and not help you hydrate.

4. **Hydration protocols work better when you're fasting.** Fasting reduces the workload on your detox pathways. And it clears the exit routes out of your body. In contrast, when you do a hydration protocol in a fed state, a lot of that water will be retained by food in the gut. Whereas, when you do a hydration protocol while fasting, more of that water is available to be used by cells and mitochondria. For these reasons, Dr. Bush starts his patients on 3–4 days of hydration protocol on day 1 or 2 of a fast.

5. **Fiber helps manage hydration.** Fiber helps the body manage water more efficiently by grabbing hold of it and escorting it slowly through the digestive tract. This allows more time for the water to get to the places it needs to go, instead of running right through

you. Fiber is also often accompanied by nutrients when it comes from a whole food. And it feeds microflora the cellulose that they thrive on. Organified silica from horsetail also aids hydration and is beneficial for the microbiome. But you do NOT want to ingest silica in a mineral form (the primary ingredient in glass) because it's super oxidative and dehydrating.

6. **Spread out your intake.** Drink small amounts throughout the day, instead of all at once. That makes it easier for the body to absorb. You may want to add a mild natural flavoring like lemon juice to pure water so the digestive tract takes longer to process it.

7. **Get more water from moisture-rich foods.** Unsweetened tea, unprocessed broths, and homemade soups are good ways to hydrate, as are fruits and vegetables with a high water content. This is how we used to get much of our water.

9. **Drink water sparingly with meals.** Water dilutes stomach acid, which neutralizes its acidity and can impair digestion. Instead, drink most of your water up to a half an hour before, or 1½–2 hours after meals.

Water quality

We've talked about the health effects of what *is* in the water you drink. Now let's examine the importance of what you want to *avoid* in water:

- Test your water supply. The most common contaminants to look for are chlorine, chloramine and fluoride, as well as residues of birth control pills, antidepressant/anti-anxiety meds, statins, beta blockers, and hormone replacement therapy such as artificial estrogen, progesterone and testosterone. Unfortunately, many municipalities rotate sources, and may mix them, so you may never know for sure what you're going to get on a given day. Consider collecting samples at different times, over a course of several weeks.

- Don't assume bottled water is pure and healthy. Most brands are sourced from municipal water systems, use fungal-promoting reverse osmosis filtration, and are contained in plastic bottles that leech toxins such as bisphenol-A. Glass bottles protect purity better than plastic.

- Spring water is usually better than city water. Water gains trace minerals, beneficial microorganisms, and subtle energies as it moves through the hydrological cycle.

- Fluoride is not your friend. Do whatever it takes to make sure there's no fluoride in your water. Filter it, or buy natural spring water. Even reverse-osmosis water is better than fluoridated water.

- Chlorine is pretty bad too. Reduce your water's chlorine content by letting it sit in an open container overnight. Since chlorine is a gas in its natural state, it off-gasses over several hours. However, chloramines (a chemical cousin of chlorine used to disinfect) evaporate much more slowly. So this trick doesn't work with them.

- Get a water filter that reduces toxins to undetectable levels, and keeps performing that way for many months. Make sure it removes the hard stuff like chloramines, heavy metals, crop chemicals, SSRIs and birth control hormones. In most cases, the bigger, the better, because small filters lose effectiveness quickly. Or change the filter frequently. Get a whole-house water filter if you can afford it.

- Even if the water you drink and cook with is bottled or filtered, you still need to consider the water you absorb bathing and showering, because any water that touches your skin is absorbed in seconds and enters the bloodstream. You can absorb up to a pound of water when you shower, bathe or swim.

Do what you can do. Testing your water can be very revealing. Consider buying an advanced water filtration system that reduces harmful chemicals to undetectable levels, while leaving the trace minerals. A whole-home system can be a sizable investment, while an under-sink one is a fraction the cost. It's impossible to avoid all toxins, so just do your best.

Water's energetic properties are the 2ⁿᵈ half of this story

Read *The Mitochondriac Manifesto* to learn how water, when exposed to natural light frequencies from in and outside the body, becomes a battery that holds energy, powers cellular activities, and allows proteins to maintain their proper shape and function.

19

MANAGING THE SYMPTOMS OF ADD
(Without fixing root causes)

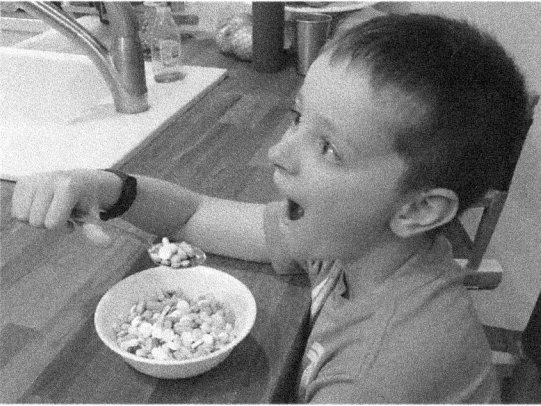

Perfecting neurotransmitter levels with drugs can be difficult and time-consuming

Finding that perfect balance of brain chemicals using drugs is complicated for these reasons:

1. **Complex interactions and counter-actions.** No drugs act in isolation. Some complement others. Some work in opposition to another. So it's very hard to predict how a drug will affect the body for the better or worse.
2. **The body doesn't have an instrument panel.** With orthodox medicine failing to keep up with worsening disease, most of us have to learn how to play detective as to why the body is doing what it's doing, and what will improve your results.
3. **Diet.** Changes in diet alter neurotransmitter production.
4. **Lifestyle choices.** Getting it right is a moving target because life happens, and you have to figure out how to stay ahead of disease.

When it comes to neurotransmitters and hormones, surpluses can throw you for a loop just as much as deficiencies, because the biochemistry of the mind and body is designed to operate within strict tolerances. If something is off just a little bit, the brain will still run, but you'll experience the difference between 'working' and 'working optimally.'

That means finding perfection through pharmaceutical intervention is like looking for a needle in a haystack – especially when you're dealing with many symptoms, multiple disorders, several drugs, and variable side effects. So, frankly, most people settle for moderate improvements in their symptoms, while tolerating annoying effects as the cost of progress.

Stated another way, it's really hard to duplicate the body's innate intelligence in balancing your biochemistry for your present situation. Your body has the instruction manual to run its own systems. And it has instruments to read the situation accurately. But you don't. Now can you can see why it's so difficult to simultaneously fix the symptoms you want to fix, create no side effects, and maintain that state of improvement, without developing a tolerance to medications?

Finding the right medications for you

In theory, there isn't any difference between brand name drugs *vs.* generic. But there certainly is. There can be substantial differences in both effects and side effects, due to slight variations in manufacturing. Drugs can affect you in different ways, depending on some of these factors:

- **Brand.** Each brand is made slightly differently, with multiple steps in manufacturing where variation can occur (as Heisenberg and Pinkman taught us). This leads to very slight differences in molecular composition and trace substances that change the way a drug affects a person's biochemistry. And going with the brand name is no guarantee it will work better, though that is often the case.

- **The pill itself.** Pill size (dosage) can make a big difference. For example, 2–10mg pills might work better than 1–20mg pill, or vice-versa. Pill size can make a difference, even when they're made by the same company. How that happens is anyone's guess. Perhaps they're made in different factories, using slightly different processes.

- **Incidental/accidental ingredients.** Colorings/dyes, coatings, and binders can make a bigger difference than you might think. Some people may react to those dyes or coatings, as Dr. Feingold suggests.

In addition to intended effects, *unintended side effects* can differ substantially between brands, pill sizes, and other ingredients. Some might give you unacceptable reactions, while another might get along much better with your system. Of course, total dosage makes a big difference, as well as interactions between drugs.

Residual "ramp down" from previous doses may complicate matters. And tolerances will usually develop to ADD drugs when taken in moderate to high dosages, thereby requiring higher and higher dosages to achieve the same effect. Foods can also interfere with a drug's effect. In particular, orange juice and foods high in vitamin C can inhibit the effects of methylphenidate. And, let's not forget, lifestyle issues can complicate matters further – including diet, exercise/lack thereof, toxins, stress, smoking, alcohol and sleep.

Dopamine and serotonin tend to work in opposition to each other

Another challenge in finding a good regimen is that when dopamine goes up, serotonin usually goes down. Stimulants raise dopamine level, while lowering serotonin. This can increase anxiety, aggression and irritability, as you raise alertness. On the other hand, taking antidepressants (SSRIs) to raise serotonin can make dopamine go down, and you're back to square one.

You need a balance of the two for your brain to function at its best. So the trick to maximizing brain function in most cases of ADD is increasing both dopamine and serotonin at the same time. Otherwise, you and your brain may operate better in some ways, but you may suffer unwanted side effects to achieve those benefits, which kind of defeats the purpose of taking drugs in the first place.☹

A few classes of drugs are known to increase both at the same time. But finding the best combo is seldom a cut-and-dry affair. Consult a knowledgeable specialist for help.

Trace amounts of some stimulants take days or weeks to eliminate

An unfortunate side effect of increased attention span, amphetamines contribute to adrenal use and exhaustion. Prescription stimulants are basically chemically-induced stress which can lead to adrenal depletion. Unfortunately, they take much longer to eliminate than people realize.

Not widely known, Adderall, Dexedrine, Vyvanse, and Desoxyn haven't completely left the body, just because you can't feel their effects any longer. After a quick ramp-up period, levels of these amphetamine stimulants seem to decline slowly over 2.5–8 hours in most people, like a gently downward-sloping plateau. Then, toward the end of a dose's effective duration, elimination organs hustle enough of it out so that your blood level dips below your conscious awareness. The remainder then trickles out slowly over about four or five days, as elimination organs remove the last traces of that dose.

Caffeine follows a similar elimination pattern, depending on the speed with which a person is genetically predisposed to eliminating it. In contrast, almost all methylphenidate (Ritalin) is gone in six hours.

Consuming certain stimulants every day without a break allows trace amounts to build-up in your system, one on top of another, like layer upon thin layer of sediment. This can make dosing and clearing tricky, because it's hard to know exactly how much residual amount is left in your system. Even worse, your adrenal system stays activated and never gets a break. It's running in an elevated state, even when you're asleep. And that elevated state of arousal, combined with conventional stress, lack of sleep, inadequate nutrition, and other stimulants like coffee, energy drinks and chocolate, run your adrenals into a state of exhaustion.

If you drink just one cup of coffee every few days, build-up never becomes an issue. But taking several powerful stimulants like these without a periodic "drug holiday" can make you feel like half a zombie, when the adrenals have spent their allowance of cortisol and adrenaline.

Weaning yourself from psychoactive drugs

Some psychoactive drugs are notorious for producing dangerous, sometimes scary, side effects when stopping them "cold turkey." Psychotic episodes of this nature can be serious cause for concern when the brain misfires so badly that the individual has suicidal, homicidal, or self-injurious thoughts. The results can be troublesome to tragic (think: school shootings).

It's thought this phenomenon is caused by neurotransmitter production getting used to these biochemicals being elevated artificially through external sources – the drug – and not being controlled by the body itself. The body then gets lazy in making its own neurochemicals. So when the drug is discontinued, the body is not geared up to make inhibitory neurochemicals, without external prompting/assistance. Hence, the brain operates grossly out of balance, and certain brain functions collapse – particularly ones that remind the person that harmful thoughts, feelings, and actions are a bad idea.

Bottom line, there is appreciable risk to starting psychoactive drugs that have these discontinuity dependencies. The individual may suffer weeks to months of disturbed psychology, while the body clears these drugs from the system, and gets used to making biochemicals on its own again.

Real sun exposure, on the eyes and skin, can help the body set its circadian rhythms and restart neurotransmitter production. Mineral-rich vegetables and fruits can supply the building blocks to make these brain chemicals. Exercise can help quite a bit. Herbal therapy is good. And meditation can be of benefit. But, generally speaking, the process can't be rushed all that much. You can only smooth out some of the bigger bumps from the process.

Good luck finding your perfect regimen and sustaining it

That is, if you can even find a medical professional willing to experiment with prescribing specific brands, dosages, and combinations of medications with which they're unfamiliar. Most people end up settling for brain function somewhere in between "better than before" and "okay," and living with side effects. Point is, the human body is infinitely better at controlling neurotransmitter levels, brain function, and all the other processes that make your body run the way that it should. It inherently knows all this stuff. What's more, it does it all automatically, when your internal ecosystem is in balance. And it does it all without a fuss.

As I've said before, your body has an incredible ability to "right itself" and reverse disease, provided you know what the real source of the problem is, and you fix that, rather than extinguishing symptoms. And, in particular, gut-based ADD is one of those reversible conditions – depending on how long a person has lived with it, and the severity of the damage already done to brain anatomy. The solution starts with asking the right questions and finding the right answers.

Medication can change a person's perception about themselves

The good news about taking prescription drugs is that if you get a good response, it can completely change the way you think about yourself. You see, we interpret the world around us through the lens of our brain. We create our own reality, and interact with it through a middleman: our brain.

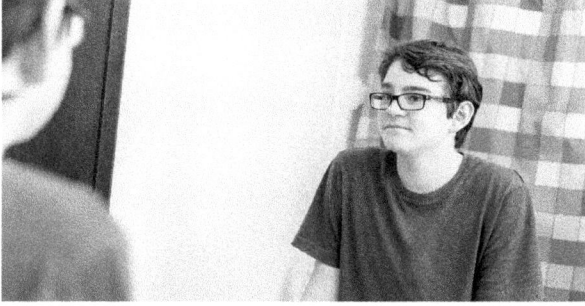

The information gathered from our senses, social interactions, learning, behavior, and progress must register in our awareness, be filtered according to relevance, and then be processed by our brain to make meaning of it all. So when brain function is imbalanced for any reason – either in collection, filtering or interpretation – it can dramatically alter our perception of ourselves. **More pointedly, when your brain is cloudy, slow, erratic or uncontrollable, you may tend to think of yourself as stupid, lazy, defective, headstrong or crazy.**

But that isn't necessarily the way it is… or has to be. It may just be a temporary, and changeable, condition that you can do something about. In many cases, drugs are the quickest way to show a person what their life could be like, when lived through a brain that works, or is simply better than it was. Drugs are usually an imperfect solution. But the stark contrast between your 'before' and 'after' can radically shift your opinion of you. If you get an excellent response from psychoactive drugs, it can literally change everything about your world and how you fit into it.

How to reset your stimulant receptors

The effect of stimulants is known to diminish over time if you don't take an occasional break. So some people resort to a "drug holiday" in which a drug's absence for 3–7 days clears trace amounts, restores neurotransmitter levels, and refreshes receptor sites. This is a big inconvenience, at best, for a lot people who have a hard time going without. Expert sources from the street say dextromethorphan in liquid cough syrup, taken before bed every two weeks or so, is able to reset stimulant receptors so their functionality never declines past a certain point. Neither the author nor the medical establishment expressly recommends this off-label use. It's just the word on the street.

Pill popping, made easier

Many children have a hard time swallowing larger-sized "horse pills," like those found in multi-vitamin supplements. My trick to swallowing just about any sized pill *whole* is to chew a mouthful of food completely. Right before you swallow it, throw the pill in. You'll never even notice the pill is there, no matter how big it is, because it's mixed in with the food and masked by the urge to swallow.

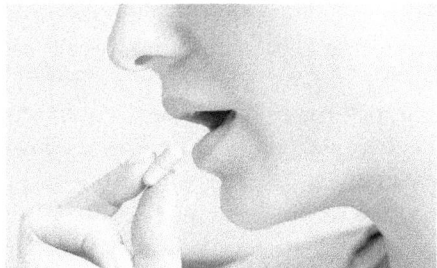

Insist and persist, until you get the results you're looking for

All that being said, if you choose to go down the pharmaceutical route, try to become more educated about the drugs you're taking than your doctor. You'd be surprised how easy that is to do with most general practitioners and even psychiatrists. Urge your clinician to let you try various drug types, brands, sizes, delivery vehicles such as extended release, timing, and combinations until you find a regimen that works well with minimal side effects.

Enlist the help of a good pharmacist to get the exact brand, pill size, etc. that you want. Don't be afraid to try the upper ranges of the recommended dosages, because the Physician's Desk Reference (PDR) tends to be conservative in its guidelines. ADD specialists often find that regimens above the recommended dosages give you additional benefit. However, only specialists who routinely deal with ADD feel comfortable prescribing outside industry standards. Once you find brands and forms that work well for you, have your practitioner write the prescription as "no substitutions." Read Dr. Daniel Amen's books to learn more.

Tools, tips and tricks to make living with ADD easier

The field is brimming with coping techniques to minimize ADD difficulties. So we'll just highlight some of the more clever ideas that practitioners have employed to help people deal with symptoms.

Externalize reminders (and free your mind). Don't rely on memory to remember deadlines and information. Instead, offload that responsibility to some sort of external device or mechanism to do it for you, such as a day planner, organizational program, or smartphone app. And then forget it, until the appropriate time. Like a computer with fewer open programs, that frees up the processing power of your mind to concentrate on the task at-hand. Use timers and alarms to put you back on track when you stray.

Exercise. Intense aerobic exercise has a powerful effect on rebalancing and restoring neurotransmitter levels, and increasing all-around energy. Better blood flow is always a good thing.

Say 'no' more often. ADD individuals are consummate people-pleasers, as well as eternal optimists. So they tend to bite off more than they can chew. Instead, err on the side of fewer commitments, as well as more time to finish them. I know, you get a squirt of pleasure chemicals by saying 'yes' to people's requests. Agreement does that. But you know you're going to pay for it down the road when you're late, or can't fulfill at all. So suffer a smaller disappointment now, for a greater avoidance of pain later. You may still use deadlines for external motivation, but now your workload will be realistic.

Move around. Consider a sit-stand desk, or treadmill desk, if you need to work off more energy.

Cognitive behavioral therapy. Many ADD individuals hold themselves back through negative self-talk. To break that chain of negativity, cognitive behavioral therapy (a special form of psychotherapy) aims to change troubling thought patterns, and counter-productive behaviors, by changing the way you think about things.

It aims to break the connection between a situation and the negative thoughts you have about it. CBT trains you to inject positive, productive thoughts/feelings into that train of thought to achieve more beneficial outcomes. For example, a woman who's having trouble at work might say to herself, "I can't seem to get to work on time. I never finish things on time. I'm always messing up. My boss hates me."

So, assuming the notion '*what you think about, you bring about*' is true, what's the likelihood that woman is attracting problems into her life? Conditioning your mind to think in the direction that you want to go will give you more agreeable outcomes. That's what cognitive behavioral therapy can help you do.

Biofeedback (aka neurofeedback, neurotherapy). Biofeedback is a therapeutic technique that trains you to have greater awareness and control over brain function in the hopes of reducing impulsivity and increasing focus. It does this by giving you feedback when brain centers are activated that trigger certain thoughts and actions. For example, it shows you on an EEG (brain wave visualizer) when inhibitory signals are being sent that block the urge to take your attention off-task, thereby heightening your awareness of which brain signal/patterns lead to which behaviors. The purpose being, through exercising the brain, you can exert greater control over your brain activity and resulting behaviors.

Conclusion: Biofeedback has helped a decent percentage of people improve their self-control. You tend to get mild-to-moderate symptomatic improvement after a fair amount of nervous system training. But it does little to address problems at the source.

Meditation, yoga, float tank. The body and mind are intimately entwined. Only temporarily does one reach a state radically out-of-sync with the other. So these three modalities entrain the brain into the same relaxed state that the body attains. They basically give the nervous system, including neurotransmitters, an opportunity to rebalance and re-center themselves back to baseline.

Meditation and floating give the brain a chance to catch up on processing backlogs of daily thoughts and emotions by giving it some downtime – a system reset, if you will. Both are great for shifting the body from fight-or-flight mode to that of rest and recuperation. In doing so, numerous processes are returned to normal functioning, instead of running in emergency operation mode. Plus, float tanks are uniquely capable of super-saturating your system with a variety of magnesium compounds that help hydrate your cells like no other source. Magnesium salts, and other electrolytes, raise the electrical charge of cells – pulling water into cells, delivering nutrients, and removing toxins.

Develop structure and flow

- Use excellent file systems. Create a folder for everything so that you (1) don't waste time thinking about where an item should go, (2) others can navigate your system, and (3) you know where anything that you're looking for went to.
- Don't let people interrupt you. If possible, set aside certain times of the day that it's okay to interrupt your flow. So unless it's an emergency, or a client calling, it can wait until those times. Tell people to use their judgment, and you'll find most things can wait without incident.
- Designate specific times in the day to do certain tasks that divert your attention, like email. Don't leave your email program open. And don't check it outside those times.
- Designate "make-up" times (flex-time) in the day to return to tasks from which you were detained.
- Don't multi-task. A lot of people think multi-tasking helps them get more work done. But, with most tasks, it both slows you down, and it diminishes the quality of your work.
- Use lists. Do the more important, more valuable tasks first. Do the inconsequential tasks later or never. Break larger tasks that you can't finish in a day into smaller chunks.
- Touch it once. When dealing with things, make a point to read it and handle it only once. Deal with it right then and there, if possible. When that isn't possible, make a decision that you can't proceed because you lack something you need. You must postpone the next step until some future occurrence, which you can define now.
- Throw things away. Ask yourself: "Can I get this again, if I need it? Will it hurt me to throw this away?"

———————— ⌘ ————————

20

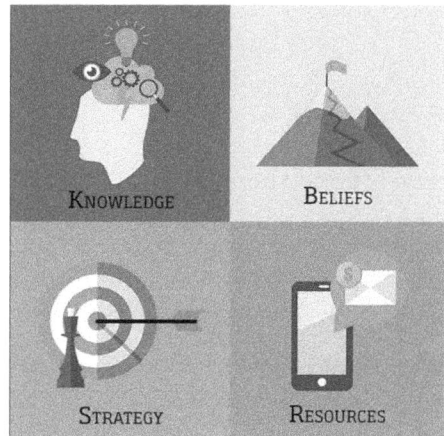

KNOWLEDGE   BELIEFS

STRATEGY   RESOURCES

TAKING CHARGE OF YOUR HEALTH

Now you have the knowledge to think and act for yourself

The main purpose of this book is not to give you all the answers to gut-brain issues. Instead, it's about empowering you and your family to take charge of your own health, and not leave it up to Big Pharma, Big Food, and the globalists whose interests seldom align with your own. This material helps you to understand the mechanisms by which your environment influences your psychological. With this knowledge, you can

1. understand the nature of gut-brain issues **(perspective);**
2. know the real source of your symptoms **(insight);**
3. find small changes in diet or lifestyle that make a big difference **(silver bullets);**
4. get back on track when your progress stalls **(course correction).**

It's about putting the dots so close together that you're never fooled from lack of knowledge, or stumped when problems arise. You always have more information and assets to deploy to overcome whatever difficulties you face. Whatever happens, you're prepared to beat gut-brain conditions that can only persist in the absence of knowledge, resources, a good team, and a willingness to act. Now these can be *your* best assets.

Get started on your healing journey by asking better questions

First, don't wait for "experts" to give you information and resources. Go get them yourself. Try searching the Internet with phrases like: "natural remedy for" + (your problem). For example, do a search for "natural remedy for diabetes" or "cure autism naturally." Using the proper search term is key to getting what you want, and none of what you don't. That means if you search for the wrong phrase, like "cancer treatment," you'll probably fall into a Big Pharma sandbox, where only FDA-approved medical treatments are permitted and promoted, among the occasional good advice and smart solutions.

On the other hand, when you choose your qualifying words more carefully, you can "un-invite" Big Pharma and mainstream medicine to the conversation, because they aren't interested in helping the body heal itself without drugs, surgery or medical interventions. Unfortunately, consumers still wed to the Big Pharma paradigm just don't demand answers to questions such as: 'what really caused my disorder' and 'how can I cure it?' They presume solutions would be welcomed into mainstream medicine with open arms. They figure if an idea were good, medical professionals would have heard about it already. Of course, you and I know that's naïve thinking. The world doesn't work that way.

Who should you listen to and trust?
Start by honing your B.S. detector to be wary of information and offerings that disempower you, create dependency, and talk in generalities, without giving specifics as to 'why' and 'how.' Be extra skeptical of stuff that takes power away from you, and gives it to someone else. Beware of those using *supposed authority* and *the collective good* (e.g., "you're being selfish") to brainwash or bully you into accepting their advice/directions/rules, rather than facts and reason. These types of people often hide behind credentials, reputation and references, which can be deceptive.

From the same socialist/Marxist playbook: Keeping you misinformed, desperate, and fearful are easy ways to manipulate you into compliance – especially when those creating problems conveniently offer you *their* solutions (posing themselves as savior). Conversely, those that empower you to find your own answers, choose for yourself, and 'do' for yourself are more likely to have your best interests at heart.

Avoid the temptation to blindly trust people simply because they make you feel good. Be suspect of people that seem to tell you exactly what you want to hear, and none of what you don't. Instead, favor advice, products, and programs that encourage you to take responsibility for your own choices and outcomes. I'm talking about those willing to sacrifice their own acceptance and income to tell you the whole truth – even when it hurts their popularity, is more involving, takes longer, costs more, conflicts with the status quo, and turns off those looking for a quick fix.

Finally, don't automatically discount those that are selling something that may cost more. Everyone has to make a living. And the fact that health insurance only pays for FDA-approved drugs and surgeries should mean nothing when deciding whether or not a therapy is right for you. The reality of being in business will always be a balancing act between helping people on one hand, and making money on the other. Everyone wants to help people, but a professional business has a lot of expenses to bring you quality solutions.

Risks of reversing attention deficit disorder
There is a legitimate risk to reversing ADD. And that is, the inclinations of the ADD brain motivate many of them toward achievement. They use it as fuel to drive them toward stimulation and reward, while at the same time escaping boredom and stagnation. This stems from the way the ADD mind is wired – you could say *powered* – in many cases. You see, at

its core, ADD is caused by an imbalance in neurotransmitter production. Dopamine and serotonin are the main pleasure chemicals that the body releases when it wants to reward the individual for certain behaviors. Thus, the feeling of enjoyment is mostly dopamine and serotonin hitting the corresponding receptors. Yet, the ADD person is habitually low in this area, and feeling "less-than" because of it.

Their system under-produces the neurotransmitters that activate reward centers, making them feel less pleasure, contentment and comfort just "being" than their nervous system should have. So the ADD mind lives in constant deficit that their psychology, actions and habits try to normalize through stimulating behavior. This results in many ADD individuals being what we call Type-A driven personalities. They can't take it easy, because that restricts the brain chemicals that give them contentment. This makes them addicted to action, and often accomplishment.

By comparison, the non-ADD person feels just fine doing boring tasks, or not doing anything at all. They're still bored doing unchallenging activities. But their tolerance level is dramatically higher, so boring tasks don't bother them nearly as much, if at all. Thus, they don't need constant stimulation to make themselves feel normal. Therefore, reversing ADD is not without risk. Its hidden danger is the potential to take away the core motivating force in these people's lives. It's not a common problem, but worth mentioning.

More frequently, extra dopamine just means the person is motivated to think and act on a higher level. Habits also tend to keep a person doing more of the same. Therefore, most people are likely to respond to more balanced neurotransmitter levels and better PFC function by gaining better power and control over their thoughts and actions, while not losing anything in terms of motivation. Simply put, strengths are increased and weaknesses are eliminated.

Detoxification and chelation
Ken Rohla was asked what is the first, best thing a person can do to improve their health
His answer: "For sure, the top #1 is detoxification, because a lot of people won't change their diet and lifestyle because they have food addictions. They have emotional connections to food. And what makes that much, much easier to change is simply by getting on detoxification programs and doing physical cleansing.

What happens is, you will flush chemicals out of your body that make you crave certain foods – in particular, sugars... You wind up developing a body of pathogens that will secrete chemicals to [cause] you to crave sugars to feed them. And so just by killing them off that will go a long way toward stopping cravings for sugar.

Then, when you get done with that, you will naturally gravitate toward healthier foods, and you will lose cravings for foods. Foods that you loved or craved in the past that weren't particularly good for you – when you eat them again – they just won't taste that good. And so you kind of just naturally lose your taste for these foods that aren't good for you, and gravitate towards healthier ones. And then you can transition your diet."

Dietary chelators *vs.* innate detoxification *vs.* chelation therapy

Detoxification is so important to staying healthy that Nature provided us with ordinary foods that chelate heavy metals on a regular basis. Some of the foods that chelate heavy metals are chlorella (algae), cilantro, garlic and raw egg whites. Even more potent, chelation with minerals and chemicals boost the body's own detox abilities with therapeutic agents. Common interventional strength chelators are zeolite, EDTA, DMSA, bentonite clay, and high dose vitamin C.

Neither approach is better than the other – dietary *vs.* supplemental. Each have their place. But the interesting thing that Dr. Natasha has found in her practice is that when you heal and seal a once-corrupted gut, and you eat foods that support chelation, the body can get rid of heavy metals by itself. You don't need to supplement your diet with chelation agents. She found this out when families came in asking if they should go on a chelation regimen to help their child recover from GAPS.

They would measure heavy metal levels. Then they did the GAPS protocol. And they found that repairing the body's own detox systems was able to lowered metal levels. Along with dramatic improvements in brain function, the GAPS Diet alone brought heavy metal levels back to normal. So they didn't have to do chelation therapy, in most cases.

For these reasons, Dr. Natasha asks her patients to wait about twelve months into the GAPS protocol before considering a formal chelation regimen. This allows the body's detox systems to come back on line (so that toxins aren't freed up and re-deposited elsewhere). At that point, supplemental chelation is often not needed.

Daily chelating agents

In today's toxic world, periodic events like a liver, bowel, or kidney cleanse can certainly help. But with our exposure level the way that it is, most people should consider taking measures to lighten the load on their detox systems. Everyone should be eating foods daily that help open up detox pathways. Everyone needs to have healthy gut flora to keep heavy metal absorption to a minimum. And the vast majority of people are in serious need of detoxifying aids to stay ahead of their everyday intake.

As we've examined in different contexts, detoxification is no longer a luxury reserved for health nuts. Now, it's a daily duty that points your long-term wellness in a positive direction. Think of the foods, micro-organisms, supplements, and practices you incorporate in your routine as an auxiliary detoxification system. Here are some front-line favorites:

- **Mineral/chemical chelators:** Zeolite, oral EDTA, activated charcoal, and bentonite clay.
- **Chelating (whole) foods:** Chlorella, cilantro, alfalfa, parsley, spirulina, wheatgrass, seaweed, apple cider vinegar, sauerkraut, kimchi, onions, garlic and dark, green leafy vegetables in general.
- **Chelating natural substances:** Acetic acid (in many fermented foods), citric acid (lemons and limes), ascorbic acid (vitamin C), lactic acid (whey, kefir, yogurt), amino acids, pectin, and natural fats (butter, lard, unrefined coconut oil, whole fats from animal products).

Daily baths get nutrients in, and transport toxins out

Not many people know how permeable the skin is in both absorbing substances inward, and in excreting substances outward. What's neat is, you can use that permeability to your advantage. Adding a therapeutic aspect to bathing gives you an opportunity to use a daily routine as another avenue to get more nutrition into the body, while pushing toxins out.

Add Epsom salt, sea salt, baking soda, vinegar, seaweed, EDTA, or other therapeutic agents to regular bathwater as a painless way to get beneficial substances absorbed directly into the bloodstream, while bypassing the GI tract, liver and detox organs that block non-food substances. To help with that, warm water causes skin pores to open up, thereby encouraging toxins to leave by soaking in chelating agents.

Juicing detoxifies and nutrifies like nothing else

"Juicing" raw vegetables and fruits with a juice extractor is one of the single best things you can do to help your body get rid of toxins, while inundating cells with minerals, vitamins, antioxidants and enzymes. Blending vegetables in a blender (and leaving the fiber in) is great too. It just offers a different set of benefits.

The reason juicing is so revered among health fanatics is that it gives you massive doses of a vegetable's best stuff, in a highly concentrated and absorbable form, minus a digestion and absorption decelerator: fiber. So instead of eating a fraction of each vegetable/fruit in a salad, with juicing, you often receive several times the nutrients and cleansing power of each in a single glass. That's why juicing supercharges the GAPS protocol.

You can juice just about any type of produce you like. But most of your juice should come from vegetables, because fruits are high in sugar and spike blood-sugar level (being in a liquid form, with fiber removed). Dr. Natasha recommends you add a raw egg white (pasture-raised is better) to your mostly-vegetable juice, along with a tablespoon of sour cream (unpasteurized, if you can get it), and mix well. This makes a wonderfully nutritious and delicious detoxifying vegetable shake that sustains you until lunch.

Health educators tell us to taste "the rainbow"

…meaning, richly-colored vegetables and fruits. Know why? It's because the pigments that produce vibrant colors in vegetables and fruits *are* its antioxidants. Their colors contain phytonutrients. That's why wellness coaches tell us to eat the colors of the rainbow. If you ever want to impress upon yourself, viscerally, how wonderful the colors of Nature are, just juice colored veggies in a slow juicer, one at-a-time, without stirring. The multi-colored juice it produces is an awesome sight.

Masticating slow-squeeze juicers outperform centrifugal juicers

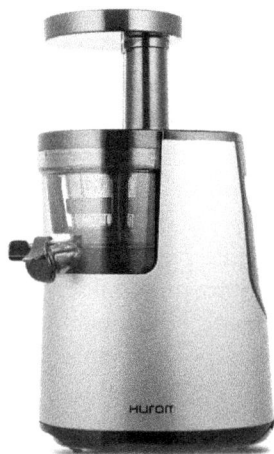

No question about it: Buy a "masticating" juicer (means to chew), instead of a traditional centrifugal juicer. Slow-squeeze juicers, as they are also described, use an auger to break down fibrous material into pulp. They then squeeze the juice out more slowly. Whereas centrifugal juicers can only shred the material and spin the juice out.

The slow-squeeze technique substantially improves the quantity and quality of juice extracted, not to mention producing more colorful juice. Kale and broccoli, as examples, can't be juiced well with a traditional juicer. But you can actually get juice out of both with a masticating, slow juicer. Overall, you get about 20% more juice from a slow-squeeze juicer. And I have no doubt the juice is better for you. You can feel that the method is more efficient because the pulp comes out much drier.

Pro tips to boost flavor, without adding sweetness. Add
- tomato for a bloody mary taste
- ¼ clove of fresh ginger for spiciness
- lemon and lime for tanginess
- part of a jalapeno or fresno pepper for some attitude
- purple cabbage rounds out the palatability.

Pulp from juicing can be used to feed gardens or pets.

Kicking up the flavor with tricks like these can go a long way toward making all-vegetable juice palatable, without resorting to fruits or sweeteners. Hurom brand juicers do a great job at reasonable prices.

Therapeutic detoxification

- Enemas and colonics.
- Detoxifying footbaths and mudbaths.
- **Intravenous chelation.** DMPS, DMSA, EDTA and DMSO are three of the most powerful agents you can employ to remove heavy metals and other toxins from the body. However, they also tend to be more expensive, involving, inconvenient, and harder on the body than oral routes because they are typically done in multiple clinic visits, under the supervision of a doctor. And they're strong.
- **Sweating in a sauna.** The skin is the largest organ of excretion, and it can remove some chemicals that can't be excreted any other way.
- **Oil pulling.**

I recommend SaunaSpace near infrared saunas because they do heat and red light therapy better than far infrared/steam saunas. Their personal "photon light" nullifies blue light hazard and spot treats with red light.

Enemas. Enemas and colonics do an amazing job of clearing the liver's primary drainage route out of the body: the bowels. Amusing as they may sound to Big Pharm believers, enemas have been used for centuries to unblock the colon and give it a gentle "power-washing." The newly opened pathway draws toxins outward. Bonus tip: Implanting therapeutic agents such as (room temperature) coffee or probiotics for a few minutes, before flushing them out, have been shown highly effective at moving toxins out, and good guys in.

Infrared saunas. Far infrared saunas have been used forever to increase sweating, which can turn skin into as big a detox channel as any. Newer technology, near infrared, can be even more effective, because its light frequencies can penetrate tissues 10–30 cm and directly charge up mitochondria and cells.

Oil pulling. Oil pulling is one of the easiest ways to remove toxins from the body – whether it be a daily practice, or in a detox program. Oil pulling is the practice of holding a tablespoon or two of a pure, healthy oil in the mouth for 1–10 minutes and swishing. This absorbs toxins like mercury from the cells of the mouth, tongue and salivary glands. Olive oil, coconut oil, sesame seed oil, or avocado oil are some preferred oils with which to do oil pulling, because they're made by Nature. But be prepared: the gunk that can come out of a person's mouth may surprise you.

Fixing a corrupted microbiome
Restoring gut health is a divine trio that normalizes heavy metal levels

1. **Border patrol.** Probiotics chelate more than 95% of heavy metals in the gut, instead of allowing them to cross the gut wall. Restoring beneficial flora keeps heavy metals out of the body, before they get in.
2. **Reducing workload.** Pathogens release toxins as waste. So increasing probiotic populations lighten the workload on the liver,

bowels, and remainder of detox pathways by reducing exposure.

3. **Packaging for export.** Heavy metals (fat-soluble) can't move through water-based blood alone. They need shuttles made from fats, cholesterol, vitamins, and minerals to package and ship them out. So, by fixing a corrupted gut, the GAPS diet supplies the nutrients needed to move toxic metals out.

You can repopulate a virtually sterile gut just by breathing

This may sound ludicrous to experienced practitioners, but Dr. Zach Bush has seen this happen to a severely emaciated pancreatic cancer patient (59 pounds) who had been passing only white, chalky stools for two years. White chalky stool indicates that there's no biological matter in them. Instead, they're made of cells shed from the gut lining.

Her digestive tract was so decimated by cancer that she couldn't eat anything, and could only sip liquids extremely slowly due to blockages in her GI tract. But four days after starting on Dr. Bush's (sterile) carbon redox molecule supplement, the woman passed her first large brown bowel movement in two years! Again, she didn't eat any solids, or take any probiotics. This means that when your microbiome's communication network comes back online, the gut grabs probiotic bacteria out of the air, and from all over your body, to repopulate the gut. Especially in the absence of pathogens which fight for territory, bacteria from the air establishes diverse microbial communities in the gut.

As a result, Dr. Bush now recommends that his patients travel to natural settings such as forests, beaches, water falls, and mountain trails to help repopulate their gut after a course of antibiotics or major infection. He tells people to stir things up in the nature, touching plants and soil, so microbes go airborne. Then inhale deeply to take in a wide variety of species from the environment. Petting animals, especially dogs, and breathing the air is particularly effective at transferring species that only they tend to host.

Similarly, naturally-made sauerkraut gets its hundreds of bacteria strains partly from the environment as well. "Wild ferments," as they're called, are made by fermenting cabbage into sauerkraut, without any starter cultures. You just add sea salt (minerals), seal the container, and let it sit.

Fecal transplants

Admit it. You're as horrified and intrigued as the rest of us at the notion of transferring fecal matter from one person to another. Understandable. However, after many years of skepticism and ridicule from the medical community, fecal transplants are becoming a treatment of choice for life-threatening infections like C. diff – mostly because drug companies have been unable to come up with anything near as fast and effective.

Fecal transplantation basically takes fecal matter from a healthy person and, after some preparation, introduces it into the colon of a person that might otherwise die from a massive pathogen overgrowth. Where medicinal antibiotics are unable to contain pathogens populations due to drug-resistance, real, naturally-occurring probiotic bacteria don't have that limitation. Their natural antibiotic weaponry continues to work.

Their innate antibiotics knock back the strongest of pathogens in hours – and without nasty side effects that medicinal antibiotics are known for. Researchers are also experimenting with fecal transplants to fix other conditions related to corrupted gut, such as obesity and mal-absorption. So it looks like traditional medicine is being forced to concede once again that Nature has a stronger, smarter solution to C. diff and other infections than orthodox medicine. Is anyone keeping score? I think Nature is winning.

Warning: Most commercial probiotics give you little to no benefit
To achieve therapeutic benefit, you need these five factors to be present – all in one supplement:

- **Quantity of organisms.** Quite a few probiotic supplements don't have enough of the critters to do you much good (you need billions of colony-forming units in each dose).
- **Diversity of species.** Most formulations have 2–8 strains of bacteria. But you need dozens, if not hundreds, to get excellent results.
- **Strain potency.** Most commercial strains (being genetically modified or poorly made) are too weak to beat resident pathogens.
- **Survival and colonization rates.** A large number are not strong enough to survive stomach acid and colonize the digestive tract.
- **Shelf life.** Some products are not viable at the time of consumption because of the way they're made, stored and delivered.

Now why would a manufacturer sell you a product that doesn't work? Do they lack the ability? Or do they just not care about your health? In this case, it probably has more to do with commercial interests, rather than dereliction of duty. You see, when your gut has too many pathogens and you take a potent probiotic, you may experience a die-off reaction in which expiring pathogens release a burst of toxins that they'd normally release in a trickle. The more pathogens killed at one time, the bigger the toxin wave. These toxins can make your symptoms worse, before they get better (typical of Nature's way). This can make you feel terrible until the poisons are cleared from your system. Natural healers know about die-off reactions, and are careful to push progress only as fast as you can tolerate.

To restate the situation, if you took a probiotic and felt crummy afterward, unsophisticated consumers wouldn't want to keep taking it, would they? Therefore, a lot of manufacturers sell weak, ineffective probiotics that provide minimal benefit in order to avoid health (or sales) consequences. They bank on the psychological benefit, rather than actual benefit. At the same time, a fair percentage of manufacturers simply don't know how to make a potent probiotic brew, or don't care. That's the reality of the marketplace.

Recommended probiotic supplements

1. In my estimation, the Natural Plus Plus brand of probiotic products, *Inner Garden* and *Turbocharged Turmeric,* are among the best you can get.
2. Many people swear by Dr. Higa's Original EM-1 brand of probiotics for people, plants, home (e.g., cleans mold and mildew), and other uses such as decontaminating soil of radioactivity.
3. Dr. Natasha Campbell-McBride recommends the Bio-Kult brand of probiotics. She helped formulate them.

GAPS Diet overview
The GAPS Diet heals and seals the gut, and fixes the microbiome

Dr. Natasha Campbell-McBride's *Gut and Psychology Syndrome Diet* (GAPS Diet) is the natural way to reverse gut dysbiosis. Corrupted gut, as I call it, involves too many pathogens, too few probiotics, leaky gut, and complications such as food allergies and autoimmunity. They go together.

Fixing gut dysbiosis undoes the mayhem that pathogens cause. It helps correct neurotransmitter and hormonal imbalances. It dampens the body's autoimmune response to inappropriate substances. It helps you extract nutrients from food more effectively. And it reduces inflammation. Together, these set the gut and its microbiome up to nourish and protect the body, instead of slowly poisoning you and causing mental disorders.

Following the diet in a consistent manner gives the gut lining a chance to replace its damaged, dysfunctional cells with healthy, productive ones. Dr. Natasha calls this "healing and sealing" the gut lining against intrusion from undigested food particles, toxins and microbial pathogens.

The younger a child is when they start the GAPS protocol, the less damage there is to undo, and the better their chances of full recovery

With gut dysbiosis, the brain and body are persistently intoxicated, producing effects from mild attention deficit to severe autism. When this happens for several years, the brain gets physically damaged. Certain brain functions can atrophy. And the child misses out on important language, cognition, and social skills that Nature instills at a certain time, in a certain order, of development.

For example, kids first learn how to eat, then crawl, then walk or talk, then play and socialize with peers, etc. When these critical time windows are missed, it is possible to catch up. But they have to sprint to catch up to classmates who are learning quickly themselves. Therefore, the sooner a child can heal their corrupted gut, the less they miss out on.

Most children under five can catch up fairly quickly because the brain has a remarkable ability to recover when a child is young and everything is new to them. But time is of the essence. Every year that their development is stunted is progressively harder to recover – both neurologically and socially. If a child falls too far behind, an accelerated learning program might be needed to fast-track their development, or else they might be considered "slow" for the rest of their lives. Full potential of their brain function might never be achieved.

An all-too common scenario: A child is brought in to assess their learning and behavioral problems. Because their symptoms don't fit neatly into any diagnostic box, as defined by the *Diagnostic and Statistical Manual of Mental Disorders*, the parents are told to bring them back in six months for further evaluation. In six months, their clinical picture is the same, so they're told to come back in another six months for re-evaluation… and another six months… or a year from now. Meanwhile, precious time is being lost when the child could have been helped.

By the time they reach their teens, their mind and body have lived with the effects of a compromised gut so long that their situation can be improved substantially by healing the gut. But they're likely to have lingering effects (e.g., habits) that they have to learn to live with.

Don't wait for a diagnosis. If a child has GAPS symptoms, start them on the GAPS Diet

If someone in your family has GAPS symptoms that haven't led to a doctor's diagnosis yet, just start them on the GAPS Diet. A formal diagnosis is not needed for a number of reasons:

1. Labeling your symptoms doesn't necessarily help you make real progress, because most psychological symptoms have a common cause: a corrupted gut.
2. All health conditions benefit from fixing the microbiome, mending the gut wall, improving digestion, reducing autoimmunity, and lowering inflammation.
3. Chronic diseases improve with better neurotransmitter levels, energy, toxin load, hormonal balance, immunity and epigenetic expression.
4. Diagnosing a person's condition involves a fair amount of guesswork and judgement. It's very unscientific. For example, a symptom such as brain fog can fit into lots of diagnostic boxes – including ADD, sleep problems, leaky gut/toxicity, autism spectrum or alcoholism. So putting a label on a collection of symptoms may help you treat a disease properly. Or it just might confuse you into *mistreating* symptoms.

On the other hand, if symptoms have the same physical origin and remedy, then the prescription should be the same: the GAPS protocol. And, indeed, that is the bulk of the answer in most cases. Therefore, the smartest course of action is to assume the most common situation is the one you're dealing with – a gut-brain condition – and apply a solution like the GAPS Diet, while at the same time staying on the lookout for exceptions to the rule.

To that end, the biggest help a doctor's diagnosis can lend to a situation is in ruling out, or ruling in, comorbid conditions that can complicate the situation or explain it some other way. Which is a fancy way of saying, 'if you've got symptoms that appear to indicate a gut-brain condition is present, then approach it using the best gut-brain solutions out there.'

This approach is far more likely to produce a satisfactory outcome in the long run than Big Medicine's mediocre-to-disappointing track record over the long term (i.e., real healing *vs.* man-made quick fixes). I submit the 1,000+ kids that have recovered from autism as evidence. Moreover, **you will never regret the plethora of benefits that a healthy gut gives you. So it's never a wasted effort.**

Why does the GAPS nutritional protocol take so long?

The GAPS protocol takes an average of 24 months to go through, depending on severity of gut dysbiosis, overall health, age, and compliance (how closely you adhere to the diet *vs.* how much you cheat). The reason it takes so long is because pathogens don't want to leave when they're being fed and sheltered. And the microbiome has built-in mechanisms to resist change. So it takes a sustained effort to create such an inhospitable environment that pathogens cede control. You have to starve them, and root them out with probiotic bacteria tough enough to unseat the undesirables.

A friend once asked me why it's so hard to heal a corrupted gut. "Can't you just blast the walls of the bowel clean with a power washer and start over from scratch?" I admit, it's an interesting concept – if only it were that simple. The reality is, there are very good reasons why you can't reset your microbiome quickly or casually. That being: a person's microbiome, like a computer's operating system, plays too many roles in running the system to be altered easily or accidentally. The microbiome takes a licking and keeps on ticking, without ever letting you know how distressed of a state that it's in. Indeed, it often takes multiple courses of antibiotics, and years of toxin exposure to corrupt the gut so that you'd notice symptoms.

On the other hand, healing can take a few years to achieve because microflora are resilient. They're constantly growing, scrapping, moving around, and dying off. This is why you can't just nuke the pathogens with some sort of pesticide and expect them to disappear. It's more about balance. To heal the gut, you have to both make life miserable for the pathogens, and encourage beneficial bacteria to proliferate.

Remember, microbes coat themselves with a mucous-y biofilm when colonizing the intestine. This gives pathogens a protective shield to hide behind when you introduce therapeutics. Another obstacle to change is the appendix. It stores bacteria from the gut, which are "out of the line of fire" to antibiotics passing through the GI tract. The appendix replenishes the gut after a major attack of cholera, dysentery, or course of antibiotics. This is why it can take 24 months, give or take, to fix a corrupted gut.

Bottom line: It often takes years, decades, or lifetimes to corrupt people's guts as bad as they are today. So we shouldn't be surprised when it takes a couple of years to reverse. Remind yourself along the way that the GAPS protocol is hardcore healing at its finest. It is true holistic restoration for those hell-bent on improving their health from head to toe.

Amount of improvement you can expect

The question is not "Can my child or I be cured of ADD or autism." That's probably the wrong question to ask because it presupposes a bunch of counter-productive assumptions. It sets up unrealistic expectations. For example, that line of thinking might suggest that diagnoses, treatments, and cures happen in isolation from motivation and commitment, lifestyle, budget, genetic and epigenetic differences, and complicating factors.

It presupposes the body is a machine... that something's malfunctioning inside it. So you're going to hook it up to a scanner, figure out what's wrong, take a pill to fix the problem, and everything will be good as new. That is simplistic thinking when, instead, we have a collage of interconnected, constantly-changing forces working for or against you. Every case of GAPS is at least a little different.

So, instead, a more productive question to ask is how much time, effort, and money are needed to achieve what level of symptom reversal? How much are the affected individual and her care providers willing to put toward the healing effort *vs.* how much improvement might they expect?

You see, there's always more gains to be had, with virtually unlimited places to look for those gains. So the secret to meeting your goals and expectations is to have a clear understanding of what you want to achieve, and what you're willing to do or not do, to get there. And that's starting to sound like a plan that achieves your goals and is very doable.

That being said, GAPS practitioners might describe their prognosis with ADD in general statements like the following:

The first 35% improvement for AD(H)D (superficial). The first 35% improvement is often achieved relatively quickly and easily – perhaps days to a few weeks. It involves eliminating the artificial colorings, flavorings, and additives notorious for triggering hyperactivity, such as red #40 and yellow #5. Similarly, lay off the foods that produce adverse reactions, such as gluten, casein and sugar. These, in particular, are responsible for driving the GALT and nervous system crazy, thereby magnifying hyperactivity. Unfortunately, this is the point – cessation of hyperactivity – at which many parents see enough improvement that they stop looking for more, as that was their chief complaint. However, it doesn't fix executive function.

Next, start doing the things that heal and seal intestinal permeability, such as the GAPS Diet and ION Gut Support. To help with these, your GAPS or Nutritional Therapy Practitioner may include probiotics, nutrient supplementation, or fast-acting detox efforts like enemas.

The next 45% improvement (real repair and healing). The next 45% improvement takes perseverance to implement the deeper healing protocols started in phase one. It typically involves a long-term elimination and gut-support diet, deeper cleansing in a detox program (e.g., zeolite, EDTA, infrared sauna), probiotic supplementation, lifestyle changes like exercise, and better sleep patterns. This level of improvement might take anywhere from six months to two years in order to heal the damage done to the: microbiome, gut lining, digestion, GALT (autoimmunity), endocrine organs, and brain/nervous system.

The final 20% improvement (maintenance). The last 20% of performance improvement can take significantly more ingenuity and effort to attain, because there may be a lot of physical injury, dysfunction, developmental delay, and atrophy to overcome – particularly with age. It often requires deeper, more comprehensive detoxification efforts. It takes a cleaner, more mineral and vitamin-rich diet, with less cheating, to realize. You'll probably need to explore modalities outside the GAPS protocol to offset genetic vulnerabilities and max out the function of your systems – for example: nnEMF shielding, earthing, Magnetico Sleep Pad, infrared sauna, hyperbarics, genetic testing, and anti-aging technologies. And, above all, your microbiome has to be faultless for you to enjoy perfect mental health.

Do you have to stay on the diet forever? Good news: You don't have to stay on the GAPS diet forever. As your gut flora become fit for duty, and your systems regain functionality, you can reintroduce some of the foods that used to cause you problems. You can indulge from time to time, as long as the majority of your diet nourishes you properly, and you help your body do what it's designed to do: heal itself, feed itself, and detoxify itself.

Fortunately, regressing to a poor diet is not as big of a temptation as you might think, because most people that have experienced the benefits of the GAPS Diet choose not to go back to the fake foods that made them sick. Most of the time, after seeing how good you feel and function when you eat well, it's hard to live any other way. So when good gut bugs are back in business protecting you, you can eat the occasional candy bar, chips, and fast food and not suffer any adverse effects. Food still impacts your health quite profoundly. But it shouldn't trigger clinical episodes the way bad food used to.

ADD summary, tremendous symptomatic improvement is often seen in the first 1–3 months. Deeper, lasting healing is often achieved from the 3-month mark to about 18 months on the GAPS diet, give or take 6 months. Incorporating other products or modalities can help the body cleanse and heal in ways difficult for the body to do itself. Emptying caches of mercury, aluminum, and old viruses are three examples.

Virtually anything is possible. You just need to (1) find out the real sources of problems, (2) determine the best ways to fix them (practitioners can help), (3) decide what you can and cannot do toward individual changes or a comprehensive plan, and (4) go and do it. That means being realistic, considering all the factors that need to be dealt with along the way. I suggest you err on the side of making fewer commitments of your time, effort, and money at first. That way, small successes will lead to greater motivation and commitment, as you see results. It's easier to put in the time and money, when you're encouraged by small, incremental successes along the way.

Success rates for autism. For autism, complete recovery is often possible if the GAPS protocol is started when the child is under the age of five. But the older they get, the more neurological damage there is to undo from toxicity, inflammation, and "mis-wiring" of the brain. They also miss out on critical psycho/social development during that time. Great strides can always be made regardless of age. But it becomes progressively harder to access full healing as the system ages and loses its plasticity to revert back to its original genetic blueprint, from changes brought about by toxicity, nutritional deficiencies, immune dysfunction, excitotoxicity, etc. Every year that goes by in a compromised state is that much harder to undo.

The GAPS Diet

The GAPS Diet is divided into three parts: the Introduction Diet, the Full GAPS Diet, and a less-restrictive "maintenance" phase of the Full GAPS Diet, where you can re-introduce certain foods as tolerated.

The Introduction Diet starts with fairly strict do's and don'ts to jumpstart healing

1. Remove foods that pathogens thrive on, such as refined carbs, sugar, and toxins (yes, some pathogens love toxins).
2. Pamper your system with unprocessed, mostly animal-based sources of nutrients that are easy to digest, and ideally suited to nourish the gut lining, so that it heals as quickly as possible. Employ foods rich in amino acids, gelatin, glucosamines, natural fats, vitamins and minerals. These mainstays of the Introduction Diet include bone broths, meat stocks, organ meats, eggs, well-cooked (non-fibrous) vegetables and homemade soups.

3. Eliminate substances that irritate the porous and inflamed gut lining. In the early stages of gut repair, indigestible fiber must be removed because it's abrasive to damaged and sensitive gut cells.

4. Healing is controlled by good gut bacteria, so the Introduction Diet calls for probiotic bacteria from fermented vegetables, and sometimes dairy, to drive pathogens out and encourage good guys to populate.

Especially important at this stage is THE nutritional powerhouse that rebuilds the gut lining fast, which is bone broth. The forgotten healer of yesteryear, bone broth, contains many of the same substances that cells of the gut lining are made from. Equally advantageous, the nutrients in bone broth hardly need to be digested at all. They're already present in a form that cells can use. What's more, bone broth is extremely gentle on wounded gut cells so healing can begin immediately.

The Introduction Diet is broken up into six sequential stages, which some people can fly through in a matter of days. Those with food sensitivities and more severe digestive problems may take several weeks to a year to complete the process. As you progress through the Introduction Diet, you'll challenge your system by periodically introducing foods and seeing how the body responds, calibrating accordingly.

Once the gut is intact and doing its job of protecting you, you can move on to supplying the body with the nutritional resources it needs to achieve deeper healing. You can continue driving pathogens out of the microbiome, and encouraging the proliferation of diverse species of probiotic critters (particularly the rare ones), with the Full GAPS Diet.

The Full GAPS Diet

Most influential of all factors is diet, because food can nourish and protect the brain and body, or it can burden you with anti-nutrients and disease-causing substances. Diet can go a long way toward removing toxins, because some kinds of foods contribute to cleansing the body as much as the best chelators. Fibrous vegetables are a good example. And fermented foods can give you concentrated, hopefully diverse, microorganisms.

The Full GAPS Diet includes many dozens of foods you can eat to your tummy's content. In general, these are nourishing whole foods that are grown or raised the way Nature intended. At the same time, The Full Diet excludes many dozens of foods to stay away from (as a new way of life). You know the categories: sweetened, refined, processed, preserved, problematic, or artificial anything.

Coming off the GAPS Diet ("The Maintenance Diet")

The subsequent "maintenance" GAPS Diet then has many foods that are allowed as-tolerated by the individual. Fortunately, when people experience how good they think and feel on the GAPS Maintenance Diet, they never want to go back to eating poorly.

Of course, there's a lot more to learn about the GAPS diet than what's presented here. I recommend you go to the source: Get Dr. Natasha Campbell-McBride's foundational book *Gut and Psychology Syndrome* to learn how to implement the diet by yourself, or with a practitioner. I also recommend Sally Fallon Morell's best-selling book *Nourishing Traditions* to get tons of super-nourishing, traditional food recipes that are also GAPS-friendly. Top experts in food-based healing swear by both.

Additional resources to accelerate your recovery and/or expand your results

The Full GAPS Diet, combined with a potent probiotic supplement, and a targeted detoxification program, give a GAPS individual the bulk of what they need to support their body on its healing journey. Other luxuries then give the body surplus resources to tell it that it's now in a state of abundance and capable of taking on new challenges:

- a quality multi-mineral/multi-vitamin supplement
- chelating agents like EDTA, chlorella or zeolite
- lots of sleep
- pure water
- detox devices like infrared sauna
- therapies such as coffee enemas
- redox molecule supplements.

No longer in conservation and compensation mode, the body then turns on its innate ability to clean house, renew damaged cells, and restore balance to dysfunctional systems on a higher level. It activates detox and healing mechanisms that only get called into action in the presence of huge nutrient excesses and wide-open detox pathways. Extra resources like these can help you get the results you're looking for faster and easier. However, they're not always needed. It depends on how much time and money you want to put into the effort. Every bit helps. But, as any practitioner will tell you, you can only do what you can do.

Diet and metabolism
Balancing blood-sugar level

Managing blood-sugar level is a high priority for the body because multiple organ systems become extremely stressed when blood sugar leaves its very narrow comfort zone. That can cause symptoms mimicking or overlapping with ADD (depending on how you define ADD). Blood sugar imbalances can be so dangerous to short-term and long-term health that the body treats highs or lows as an emergency, and employs potent mechanisms to bring levels back into a normal range.

Here are the basics: Insulin, released by the pancreas, is the hormone that shuttles glucose into cells. Conversely, glucagon, released by the liver, is the hormone that raises blood-sugar level. When sugar and refined carbs enter the bloodstream (molecularly very similar), the pancreas receives the call to release insulin so that blood sugar doesn't get too high and cells receive fuel. Unfortunately, the organs that sense the rise in blood sugar can't tell exactly how much sugar has yet to be released into the bloodstream as the stomach and intestines release the food they were working on.

So the pancreas, sensing the rapid rise in blood sugar, errs on the side of releasing too much insulin, rather than not enough. This typically results in a sudden drop in blood sugar about 45 minutes to an hour and a half after a sugar high. This sudden drop is taxing on the mind and body. It can cause sleepiness and brain fog. And it pushes your "hunger button" prematurely, which encourages you to consume more sugar, thus repeating the cycle. Some call these wild fluctuations in glucose the blood-sugar roller coaster.

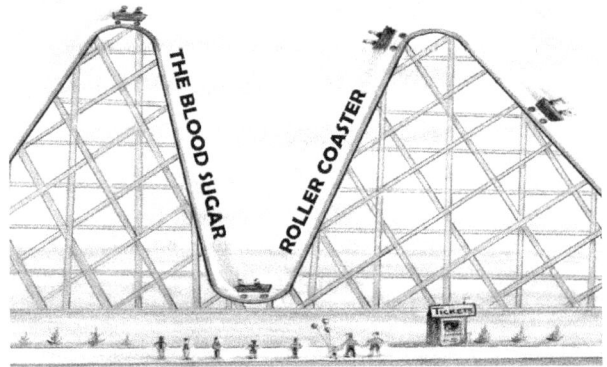

Blood sugar swings can cause ADD symptoms

Often associated with ADD: high blood sugar (hyperglycemia) can induce hyperactivity, manic episodes, and self-stimulation in autistics. While low blood sugar (hypoglycemia) can cause inability to concentrate, low energy, headache, excessive sweating, bad mood, tantrums, aggression, and a highly unsettled feeling. In short, the blood sugar roller coaster can cause problems typical of ADD – including those related to hyperactivity, behavior, social interactions, learning and concentration. Therefore, glycemic index – which is the propensity for a food to raise blood-sugar level – is a primary consideration when choosing which foods to eat in a healing protocol, when, and how much.

Fats, protein and fiber smooth out the blood-sugar rollercoaster

Healthy fats don't cause any rise in blood sugar. This makes them the most efficient source of energy for the body. Next best is a slow, steady release of glucose into the bloodstream with low glycemic-index foods, such as fibrous vegetables and fruits, nuts, and protein.

Whole foods are best at this "timed release" of energy, because their structure takes longer for the digestive system to unbundle and transport into cells. Healthy fats and protein (particularly naturally-raised animal fats) are an excellent way to moderate glycemic highs and lows. But don't listen to the food companies: Saturated animal fats are the bulk of what you should be eating in that effort, not seed oils. Naturally-crafted butter, for example, is much healthier for you than fabricated vegetable oils, such as margarine and butter substitutes.

Reduce craving for sweet foods by eating more bitter foods

One way to curb a sweet tooth is to reset your palate with fermented foods. Fermented foods are naturally sour. And the more of them that you eat, the greater your taste for them. At the same time, you tend to crave sweets less. However, the transition to bitter foods can shock the taste buds of those indulging in super sweet, salty, spicy, and unnaturally powerful flavors.

Fortunately, within a few days of taking up sour fermented foods, most people start to lose their craving for salt, sugar and glutamates while, at the same time, gaining an appreciation for tangy fermented food. Of course, the food has to be eaten in its natural, unflavored state – without sugar or flavorings – to get this effect. Eating fermented foods has the additional benefit of denying pathogens their favorite foods – sugar and carbs – while bringing in probiotic bacteria to suppress the pathogens.

Ferments helped our ancestors stay healthy, before refrigerators and preservatives. Eskimos even discovered that fermenting gave them access to hidden nutrition – coming in huge handy with their sled dogs. So, if you want to make it easier for your family to eat healthier and lose their sugar cravings, introduce them to tart, fermented foods. (Unflavored) fermented foods are powerhouses of nutrition that can do wonders for the body.

Eating healthier also reduces cravings for junk food

In the same way that sour foods reset your palate, eating healthier quashes your cravings for junk food. The big bonus is that you tend to lose weight if you're overweight, or gain weight if you're underweight. You see, when you eat empty calories, hunger subsides for a while, then returns prematurely. On the other hand, when you eat nutrient-dense, bio-available foods, you don't get hungry as much. Consistently eating whole foods, the way Nature made them, is the key to getting all the nutrition you need, while avoiding junk food cravings.

To illustrate with animals (that don't eat for emotional reasons), soil microbiologist Dr. Elaine Ingham recounted that clients of hers were concerned that their cattle were only eating ¼ of what they used to eat before she helped them transition to bio-friendly farming techniques. Using her methods, the protein level in their grass quadrupled. Their cattle then got all the nutrition they needed, so they didn't need to eat as

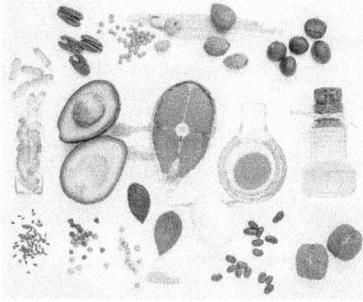

much. So that's two steps in a pro-life direction: High quality food both adds nutrition and subtracts empty calories. Humans and animals get all the benefits good nutrition brings, while weight tends to normalize, without demanding diets.

Essential fats, chronic inflammation and "vagal nerve tone"

The body has the ability to manufacture many fats that it uses. But there are a class of fats that are both essential to many bodily functions, and which the body cannot make on its own. So we have to get them from food. These are called essential fatty acids (EFA).

Our cells are made from EFAs – particularly cells of the brain and nervous system. Many functions of the brain, hormones, and immune system depend on fats to run properly. For these reasons, essential fatty acids are important in treating neurological and degenerative conditions such as autism, ADD, depression, Alzheimer's, cancer and diabetes.

Specifically, there are two "master fats" from which all others are made: omega-3 "alpha-linolenic acid" (ALA), and omega-6 "linoleic acid" (LA). The main fats made from ALA are eicosapentaenoic acid (EPA) and docosahexaenoic acid (DHA). Omega-3 oils are abundant in fatty fish such as salmon, mackerel, herring, tuna, sardines and cod liver, as well as walnuts, flaxseed, chia seeds and oysters.

The fats derived from LA are: gamma-linolenic acid (GLA), dihomogamma-linolenic acid (DGLA), and arachidonic acid (AA). We get omega-6 oils predominately from vegetable and seed oils of soybean, corn, sunflower and safflower. Arachidonic acid, in particular, not only makes up the largest component of brain matter, it's also used in the production of tight junctions that hold barrier membranes together.

Just as influential in GAPS, arachidonic acid is used to maintain vagal nerve function – enabling the brain to communicate with the gut via this so-called "gut-brain axis." The vagus nerve – a large bundle of nerves that interconnect internal organs from the brain to the colon – is the main superhighway of the parasympathetic nervous system (rest and digest). The vagus nerve coordinates: stress response, digestion, anxiety, depression, immunity, motor and sensory nerves, as well as autonomic functions such as breathing and heart rate. When messaging along the vagus nerve is unclear, many involuntary processes become glitchy – including your mood, ability to de-stress and shut down inflammation, immune response, gut motility – even executive function of the PFC and emotional connection to others.

Unfortunately, many GAPS individuals are deficient in AA and other fats, and therefore benefit tremendously from eating meat, eggs and dairy, and/

If inflammation from linoleic acid contributes to sunburn, then it probably contributes to wrinkles and skin cancer as well by depleting our antioxidant reserves.

or supplementing, to reach therapeutic levels of AA. The problem being, linoleic acid is pro-inflammatory, which can be helpful or it can be harmful, depending on how much omega-3 fats you have to offset inflammation from omega-6s. Similar to oxidative stress (i.e., too much oxidation, not enough reduction), Dr. Joe Mercola believes linoleic acid is probably *the* worst thing about processed food because we consume way too much of these inflammatory omega-6 fats in our diet relative to anti-inflammatory fats/foods. He says inflammation from linoleic acid greatly reduces one's ability to tolerate (ionizing/oxidative) UV light, thus promoting sunburn.

You see, nutritional science doesn't distinguish between omega-6 fats in their natural state, and those that have been oxidized by heat in the refining process. Refining makes seed oils more problematic for our systems to handle. In contrast, omega-6 oils in walnuts, hazelnuts, pecans and Brazil nuts are a healthier way to get linoleic acid.

Nutritionists recommend an omega-6 to omega-3 ratio somewhere between 4:1 to 1:2, in order to minimize inflammation. This isn't hard to do when you eat what grows in your environment. But the Standard American diet heavily favors linoleic acid from refined vegetable/seed oils in fried and convenience foods – often reaching 10 or 20 to 1 in people – endlessly fueling inflammation.

Another complication in converting parent fats into juniors is that the body needs vitamins B_3, B_6 and C, magnesium, zinc, and enzymes to make the conversion. However, GAPS patients are routinely deficient in these nutrients – leading to all sorts of problems with digestion, brain function, hormones, sensory processing and immunity. Many experts believe this is major mechanism through which a corrupted microbiome (nutrient deficiencies) turns into GAPS conditions (fatty acid dysfunction dysregulating the gut-brain axis through the vagus nerve).

Bottom line: Get your essential fatty acid picture right, and GAPS/ADD is easier to solve. Please see Dr. Natasha's GAPS book, a GAPS practitioner, or an NTP to learn how to incorporate EFAs, therapeutically or preventively, to reverse brain and body dysfunction.

Green Pasture's fermented essential fat products (rich in omega-3s)

I work out regularly. Have for decades. And I don't drink coffee. So I'm acutely aware of how energetic or tired I feel when I work out. Recently, I stopped taking Green Pasture's fermented fish-oil products (as I have for several years) to try another maker's essential fatty acid multi that claims to be the ultimate source of vitamins K_2 MK-4, A, D, E and omegas.

Unexpectedly, I experienced the same dramatic difference in energy that the Eskimos noticed when they fed their sled dogs fermented fish versus unfermented. I believe the abundant and bioavailable vitamins A, D, E and K found in Green Pasture products enables other vitamins and minerals to do their jobs, making the whole body work better. The empirical proof is that I notice a difference in athletic performance.

Off them, I feel more tired and weak when I work out. And I recover slower. But, on Green Pasture products, I don't get tired. And I don't need any time to recover. Bottom line: I don't need published studies and a health agency's seal of approval to know if something is good for me. The noticeable difference in (real) energy is all I need to know.

What's more, many practitioners swear by Green Pasture products as a go-to source for essential fatty acid products – including GAPS practitioners, Nutritional Therapy Practitioners, and the Weston A. Price Foundation. Find them at: www.greenpasture.org.

The importance of balancing pH levels

Body fluids such as blood, lymph, saliva, and stomach need to be maintained within a very narrow pH range. Too high or too low each can cause serious problems. Most important of all, *blood* pH must be kept between 7.35 and 7.45, which is slightly alkaline.

The problem for those eating a standard American diet is it acidifies the blood. This requires the body to pull highly-alkalizing minerals such as calcium and magnesium away from bones, teeth, and other processes in order to raise blood pH into the alkaline range. Acidifying diets force the body to steal minerals from places and processes where they're badly needed, in order to balance blood pH and keep the body functioning. That's a big reason why processed foods rob you of health in so many ways. And it is why special diets place so much emphasis on pH level – *eating right for your blood type* is one such diet.

Measure nutrient levels in produce with a "brix meter"

For about $30–100, you can get a simple, hand-held device that tells you how much nutrition is in the juice of a fruit or vegetable. Just squeeze a few drops of their juice onto to a brix meter (aka a "refractometer"), and the degree to which light bends through the sample tells you how much sugar and dissolved solids are in it. Compare that reading against known ranges on a brix chart, and you'll have a very good idea how much nutrition is in that fruit, vegetable, wine or beer. The higher up the brix scale it reads, and the fuzzier the dividing line, the more dissolved solids are present in the sample.

Measuring primarily sugar content, a brix score is a good indicator of mineral content, specific gravity, enzyme level and protein. Interestingly, vegetables with a high brix score also stay fresh longer (don't ask me how).

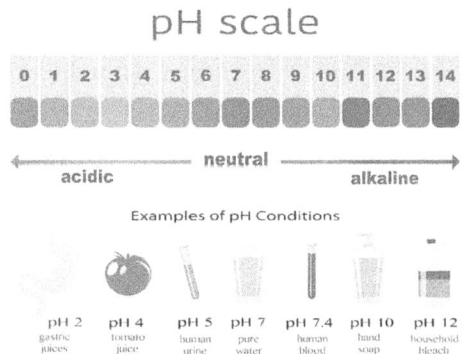

pH scale

0 1 2 3 4 5 6 7 8 9 10 11 12 13 14

acidic — neutral — alkaline

Examples of pH Conditions

pH 2 gastric juices | pH 4 tomato juice | pH 5 human urine | pH 7 pure water | pH 7.4 human blood | pH 10 hand soap | pH 12 household bleach

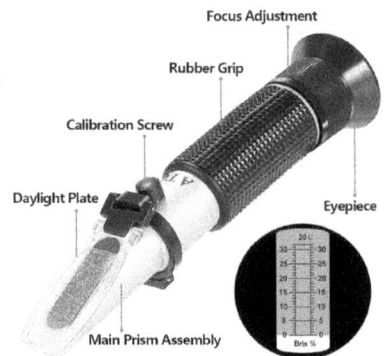

Focus Adjustment
Rubber Grip
Calibration Screw
Daylight Plate
Eyepiece
Main Prism Assembly

MINERALS
(per 100g)

ENERGY ⚡ 18 kcal
(per 100g)

237 mg K
Potassium

24 mg P
Phosphorus

11 mg Mg
Magnesium

10 mg Ca
Calcium

5 mg Na
Sodium

0.27 mg Fe
Iron

0.17 mg Zn
Zinc

0.114 mg Mn
Manganese

0.059 mg Cu
Copper

CARBOHYDRATES
3.89 g

FAT
0.2 g

PROTEIN
0.88 g

VITAMINS
(per 100g)

C 13.7 mg
Ascorbic Acid

B₄ 6.7 mg
Choline

B₃ 0.594 mg
Niacin

E 0.54 mg
Alpha-Tocopherol

B₅ 0.089 mg
Pantothenic acid

B₆ 0.08 mg

B₁ 0.037 mg
Thiamine

B₂ 0.019 mg
Riboflavin

A 42 µg

B₉ 15 µg
Folate

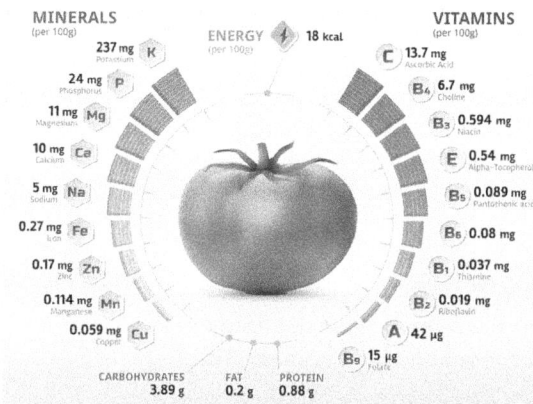

This is how some people in the supply chain do in-field tests prior to doing elaborate lab testing. For consumers, brix meters are a neat tool to compare actual nutrient levels present in produce to theoretical quantities on the Internet, or historical levels on nutrition labels. Now you don't have to guess. You can test that veggie yourself. However, produce managers might think it a bit odd.

Stop thinking about weight, and start fixating on nutrition

Millions want to lose weight. But whether you want to lose weight for looks or health, weight is not the right metric to focus on. It's somewhat of a false idol. That's because weight is only a symptom (objectionable as it may be) of inadequate nutrition. Weighing too much or too little is a consequence of poor nutrition. And nutrient deficiency typically makes you susceptible to imbalance and dysfunction.

Hunger is designed to be a mechanism that regulates nutrient intake. When you need minerals, vitamins and other nutrients, hunger is supposed to suggest which foods you should eat, when, and how much. Later, when those nutritional requirements have been met, hunger stops. On the other hand, if the food you ate lacks the nutrients your system needs, your hunger mechanism gets turned back on prematurely. Therefore, obesity is a reflection of your nutritional state. It's far more of a symptom than a cause. As important as any concept you learn here, nutrient deficiencies are a foundational element of disease and dysfunction.

Therefore, nutrition is the smarter metric to focus your efforts on, not weight or calorie count. Unfortunately for most modern humans, nutrient deficiency shows up as obesity, because our food, on average, is low in nutrients, relative to calories. So instead of trying to lose weight, increase your nutrition and the weight tends to take care of itself (many complications, such as toxin load, hormonal, thyroid and adrenal function notwithstanding). That's the smarter way to frame the conversation about nutrition and weight in your head.

Healing on a budget

Why does organic food cost more?

Organically-grown meat and animal products cost more because animal farmers have to feed their livestock organic feed, which is more expensive. And naturally-raised livestock often yield less milk, meat, eggs, etc. than commercial "frankenfood" methods. It costs growers more to yield less. That's in addition to the core cost of obtaining and maintaining organic certification. Organic vegetables and fruits cost more primarily because growers typically have to pay workers to pick weeds by hand. Fortunately, there are strategies to help shallow-pocketed consumers who are making their family's health a priority.

Strategies to keep costs down

1. **Buy meat direct.** Buy your meat in bulk, directly from a conscientious, local meat producer so you can learn how the animals were raised. Have them butchered by an independent butcher. And store the meat in a dedicated freezer.
2. **Asian markets are great for produce.** Buy your vegetables and fruits from local Asian markets. They often deal directly with local farms, and in smaller quantities. In doing so, the produce you get may not be as pretty and perfect as what you'd find in a major grocery store. But their priorities are often in closer alignment with your health goals than the chain stores. The produce is often higher in nutrients, lower in toxins, and cheaper than premium grocery stores. Look for (or ask for) deals on ugly or already-ripe produce. Produce managers are happy to get anything for produce that they might have to throw out.
3. **Join a food buying club.** There's purchasing power in numbers. Join a healthy food buyer's club. These go by many names, such as community supported agriculture (CSA). Most memberships will get you better quality food for just the cost of a little planning and preparation. And most locales have many to choose from.
4. **Grow your own food.** Most people have some room to grow their own fruits or vegetables, if only a few tomatoes or berries indoors.
5. **Prepare meals in advance.** Prepare a week's worth of meals in advance and freeze them.

You pay for the comfort and convenience of modern living, one way or another

Either you pay upfront for good quality food that contributes to your health bank account. Or else you'll pay later in the form of health problems, insurance co-pays, and dreams left unlived. Think of this as owing money on your health credit card. It's your choice.

Also worth mentioning

Getting buy-in

You've heard the old adage 'A man convinced against his will is of the same opinion still.' Well, same thing goes for healing. Getting the permission and involvement of the affected individual(s) is essential in aligning their energy and efforts toward ideal outcomes. Whether that means avoiding the temptation to cheat on a special diet, or selling an idea to friends and family, or even harnessing the placebo effect – true change begins in the mind. So unless/until you get the individual on-board with their own healing journey – meaning an active participant – your efforts may be resented and even sabotaged.

Reinforce natural healing successes with *challenge-rechallenge* testing

Whether food, supplement, practice or protocol – people tend to dismiss and abandon natural healing methods that once worked well for them. That's because it's human nature to discount things that aren't blessed by "authorities" and supposed "experts" as the right thing do to. In other words, "they" tell you what to do and, most of the time, you do it without a second thought.

On the other hand, when you arrive, through your own volition, at something that works for you, there's a tendency to downplay and doubt your own intellect and experience, because you trust authority figures more than you trust yourself. In effect, you doubt your own reality and, instead, believe the reality that others craft for you.

As a result, people tend to forget to reorder a supplement that worked well for them. They stop doing the therapy that helped them manage an area of their life better. They get busy, stressed, and sidetracked and go back to eating the diet that made them sick, because it's cheaper and easier than living life as your own health authority. Life happens.

It's for these reasons that you need to incorporate challenge and rechallenge testing into your process. Purposely take a mental snapshot of what that helpful thing is doing for you (the "before" picture) in phase one. Then, stop doing it to compare and contrast the difference (the "after" picture). And then resume the therapy to confirm or deny your results. Many times, you'll find that you underappreciated its effectiveness when you don't have medication-style side effects to convince you that it's doing something.

Action items: First, realize that natural healing methods are not jarring on the body the way that modern medicine is designed to be. Natural healing is invisible, so you don't notice it. Therefore, the benefits and advantages may escape your conscious awareness, were you to overlook their benefits. Then, analyze the positive effects a healing tool has on you *vs.* its side effects and disadvantages, such as cost or convenience.

Consciously decide if it's worth "hiring" in your life or "firing." Do not leave it up to the mood of the day or happenstance, because that's guaranteed to limit your success in health (and life). And then, of course, do what your analysis suggests. Sometimes, you'll need to test and retest several times before you accept that your initial conclusions are valid. Finally, make the therapy an automatic part of your regimen unless/until it stops serving you.

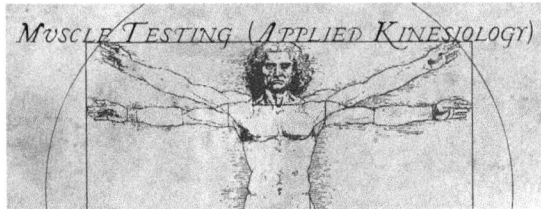

Muscle testing tells you if your body likes a substance or not

Your body can tell whether a substance complements your biology or not, just by sensing its energetic field. You don't even have to taste, smell, touch, or even see it to know whether it's good for you or not. Just hold a substance close to your body and see whether it makes your muscles go strong or weak, using a simple muscle-testing technique. You could even put it in a paper bag, completely "blinded" to it, and your body will react to its energetic field.

This phenomenon, which started out being called "applied kinesiology" by the alternative community, and now more commonly referred to simply as "muscle testing," is now a widely-accepted method to test how your body will respond to a substance – whether that be a food, supplement, herb, medicine, food constituent such as artificial sweetener, household cleaner, personal care product or chemical. Whatever it may be, life-enhancing substances make muscles strong when tested this way, while health-stealing substances make your muscles go weak.

I couldn't tell you precisely how the science works. But the general idea is that when a substance's energetic frequency interacts with that of your own biology, the resulting waveform can increase or decrease. When the frequencies are harmonious, the heightened waveform manifests as strength, which means the substance supports you physically, mentally and spiritually. But, when the rate or intensity of vibration runs contrary to your biology, it saps you of strength. That might mean the substance is artificial, an allergen to you, genetically modified, wrong for your blood type, or just plain toxic.

Muscle testing is one more instance of phenomena once-considered woo becoming widely accepted because it works. It's a cheap, fast and reliable way to determine how good or bad something is for you. However, you won't hear about it from mainstream sources.

Search YouTube for "muscle testing" to see it in action. Or read the best-selling book Power vs. Force *by David R. Hawkins PhD to learn more.*

Secret health saboteurs to watch out for

Here are some common conditions that can smolder along inside of you, chronically undermining your energy level, inflammation and resiliency. Eliminating these hidden health saboteurs can catapult you out of deficiency and on the road to optimal wellness:

- lingering infection after root canal or improper extraction
- chronic mold exposure
- Lyme's disease
- Epstein-Barr virus
- dental amalgams.

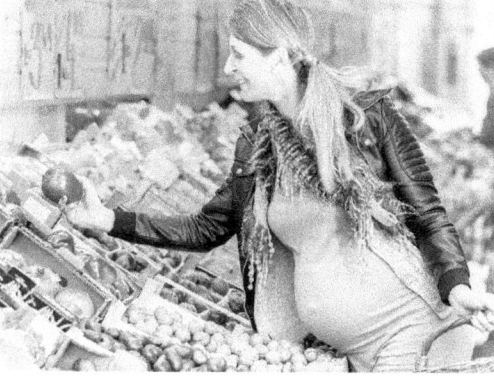

Preconception protocol

What a novel idea: How about *preventing* GAPS conditions from happening entirely. To that end, indigenous cultures through the ages have placed far greater importance on preparing women's bodies for pregnancy than our modern medicine. Today, our healthcare system recommends abstaining from smoking and drinking (alcohol), eating "healthy" (by Western standards), prenatal vitamins, staying hydrated, and fetal ultrasound checkups. That's about it.

In contrast, women in traditional cultures might prepare their bodies for up to two years before they even conceived, in order to make absolutely certain they have a healthy baby. Men might do the same with a less rigorous protocol. Part of the reason they seemed to over-prepare by today's standards is, having very little to fall back on, families couldn't afford to have unhealthy children. Raising a handicapped or retarded child in an unforgiving society with no social services could ruin a family in many ways. In Asian cultures, for example, it brought shame to a family that had irregular children – past and present.

For more information on how to eat well in preparation for optimal baby health visit the Weston A. Price Foundation website: westonaprice.org.

The other half of the story is they knew nutritional protocols work

They knew that eating properly could prevent birth defects and health problems, throughout a person's life. Radical differences in culture aside, indigenous cultures did not accept mental and physical handicaps as normal and unavoidable. Instead, they understood that there was a great deal a couple could do to produce healthy babies, which boiled down to this: no processed foods (they were lucky that way), plenty of organ meats such as liver, and fermented foods like kimchi – if they had them. Basically, they loaded up on concentrated, natural sources of minerals and vitamins. They took steps to detoxify as best they could. And they stayed away from foods that are hard to digest and eliminate.

———— ❦ ————

PARTING WORDS

Some people have the good fortune to be gifted excellent health through-out their life and don't have to work very hard for it. Unfortunately, those people are quickly becoming an endangered species. The majority of people will now have to fight at some point in their lives for the right to be healthy and live the life they desire. But although the health challenges facing us all may seem daunting, be assured there are solutions to fix them. The alternative community knows what causes ADD, GAPS conditions, and the chronic, degenerative diseases we all know by name.

So the principles and practices you need to reverse gut-brain issues are understood by a growing number of professionals and patients. The roads have been travelled, but the trip may be different for each person. The solutions may not be as quick, cheap, and easy as we would like them to be. But they're almost always quicker, cheaper, and easier to fix health problems than it was to create them. So keep your expectations realistic short-term, and your outlook on health and life optimistic long-term.

In other words, don't accept anything less than excellent health, a fully-functional brain, and robust energy in your life, because you now have a choice. It is with these thoughts in mind that this collection of cutting-edge principles and practices is offered to you, your family, and your loved ones.

The End

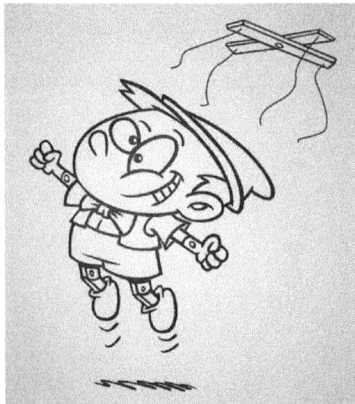

GLOSSARY

Acetaldehyde highly toxic metabolite responsible for giving heavy drinkers a hangover.

Aerobic with oxygen.

Anaerobic without oxygen.

Aromatic amino acid a building block of neurotransmitters.

ATP adenosine triphosphate is an energy storage molecule made in mitochondria that drives dozens of cellular processes crucial to running the body.

Biophysics the physics that controls biology.

Campbell–McBride, Dr. Natasha pioneer in connecting gut health to brain function – particularly autism, attention deficit, and what wellness experts call "GAPS" conditions (short for Gut and Psychology Syndrome).

Circadian rhythm biorhythm lasting about 24 hours, such as daily cycles of sleep and waking.

Epigenetics environmental factors control the way our genes turn into physical traits and behaviors.

Extracellular matrix supportive structures and biochemicals outside of cells (e.g., collagen, enzymes, glycoproteins and minerals).

GAPS coined by gut-brain health pioneer Dr. Natasha Campbell-McBride, Gut and Psychology Syndrome conditions are gut imbalances, such as leaky gut and gut dysbiosis, that cause impaired brain function, such as ADD, autism, anxiety and depression.

Gene snippets of DNA coding that tell the nucleus of cells how to make proteins, organs, systems, and the organism. Genes are instructions to produce physical traits and (indirectly) behaviors.

Hypoxic low oxygen.

Ingham, Dr. Elaine world's leading soil biology researcher, characterized "The Soil Food Web," author of the USDA's Soil Biology Primer.

Intracellular space collagen–connected space between cells.

Mitochondria microscopic powerplants of the cell. They convert sugar, fat and protein from food into energy that the body can use (ATP).

nnEMF non–native electromagnetic frequencies (i.e., man–made electromagnetic frequencies).

Normies unawakened member of the general public who believes official narratives because they trust authority figures more than themselves.

Tight junctions filaments between cells of the gut lining that open and close on–demand to let food particles and immune cells through. When these break, undigested food particles enter the bloodstream and cause food sensitivities, autoimmunity and toxicity issues.

Zonulin protein that modulates permeability of tight junctions of cells lining the intestinal tract.

———————⟲∽⟳———————

INDEX

ABOUT THE AUTHOR

Randy (The Mito Man) is an independent researcher, author, and citizen scientist who's both blessed and cursed to have been born with a fanatical need to know. Today he's a reality/false-reality decoder. But he must have been an inventor or reporter in a previous life, because he loves searching for the perfect way to say and do things.

His idea of fun is to learn how the body really works, and impart that knowledge to others so fear and uncertainty lose their power over you. His greatest assets in helping people arrive at a place of accurate thinking are a bountiful perspective, a talent for seeing how dots connect to each other, and an obsession with polishing ideas so others can see them in the best light. In doing so, he presents ideas nearly as well as the experts themselves, sometimes better, so your time and attention are rewarded with a proper understanding you can use to great benefit.

The sequel to *Gut-Brain Secrets, The Mitochondriac Manifesto,* aims to overturn our old beliefs about where health or sickness comes from, in light of what we now know about mitochondria, seasonal cycles, and energies in and around the body. Together, they give health professionals and consumers a cutting-edge perspective into the factors that contribute to your health bank account, as well as the modern exposures that deplete your bucket of life force.

NOW WHAT?

Get expert help on your healing journey

Consult with a certified GAPS practitioner, or a Nutritional Therapy Practitioner (NTP or NTC) from the Nutritional Therapy Association to assess your situation and help you create a plan that accomplishes what you want, and is realistic in terms of budget, commitment, health condition, resources and limitations. They can give you an extra measure of guidance and support you would not have on your own. Specifically, they can be as much a motivator as they are an educator and problem solver. For best results, get the best people on your team.

To find a GAPS practitioner to talk to or work with go to: www.gaps.me and click on the link "Find a GAPS Practitioner." To find a NTP in your neighborhood to talk to or work with go to: www.nutritionaltherapy.com and click on "Provider Listings."

Take action

Now it's time to start saying goodbye to temporary symptom relief using "biochemical band-aids" and, instead, start getting the real, lasting results you're looking for. It's time to let the real progress begin by

- healing and sealing the gut lining
- righting the microbiome
- supplying nutrient-dense foods, so the body can heal and protect itself
- removing the toxins that impair both mind and body.

Stop being exploited by society's conveniences and constructs… and start putting the information you've learned to good use. You're now much better equipped to make small changes seeking incremental improvement, or sweeping changes bent on complete recovery. Remember, life favors decision and action. So if you or a member of your family are unwell, any action is likely to be a step in the right direction.

Help spread the word

If you found this information valuable to your health and life(style), go to Amazon.com and leave an honest review. Total number of reviews helps Amazon and prospective readers determine a book's worth.

———— ❦ ————

RECOMMENDED RESOURCES

Recommended reading

- *The Mitochondriac Manifesto,* by R. D. Lee.
- *Gut and Psychology Syndrome,* by Dr. Natasha Campbell-McBride.
- *Nourishing Traditions,* by Sally Fallon Morell.
- *Healing the Symptoms Known as Autism,* by Kerri Rivera.
- *Healing ADD;* and *Change Your Brain, Change Your Life,* by Dr. Daniel Amen.
- *Your Body's Many Cries for Water,* by Fereydoon Batmanghelidj, MD.

Magnetico Sleep Pad

Full disclosure: I have an affiliate relation with The Magnetico Company, and may earn a commission on purchases.

- www.magneticosleep.com
- 1.800.265.1119 (North America only). Direct: 1.702.952.5243.
- Use promo code **TheMitoMan** to receive a small price break.

Sauna Space faraday saunas and personal near-IR "photon lights"

- https://sauna.space/
- 573.667.2862
- hello@sauna.space

Products to detox from radiation poisoning

- Apple pectin powder.
- Liposomal vitamin C from LivOn Labs.
- Ken Rohla sells the following at his website: freshandalive.com:
  - "Illumodine™" is monoatomic iodine programmed with anti-frequencies to radioactive elements.
  - "Rad D-Tox," from Liquid Manna, contains ORMES elements programmed with anti-frequencies.
  - "No-Glo Radiation Detox" from Dr. Morse.

Food, farming, and the healing arts

To learn more about how good food supports our biology, and bad food wrecks it, visit the Weston A. Price Foundation: www.westonaprice.org.

www.ingramcontent.com/pod-product-compliance
Ingram Content Group UK Ltd.
Pitfield, Milton Keynes, MK11 3LW, UK
UKHW011010270125
4300UKWH00008B/90

9 798218 079574